HEARING
AID
EVALUATION

HEARING AID EVALUATION

Margaret W. Skinner

Washington University
School of Medicine
St. Louis, Missouri

PRENTICE HALL   ENGLEWOOD CLIFFS, NEW JERSEY   07632

Skinner, Margaret W.
    Hearing aid evaluation.

    (Remediation of communication disorders series)
    Bibliography: p. 361
    Includes index.
    1. Hearing aids—Fitting. I. Title. II. Series:
Remediation of communication disorders. [DNLM:
1. Hearing Aids—standards. WV 274 S628h]
    RF300.S57 1988 617.8′9   87−11422
    ISBN 0−13−385717−4

Printed in the United States of America
10 9 8 7 6 5 4 3 2 1

ISBN 0-13-385717-4   01

Prentice Hall International (UK) Limited, *London*
Prentice Hall of Australia Pty. Limited, *Sydney*
Prentice Hall Canada Inc., *Toronto*
Prentice Hall Hispanoamericana, S.A., *Mexico*
Prentice Hall of India Private Limited, *New Delhi*
Prentice Hall of Japan, Inc., *Tokyo*
Prentice Hall of Southeast Asia Pte. Ltd., *Singapore*
Editora Prentice Hall do Brasil, Ltda., *Rio de Janeiro*

To my husband,
Milton,
and to my sons,
Geoff and Jonathan,
with love.

CONTENTS

FOREWORD

The information explosion of recent years has brought a proliferation of knowledge of both scientific and social inquiry. The specialty of communicative disorders has been no exception. Two decades ago a single handbook might have sufficed to provide the aspiring or practicing clinician with enlightenment on an array of communication handicaps. This is no longer possible—hence the decision to prepare a series of single-author texts.

As the title implies, the emphasis of this series, *Remediation of Communication Disorders,* is on therapy and treatment. The authors of each book were asked to provide information relative to anatomical and physiological aspects of each disorder, as well as pathology, etiology, and diagnosis to the extent that understanding of these factors bears on management procedures. In such relatively short books this was quite a challenge: to offer guidance without writing a "cookbook;" to be selective without being parochial; to offer theory without losing sight of practice. To this challenge the series authors have risen magnificently.

Dr. Margaret Skinner was an obvious choice to write about the selection of hearing aids. Her highly regarded research publications and her broad clinical experience make her unique among her colleagues. This book, the product of her current work, is a state-of-the-art presentation on the most important subject of helping patients to hear better by using amplification. It is both scientific and humanistic and will undoubtedly prove highly beneficial to its readers.

Frederick N. Martin
Series Editor

PREFACE

The major focus of this book is on how to choose and adjust the characteristics of a hearing aid and earmold so that the amplified sound, particularly conversational speech, is matched to the residual hearing of a hearing-impaired individual. The basic premise is that the setting of the frequency response, gain, and maximum acoustic output of the hearing aid does make a difference in the amount of benefit the aid provides. Although most of the book is devoted to technical aspects of hearing aid evaluation, part is devoted to human dimensions that are of key importance in the successful use of a hearing aid.

In writing this book I have referred to the work of many researchers, clinicians, and manufacturers, much of it published in the last fifteen years. These people have addressed many of the points that should be considered in selecting and fitting a hearing aid and in counseling the person who is going to wear it. The organization of the book reflects a synthesis of this information to answer questions that I, as a clinician, believe are most important. For example:

- What sounds should I use, and how do I produce, control, and measure them?
- What procedures will enable the individual to respond most reliably at threshold, comfortable listening levels, and uncomfortable listening levels?
- What procedures are available for prescribing the real-ear gain and maximum acoustic output of a hearing aid, and on what basis might I choose one instead of another?
- What factors should I consider in choosing the appropriate type of aid(s) plus earmold, and how can I estimate what frequency response, gain, and maximum acoustic output characteristics (measured in a 2 cm^3 coupler) will provide the prescribed real-ear gain and output?
- How can I verify that we have obtained the prescribed characteristics, how can I adjust the aid if I have not obtained them, and do I need to make further adjustments to make the sound acceptable for the individual?
- What do I need to know to effectively help this individual use the hearing aid in everyday life?

The emphasis is on providing a conceptual framework and a wealth of facts that it is hoped will enable those who manufacture, fit, and dispense hearing aids make thoughtful, rational choices from among a myriad of alternatives. No one choice or set of criteria will necessarily be the "correct" one—including the ones in this text. Most choices involve compromise among a number of factors; however, we should know why we have made them. To make these choices most beneficial to the hearing-impaired individual, the criteria for making them must be constantly updated as new information and technological advances become available.

Many tables and figures have been included with the text to summarize relevant data, to illustrate concepts, and to give specific examples of how they can be implemented clinically. Among these examples are applications of fitting procedures based on actual data from hearing-impaired individuals. There are also tables that have proved valuable as reference sources for calibration of equipment, preselection of a hearing aid and earmold, and information about hearing aids. Although it is beyond the scope of this book to describe the computer programs that are available for cataloging hearing aid specifications, choosing from among available hearing aids, or choosing frequency-gain and maximum-acoustic-output characteristics according to a prescriptive procedure, such programs can be evaluated (or new ones created) based on relevant information in the text, tables, and figures.

In the last few years vibrotactile aids and cochlear implants have become clinically available for profoundly deaf people. These hearing aids give a number of people significant benefit. Although the concept of fitting the sounds of everyday life between an individual's threshold and discomfort levels is the same for these devices as it is for conventional hearing aids, the sound-processing strategies are often much more complex. For this reason, a description of vibrotactile aids and cochlear implants has not been included.

This book is intended for clinicians who fit and/or dispense hearing aids, for students enrolled in courses on hearing aids and the professors who teach them, for manufacturers of hearing aids and related sound-measurement systems, and for people who repair hearing aids and the equipment used for the evaluation of aids. Some sections, such as those on audiometric equipment, test rooms, sound measurement, sound-field testing, and the effect of the frequency-gain characteristics on speech recognition by hearing-impaired individuals, may be of interest to students and professors in courses other than those devoted specifically to hearing aids. In writing this book I have followed the same organizational principles that proved effective during the six years I taught a three-semester course on hearing evaluation for master's-level audiology students.

I am indebted to many people who have helped shape my understanding of hearing aids. At the Cleveland Hearing and Speech Center (1958 to 1961) Earl Schubert and Martin Schultz showed me how important it was for speech to be audible in all frequency regions, and my work with Ruth Bender and the hearing-impaired children in her nursery program convinced me of the efficacy of binaural hearing aids placed on the head. During this same time Marcia Rosenthal Valente, Marilyn Heasley Giolas, and Phil Yantis all gave me excellent clinical supervision, and Joe Millan, Raymond Rich, and Pat Clark shared their expertise gained from fitting and dispensing many hearing aids. At the University of Michigan Medical Center (1962–66) I learned much about otologic disease from the attending staff and residents and their patients, and I had an opportunity to evaluate hearing aids for many patients.

My years at Central Institute for the Deaf (1969–83) were special in many respects. The first two years I worked closely with David Pascoe and Irv Shore, who with Roy Gengel had developed a frequency-specific fitting procedure for adjusting hearing aids. After five years of doctoral work under the tutelage of Chuck Watson, Jim Miller, Ira Hirsh, and other fine professors, I became a research associate and member of the hearing aid research team. This team included Jim Miller, David Pascoe, Art Niemoeller, Maynard Engebretson, Jerry Popelka, and Arnold Heidbreder. For six years we met, shared ideas, planned research, and analyzed the results together. This was an incredibly rich environment in which to learn and explore new ideas, and my vantage point in writing this book strongly reflects our collaborative work.

Much of the book has been written since I became a member of the Department of Otolaryngology—Head and Neck Surgery at Washington University School of Medicine. The audiologists with whom I work have found the Pascoe prescriptive procedure an effective basis for fitting and dispensing hearing aids. I am grateful for our discussions, from which I have gained new insights.

David Hawkins, Robyn Cox, Mead Killion, Denis Byrne, and Arne Leijon have given me manuscripts of their work prior to publication and discussed various aspects of the book with me. Fred Martin, David Pascoe, Jerry Popelka, Roanne Karzon, Jim Miller, Art Niemoeller, J.P. Gagne, Debbi Servi, Bob Loomis, Tina Wood, Max Wood, Maureen Valente, Mike Valente, Mead Killion, Denis Byrne, and Sam Lybarger have critiqued one or more chapters of the book, for which I am very grateful. Substantive changes or additions were made based on their suggestions. Preparation of this manuscript was supported in part by Program Project Grant NS03856 from the National Institute for Neurological and Communicative Disorders and Stroke to Central Institute for the Deaf and in part by the Department of Otolaryngology at Washington University School of Medicine.

The love and encouragement my husband, Milton, has given me at every bend of the road have made it possible for me to finish this book. He had the foresight to buy a computer and word-processing software with which I wrote and edited the manuscript, and he developed a computer program with which many of the figures were produced. This has truly been a joint project! Throughout the four years my children, Geoff and Jonathan, and friends have cheered me on, and Fred Martin, who invited me to write this book, has shared his wisdom and given me support. I am thankful for all that they have given me.

Margaret W. Skinner
St. Louis, Missouri

Chapter One

HUMAN AND TECHNICAL DIMENSIONS OF A HEARING AID EVALUATION

HUMAN DIMENSION
Reasons for Seeking Help
Medical and Audiological Assessment of Hearing
Counseling and Orientation
TECHNICAL DIMENSIONS
Effect of Hearing Impairment on Speech Recognition
Room, Equipment, and Stimuli
Measuring Sound
Criteria for Prescribing Hearing Aid Characteristics
Preselection of a Hearing Aid and Earmold
Measurements for a Successful Fit
SUMMARY

There are two major dimensions of a hearing aid evaluation—the human and the technical. A thorough understanding of both dimensions is essential to provide the best care for someone with a hearing impairment that cannot be alleviated medically. Although most of this book is devoted to the technical dimensions, I hope the information given on the human dimension will encourage clinicians to develop their skills in this area as well. This chapter is an overview of the topics that will be described in greater detail in subsequent chapters.

HUMAN DIMENSION

The human dimension includes people who seek help, clinicians who give help, and the ways they work together to alleviate the communication problems caused by hearing impairment.

Reasons for Seeking Help

Adults who seek help do so because they can no longer ignore the difficulty they are having hearing speech and other sounds. Attempts to communicate with family, friends, and other people are often frustrating because of the inaccurate reception of what is said, and this can lead to feelings of inadequacy, isolation, and depression. Those who are able to face this uncomfortable situation by looking for possible solutions will seek help independently. Others, who deny the problems they are having, seek help because their family or friends, who recognize the problems, exert enough pressure to convince them to at least seek an evaluation. Children are brought in for evaluation because their parents and/or teachers notice that they are not hearing sounds or that speech and language are not developing normally. In all cases, a need has prompted them to seek our help as professionals and this need must be carefully assessed to determine whether a hearing aid is appropriate.

Medical and Audiological Assessment of Hearing

It is important for anyone who has difficulty hearing to have a medical examination by a physician who specializes in diseases of the ear, because there may be a condition that needs treatment. In some cases, treatment may restore hearing to normal and eliminate the need for a hearing aid. If treatment is not needed or does not restore hearing to normal, then a hearing aid may provide significant benefit.

Because the person with difficulty hearing may need treatment, the U.S. Food and Drug Administration (FDA) ruled in 1977 that persons who purchase a hearing aid should be examined by a licensed physician within 6 months prior to the fitting of the aid. Medical clearance is compulsory for anyone under eighteen, whereas adults may sign a waiver if they do not want to be examined. However, if any of the following conditions exists, the hearing aid dispenser must advise the person to seek medical attention:

1. visible congenital or traumatic deformity of the ear,
2. history of active drainage within the previous ninety days,
3. history of sudden or rapidly progressive hearing loss within the previous ninety days,
4. acute or chronic dizziness,
5. unilateral hearing loss of sudden or recent onset within the previous ninety days,
6. an audiometric air-bone gap equal to or greater than 15 dB at 500, 1000, and 2000 Hz,
7. visible evidence of significant cerumen accumulation or a foreign body in the ear canal,
8. pain or discomfort in the ear. (FDA 1977).

An audiological evaluation is necessary to determine whether hearing thresholds are abnormal, to measure the amount of conductive hearing loss if it exists, and to assess the ability to recognize speech both at threshold and at a comfortable listening level. Other audiological tests, such as tympanometry and measurement of acoustic reflex thresholds or auditory brainstem evoked potentials, may be indicated to help diagnose the site of lesion. The results of this evaluation are an integral part of the data on which a medical diagnosis is based. Audiologic results also contribute information for planning rehabilitation for the hearing-impaired individual. (See table 1.1 for one classification of the degree of hearing impairment as a function of average hearing level and the predicted effect on unaided understanding of speech.) If the average hearing levels (500, 1000, and 2000 Hz) are poorer than normal, if there is a significant hearing loss at 2000 Hz and above and if

TABLE 1.1. General Guide to the Relation of Hearing Impairment Based on Average of Pure-Tone Air-Conduction Thresholds (dB HL; ANSI 1969) at 500, 1000, and 2000 Hz to Typical Unaided Speech Understanding.*

MEAN THRESHOLD (dB HL)	DEGREE	TYPICAL UNAIDED SPEECH UNDERSTANDING
0–15	Normal	No significant limitations
16–39	Mild	Difficulty with faint speech, especially from another room
40–54	Moderate	Frequent difficulty with normal speech
55–69	Moderately severe	Frequent difficulty even with loud speech
70–89	Severe	Loud (or amplified) speech might be understood depending on factors such as type of impairment
90 and above	Profound	Understanding of speech severely limited even with amplification

*Information based in part on table 2.1 from J. Katz and T.P. White 1982. "Auditory impairment versus hearing handicap." In *Rehabilitative Audiology*. Ed. R. H. Hull. Reprinted by permission of Grune and Stratton, Inc. and the authors.

the hearing impairment is not amenable to medical or surgical treatment, a hearing aid is a key part of the total rehabilitation program.

If a hearing aid is indicated and the individual decides to try one, it is important to do further audiological tests to determine where sounds of different pitches (250–6000 Hz) are comfortably and uncomfortably loud and where speech is uncomfortably loud. Together with the thresholds for tones and speech, this information defines the individual's area of residual hearing. For an aid to be most effective, the most important sounds in everyday life, particularly speech, must be amplified to fall within this area.

Counseling and Orientation

The major goals of counseling prior to a hearing aid evaluation are, first, to determine the hearing and communication problems of the individual and, second, to create an environment in which solutions to these problems are sought by the individual with the guidance and support of the clinician. Guidance includes communicating information about hearing loss, its effect on communication, appropriate hearing aids, and aural rehabilitation. This approach is different from the traditional, authoritarian one in which the physician, audiologist, or hearing aid dispenser *tells* the person with the hearing impairment *what to do*, based on the professional's expertise. This traditional approach (coupled with insufficient guidance) may be one reason why in the most recent National Hearing Survey in the United States (see figure 1.1) only 12 percent of people three years of age and older who had a significant hearing impairment were wearing a hearing aid at the time of the interview. One important step to change this trend is to recognize that the hearing aid is an integral part of an aural rehabilitation process in which the person with the hearing impairment and family members are key participants.

The primary responsibility of the clinician is to create an accepting situation in which people with hearing impairment are encouraged to talk about the difficulties hearing loss causes in their everyday lives, their feelings about having a hearing loss, and what they would like to do to resolve their communication problems. Sometimes it is difficult for us as clinicians to listen with a caring attitude, particularly with people who are defensive about their inability to cope and who blame others for their problems. However, if we remember the moments when we have felt defensive, we realize how much it means to be accepted rather than judged. Growth occurs in our own lives when we gain a new insight through experiences we have and decisions we make, rather than doing what someone else tells us to do. Furthermore, growth cannot be hurried; it takes time and patience to change old patterns, and each person follows a different path and pace. With this in mind, it is clear that we can be most helpful to those whom we counsel by intertwining information and support with genuine acceptance.

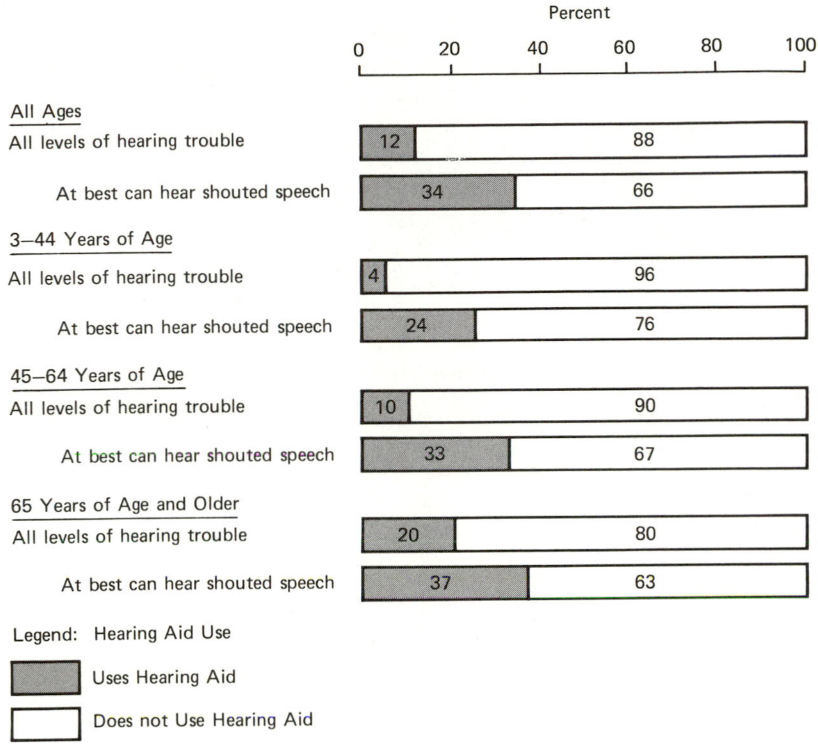

Percent

| | 0 | 20 | 40 | 60 | 80 | 100 |

All Ages

All levels of hearing trouble — 12 | 88

At best can hear shouted speech — 34 | 66

3–44 Years of Age

All levels of hearing trouble — 4 | 96

At best can hear shouted speech — 24 | 76

45–64 Years of Age

All levels of hearing trouble — 10 | 90

At best can hear shouted speech — 33 | 67

65 Years of Age and Older

All levels of hearing trouble — 20 | 80

At best can hear shouted speech — 37 | 63

Legend: Hearing Aid Use

▨ Uses Hearing Aid

☐ Does not Use Hearing Aid

FIGURE 1.1. Percent of individuals three years of age and over who had trouble hearing and were wearing a hearing aid at the time of an interview during the 1977 National Health Survey in the United States. Adapted with permission from J. D. Schein 1985. Based on data from "Hearing ability of persons by sociodemographic and health characteristics: United States." *Vital and Health Statistics*, ser. 10, no. 140 (August 1982).

Many factors affect an individual's reaction to a hearing impairment; these are summarized in table 1.2. Although the magnitude, type, and configuration of hearing impairment are major factors, one cannot use these alone to predict the interference, or *handicap*, that this impairment will cause in a person's life. For example, a hearing impairment that occurs gradually and allows the individual to learn skills to compensate effectively will not interfere as much as one that occurs suddenly or fluctuates. An individual who (1) accepts the impairment, (2) is highly motivated to wear a hearing aid and compensate for the difficulties in communication, and (3) has an understanding, supportive family will have less of a handicap than someone who (1) denies the impairment, (2) finds many excuses not to adjust to or wear a hearing aid, and (3) has a family that responds by perpetuating communication difficulties.

An infant who is born with a moderate hearing impairment will need appropriately fitted hearing aid or aids and intensive speech and language

TABLE 1.2. Variables Affecting Reaction to Hearing Loss.*

AUDITORY

A. Degree
 1. Mild
 2. Moderate
 3. Severe
 4. Profound
B. Type
 1. Conductive
 2. Mixed
 3. Sensorineural
 4. Central
C. Configuration
 1. Degree of slope
 2. Unilateral vs. bilateral
 3. Symmetry
D. Speech perception
E. Recruitment/loudness discomfort
F. Etiology
G. Permanency
 1. Temporary
 2. Fluctuating
 3. Progressive
 4. Permanent
H. Temporal factors
 1. Duration of loss
 2. Rate of onset

PERSONAL

A. Age
B. Sex
C. Race
D. Intelligence
E. Education
F. Occupation
G. Socio-economic status
H. Health
 1. Tinnitus
 2. Vestibular disorder
 3. Visual acuity
 4. Illness
 5. Other physical
  problems
I. Psychological adjustment

COMMUNICATIVE DISTURBANCE

A. Degree
B. Duration
C. Frequency

INTERPERSONAL SUPPORT

A. Family
B. Friends
C. Business or work associates

COMPENSATORY ABILITIES

A. Use of amplification
B. Use of visual cues
C. Willingness and ability to ask for help
D. Environmental manipulation skills

**METHODS OF MEASURING
REACTIONS**

A. Instrument used
 1. Observation
 2. Self-report scales
 3. Standardized test
 4. Daily log
B. Reactions studied
 1. Personality
 2. Social competence
 3. Fears
 4. Adjustment
C. Respondents
 1. Hearing-impaired person
 2. Spouse, significant other

*From J. G. Alpiner 1982. *Handbook of Adult Rehabilitative Audiology*, 2nd ed. Adapted from table 5.1 in M. A. Wylde. "The remediation process: Psychologic and counseling aspects." Copyright 1982, Williams & Wilkins, Co., Baltimore. Reprinted with permission of the publisher and the author.

training to develop normal communication, whereas an adult with an acquired hearing loss, who already knows the language and speaks intelligibly, will need to compensate far less for the hearing impairment. An elderly person who is ill or has physical problems will have more difficulty than a younger person who is healthy and more adaptable. In addition, certain jobs and lifestyles are much more demanding of accurate recognition of sound, particularly speech, than others. For example, a librarian, who needs to hear people who speak softly, will probably benefit more from a hearing aid than someone who is retired, lives alone, and rarely talks with other people.

Before recommending a hearing aid evaluation, it is essential to assess which of these factors are contributing to the communication problems. If hearing impairment is interfering with normal communication, the individual should have an opportunity to try a hearing aid or aids. This includes people who may have been told that a hearing aid will not be helpful, such as those with high-frequency hearing losses (at 2000 Hz and above), profound hearing losses, or severe difficulty understanding speech. For infants and children, we need to help parents understand how critical a hearing aid and special education are to their child's development of speech and language. For adults, we need to assess whether the individual finds that the hearing impairment interferes enough with their lives to warrant the time, energy, and money to try a hearing aid and learn ways to communicate more effectively.

Although it is most helpful to small children to fit hearing aids as soon as a hearing impairment is definitely established, the hearing aid will be only as effective as the care the parents give in helping their child adjust to it. The parents need to make sure it is functioning properly each day, replace dead batteries immediately, and guide their child in wearing it consistently. Unless they understand the effect of the hearing loss and the value of the aid to their child, it is likely that they will not make this effort. Furthermore, children are quick to sense parents' lack of acceptance and, consequently, refuse to wear their aids. Therefore, it is better to wait to fit hearing aids until parents or caregivers are ready to accept responsibility for helping their children to use them effectively. If the parents participate in a parent–infant program, this should give them the guidance and experiences that will enable them to accept responsibility for their child's hearing aid.

If an adult is strongly resistant to trying a hearing aid, it is important to respect this desire. Despite the unwillingness to try a hearing aid, s/he may be willing to attend an aural rehabilitation group with other people who are learning new ways to compensate for their hearing losses and communicate more effectively. This experience may provide the opportunity to discover that s/he is not the only person having problems and that new skills can be helpful in easing the stress of communication. With this discovery s/he may now be willing to have a hearing aid evaluation. Those who do not want either a hearing aid or aural rehabilitation may want to try these later if their needs change. They will be more likely to seek help later if the clinician accepts their decision and offers the opportunity to return in the future rather than urging them to try a hearing aid now.

For people who are willing to have a hearing aid evaluation, clinicians can demonstrate to them and their families what intensity levels are necessary for them to hear speech comfortably without an aid and how well they can recognize speech with a well-fitted hearing aid. This experience almost always leads to a new appreciation of the problems they have had and the benefit a hearing aid will provide. It is equally important to talk about the limitations of a hearing aid and situations in which it will be less useful. Unlike eyeglasses, which compensate for inaccurate focusing of light on the retina, a hearing aid cannot compensate fully for missing or dysfunctioning cells in the inner ear. Consequently, the benefit that can be expected will be in relation to the residual hearing. If the individual's family understands about the hearing loss, its effect on communication, and the benefits and limitations of a hearing aid, they can provide valuable support as the individual learns to use the aid.

Many people who are evaluated with a hearing aid for the first time want the smallest, least conspicuous instrument. The attitude of many in our society is that people with hearing losses are physically handicapped, and therefore such people are sometimes less accepted. As a result, those with a hearing loss want to hide their hearing impairment because of vanity or because they fear being ostracized. These are legitimate concerns and must be respected. Our responsibility is to show them that they communicate best when the hearing aid is selected to match their residual hearing. If this happens to be a bigger aid than they will wear, it is better to have them wear a smaller aid than none at all. Perhaps at a later date they will be willing to shift to a more appropriate aid.

After a hearing aid and earmold are selected and adjusted to amplify speech to comfortable loudness levels and to limit sound so that it is not uncomfortable, further guidance and orientation in the care and use of the hearing aid are given. This and other aspects of counseling are described in chapter 10. This guidance is most effective when it is incorporated in an aural rehabilitation program. Although suggestions for improving communication skills are included in chapter 10, a description of aural rehabilitation is beyond the scope of this book.

TECHNICAL DIMENSIONS

In recent years we have come to a much better understanding of the technical factors that must be considered to successfully match the amplification characteristics of a hearing aid to an individual's residual hearing. The goals are to make speech and other important sounds comfortably loud in the frequency region between 250 and 6000 Hz and to limit the maximum acoustic output so that the sound does not become uncomfortably loud.

Effect of Hearing Impairment on Speech Recognition

Hearing impairment can be caused by malformation or disease at any point along the auditory pathway. The sound can be blocked before it reaches the inner ear, resulting in a conductive hearing loss. The major effect of this impairment is a reduction of sound intensity; amplification from a hearing aid can effectively compensate for this type of hearing loss. If cells in the inner ear that change sound to neural energy are lost or damaged, low-intensity sounds are not heard, but high-intensity sounds are often heard at a normal loudness level. With this type of cochlear hearing impairment, the hearing loss is often greater at some frequencies than at others, so the gain of the hearing aid has to be adjusted to compensate for this. Furthermore, the maximum sound levels have to be limited to prevent sound from being too loud. If a hearing aid is appropriately fitted, it can give significant benefit to a person with cochlear hearing impairment even though there still may be distortion of speech. If nerve cells that carry the sound signal from the inner ear to the brain are lost or damaged, the sound is not transmitted or analyzed accurately and usually does not seem as loud as normal at high intensities. At the present time hearing aids cannot compensate for this loss of nerve cells, except to increase the intensity of the sound. In fitting a hearing aid it is important to know where in the auditory pathway there is dysfunction and what effect this dysfunction has on the ability of the individual to recognize speech. This is discussed in chapter 2.

Room, Equipment, and Stimuli

The gain and output of a hearing aid measured in a 2-cc coupler are *not* the same as the gain and output when a person is wearing the aid. These parameters are significantly affected by the earmold configuration, the microphone placement, the residual earcanal volume, and the acoustic immittance of the individual's middle-ear system. Consequently, it is essential to verify whether the prescribed real-ear characteristics have been obtained by measuring the unaided and aided thresholds in the sound field (functional gain) or by measuring the sound pressure level (SPL) in the ear canal with and without the hearing aid in place (insertion gain). Both of these measurements must be made in a relatively quiet space, such as a sound-treated room. Equipment is needed for generating these sounds, amplifying them, and presenting them to the hearing aid. Sound-level meters are needed to measure the sound in the field, and a hearing aid test box is needed to measure the amplification characteristics of hearing aids. This is discussed in chapter 3.

Measuring Sound

Measuring sound is a fairly complicated matter, particularly when you want to compare measurements made at several different reference points. Ideally, all measurements should be referred to an individual's eardrum, but this is not clinically feasible. In reality:

1. earphone sound levels are referred to measurements made with a microphone in a 6-cc coupler,
2. sound-field levels are referred to measurements made at a point in space that represents the midpoint on a line between the listener's two ears,
3. probe or probe-tube microphone sound levels are referred to measurements made at a point at least 5 mm toward the eardrum from the tip of the earmold, and
4. hearing aid output is referred to measurements made with a microphone in a 2-cc coupler or an ear stimulator.

Ways to relate measurements to a single reference point, so that the output of the hearing aid can be directly compared with the individual's residual hearing, are described in chapter 4.

The position of the listener in relation to a loudspeaker strongly affects the sound reaching the eardrum. Small movements of the head can cause relatively large changes in the sound level, depending on the distance of the person from the loudspeaker and the reverberation patterns in the room. These effects on tonal and speech stimuli are described in chapter 4.

Manufacturers publish specifications for each model hearing aid that they produce. The American National Standards Institute (ANSI) has adopted standard methods for measuring hearing aids; these are used to determine whether a hearing aid is functioning properly. The aid may be new, used, or repaired. In addition to the standard measurements, the output of the aid is measured where it was set for aided testing in the sound field (i.e., at use-gain). These data are used to monitor changes in use-gain and to compare sound levels between the 2-cc coupler and the sound field. The standard measurements of hearing aids are described briefly in chapter 4.

Criteria for Prescribing Hearing Aid Characteristics

A hearing aid will provide the greatest assistance to communication if:

1. it amplifies conversational speech in specific frequency regions between 250 and 6000 Hz to a comfortable listening level for the individual,
2. the overall level of speech can be adjusted so it is comfortable for various listening situations,
3. the sound quality is acceptable, and
4. the maximum output does not allow the amplified sound to surpass the individual's discomfort level.

To achieve these criteria, the amount of real-ear gain (that is, the difference between the unaided and aided condition in the sound field) and maximum acoustic output in specific frequency regions need to be specified. These specifications are based on data obtained from the person being evaluated. These data, which define the boundaries of the individual's residual hearing, include thresholds, comfortable listening levels, and un-comfortable listening levels for frequency-specific sounds and speech. Several procedures for obtaining these data are described in chapter 5. In chapter 6 and 7 the use of these data to prescribe the real-ear gain and maximum acoustic output is described and compared for six different procedures.

Preselection of a Hearing Aid and Earmold

There are several different types of hearing aids and hundreds of different models from which to choose. In addition, there are a number of different types of earmolds, tubing, and venting that can markedly affect the acoustic output of the hearing aid. The types of hearing aids and ear-molds are described, including their advantages and disadvantages, in chapter 8. After weighing and balancing these, a hearing aid(s) and earmold are chosen based on the acoustic and nonacoustic needs of the individual.

Given the prescribed real-ear gain and estimated maximum acoustic output, it is *impossible* to predict exactly what the 2-cc coupler gain and the saturation sound-pressure level for an input of 90 dB SPL (SSPL90) of hearing aid should be. However, average values, which take into account microphone placement, earmold effects, effects of the residual earcanal volume and acoustic immitance at the eardrum, can be used to give an approximation of the needed output. Tables of these values are given in chapter 8. In addition, one prescriptive procedure was chosen to show how the residual hearing data from three people and values from these tables were used to select an earmold and estimate the needed 2-cc coupler gain and SSPL90.

Measurements for a Successful Fit

The only way to determine whether the preselected hearing aid(s) (or the person's own hearing aid) and earmold are comfortable, provide accept-able sound quality, give the prescribed characteristics, and are useful to the individual is to put the aid(s) on and make a number of measurements and observations. It may be necessary to adjust the hearing aid, the earmold, or both to obtain the prescribed characteristics, after measuring the real-ear gain and determining whether loud sound is limited before it becomes uncomfortable. If the aid cannot be adjusted, another one should be tried. *Once the prescribed characteristics are obtained*, the person who is wearing the aid(s) evaluates the sound quality and the clarity of amplified speech. Tests of speech recognition may also be done. Further adjustments may be needed to make the amplified sound most helpful and acceptable, particularly in listening conditions outside the test room. These measurements, adjustments, and observations are described in chapter 9.

SUMMARY

The human and technical dimensions of a hearing aid evaluation both must be considered for the aid(s) to provide maximum benefit. The major goals in the human dimension are: (1) to determine the hearing and communication problems of the individual and (2) to create an environment in which solutions to these problems are sought by the individual with the guidance and support of the clinician. This guidance, which includes information about hearing impairment, its effect on communication, appropriate hearing aids, and aural rehabilitation, needs to start before the hearing aid evaluation begins and continue after the hearing aid has been fitted. Ultimately, it is the responsibility of the hearing-impaired individual to enhance communication by using a hearing aid and learning compensatory skills.

The major technical goal is to select and adjust a hearing aid or aids that provide the *best hearing function* given the underlying hearing impairment and the acceptability of the sound quality. No matter how well we achieve this goal, the hearing aid will provide no benefit unless the person wears it. Consequently, it is essential to consider both the human and the technical dimensions in a hearing aid evaluation.

Chapter Two
EFFECTS OF HEARING IMPAIRMENT ON IDENTIFICATION OF SPEECH SOUNDS

Speech is the most important sound human beings hear. To amplify speech so that it is maximally intelligible as well as comfortable, it is important to know something about its physical dimensions and what factors affect its identification by hearing-impaired individuals. An understanding of this material is essential for choosing the appropriate criteria for fitting a hearing aid.

ACOUSTIC PARAMETERS OF SPEECH

Speech information is carried by the changing pattern of sound energy, which varies in frequency and intensity as a function of time. The spectrogram of the sentence shown in the lower half of figure 2.1 illustrates this

FIGURE 2.1.   Lower panel: Spectrogram of the sentence "Teak is more expensive than wheat," spoken by a male talker. In this display, frequency is represented on the ordinate, intensity by the darkness of the trace (that is, the darker the trace, the more intense the sound), and time on the abscissa. Upper panel: Relative intensity trace as a function of time for this sentence. From M. W. Skinner 1978. "Hearing of speech during language acquisition." *Otolaryngologic Clinics of North America* 11:631−50, figure 1. Reproduced with permission of the publisher.

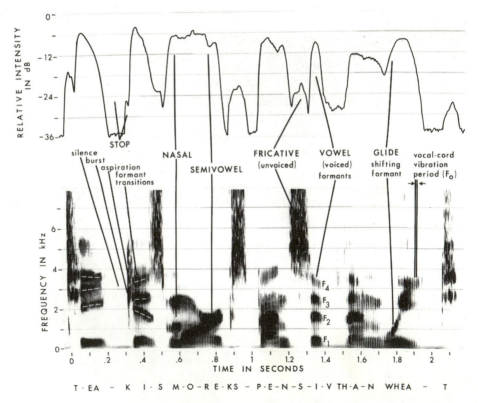

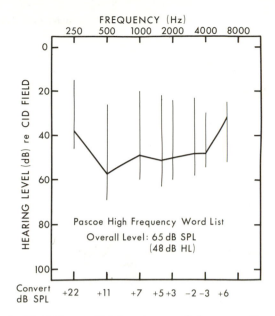

FREQUENCY (Hz)

FIGURE 2.2.
Measurements of the intensity levels in specific frequency regions (one-third octave wide) for fifty monosyllabic words (Pascoe High-Frequency Word List, Pascoe 1975). Spoken by a male talker. One root-mean-squared (rms) level (dB SPL) was sampled every 20 milliseconds; the vertical lines represent the range of levels for the entire word list. The heavy line depicts the one level in each frequency region exceeded by 10 percent of the samples.

Pascoe High Frequency Word List
Overall Level: 65 dB SPL
(48 dB HL)

| Convert dB SPL | +22 | +11 | +7 | +5 +3 | -2 -3 | +6 |

changing pattern. In the upper half of figure 2.1 is a trace of the overall intensity of the speech as a function of time. Note that the voiceless consonants such as /k/, /s/, and /th/ are less intense than the voiced consonants and vowels. When the overall intensity of this sentence or of a list of words is measured, it is an average of these momentary fluctuations in intensity level.

The sound energy of speech in specific frequency regions can also be measured. The intensity level in these regions will fluctuate as a function of time. If successive measurements are made at short time intervals, a range of levels are obtained. This range of levels is shown in figure 2.2 by the vertical lines. The heavy line connecting them represents one level in each frequency region chosen to represent an average of this range. Note that the range of levels is approximately 12 dB above this line and 18 dB or more below this line (except for the 6000-Hz band). The total range of intensity levels in one frequency region is 30 dB or more for this word list spoken at one overall level (65 dB SPL in the field).

In everyday life people speak with vocal efforts that range from casual to a shout. An example of the change in spectral energy as a function of vocal effort is shown in figure 2.3. Note that the low-frequency energy is more intense than the high-frequency energy for the casual and normal vocal efforts, but for loud speech the mid-frequency energy is most intense. The range of overall levels is 54 to 81.5 dB SPL. Although the range of overall levels is approximately the same for men and children, the spectra are somewhat different. The men, who speak with more low-frequency energy, are often easier for hearing-impaired listeners to understand.

Since people seldom shout, the normal range of overall levels for conversational speech is about 20 dB (55 to 75 dB SPL at 1 m). However, this range needs to be expanded to 25 dB to include the level (approximately 80

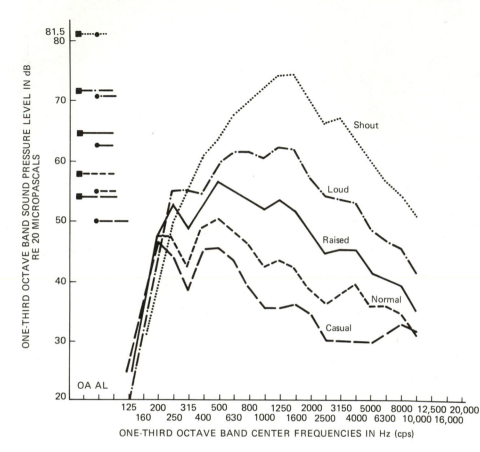

FIGURE 2.3. Average speech spectra for females at five vocal efforts measured 1 m from the talker. The overall level (dB SPL) for each vocal effort is depicted by the square symbols at the far left side of the graph. From K. S. Pearsons, R. L. Bennett, and S. Fidell 1976. "Speech levels in various environments." *Bolt Beranek and Newman Report No. 321.* Reproduced with permission of Bolt Beranek and Newman, Inc.

dB SPL) at which our own voices reach our ears. If this 25 dB range is added to the 30 dB range of the momentary fluctuations in specific frequency regions, hearing-impaired individuals will function best if they have at least a 55 dB range within which to receive amplified speech.

LISTENING CONDITIONS

Speech in Noise

The overall intensity at which people speak varies as a function of the background noise. Measurements made in several environments (see figure 2.4) indicate that on the average people speak at 55 dB SPL for noise levels

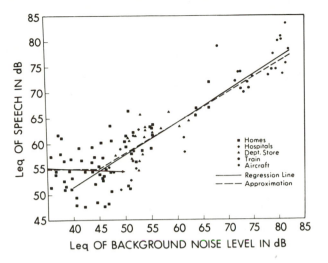

FIGURE 2.4. Conversing speech level for face-to-face communication as a function of background noise in several environments. The level equivalent (Leq) of speech (and noise) is the same as the long-term rms level measured over an extended period of time. An A-weighted filter on the sound-level meter was used for this measurement, and the speech levels were subsequently normalized to the level at 1 m. From K. S. Pearsons, R. L. Bennett, and S. Fidell 1976. "Speech levels in various environments." *Bolt Beranek and Newman Report No. 321.* Reproduced with permission of Bolt Beranek and Newman, Inc.

up to 45 dB SPL. The speech-to-noise ratio is approximately +10 to +20 dB in this range. When the background noise increases above 45 dB SPL, people raise the level of their speech and move closer to the person with whom they are talking to keep the speech level higher than the noise level. In high-level noise the speech-to-noise ratio may be 0 dB or less.

In quiet places, such as a living room, where the speech-to-noise ratio is +10 dB or higher, adults with mild or moderate hearing loss and well-fitted hearing aids can understand what is said with little difficulty. Those with severe sensorineural hearing loss need higher speech-to-noise ratios (+15 or +20 dB) to understand speech optimally. As the speech-to-noise ratio decreases, all hearing-impaired individuals experience difficulty understanding what is said. Individuals with a significant neural component to their hearing loss seem to have more difficulty understanding speech in noise than those with a cochlear hearing impairment.

Many environmental sounds have high energy in the low frequencies (approximately 100 to 500 Hz) and less energy in the high frequencies (above 1000 Hz). Normal-hearing individuals take advantage of the high-frequency cues of speech to understand in noisy places. Those with normal low-frequency hearing and a high-frequency sensorineural hearing loss

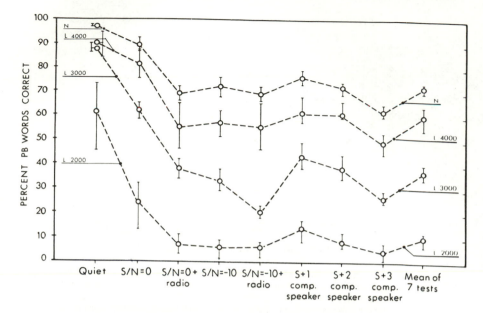

FIGURE 2.5.   Mean score (and 95 percent confidence interval) for normal-hearing individuals (N), for individuals with bilateral sensorineural hearing loss of 50 dB or more at 4000 and 6000 Hz and normal hearing at 3000 Hz and below (L4000), for individuals whose hearing loss began at 3000 Hz (L3000), and for individuals whose hearing loss began at 2000 Hz (L2000). The individuals, who were from twenty-four to forty-nine years old, identified Swedish, phonetically balanced monosyllables presented at 60 dB(C) in the field both in quiet and in six different competing noises. In quiet those with significant losses at and above 3000 Hz performed almost as well as those with normal hearing. In noise all the individuals with high-frequency hearing losses, even those where the loss started at 4000 Hz, obtained scores significantly lower than those for the normal-hearing individuals. From G. Aniansson 1974. "Methods for assessing high frequency hearing loss in every-day listening situations." *Acta Otolaryngologica* (Stockholm), supp. 320, 1–50. Reproduced with permission of the publisher.

(and no hearing aid) have more difficulty understanding speech in noisy conditions than those with normal hearing (see figure 2.5).

Speech in Reverberant Rooms

When someone speaks outdoors, for example, in a meadow, there are no hard surfaces to reflect the sound. This is called a free-field condition. In this case the speech is only as intense as the speaker makes it, and the level decreases as the listener moves away from the person speaking. When someone speaks indoors, the sound is reflected from the ceiling, floor, and walls. The amount of sound reflection (reverberation) is dependent on the size of the room and the absorption its surfaces provide. Rooms with heavy carpeting, acoustically treated ceilings, and draperies are much less reverberant than spaces completely enclosed by hard walls such as subway corridors or caves. One measure of the reverberation of a room is the time it takes for the sound-pressure level to decrease 60 dB after a steady-state sound stops; this is called the reverberation time (RT). The longer the reverberation time, the more sound will seem to echo in the space.

Some reverberation is desirable, especially that which occurs within 200 msec. after the person speaks, because it increases the intensity of the received speech signal. This increase in intensity can be associated with more intelligible speech. Too much reverberation (rooms with reverberation times longer than ½-sec.) can cause speech to be less intelligible. This decrease in intelligibility is caused by the later reflections "time smearing" the speech patterns. An example of this "smearing" is shown in the spectrogram in the right panel of figure 2.6.

Individuals with mild or moderate sensorineural hearing impairment understand speech better in reverberant rooms when the high-frequency energy is audible and when they listen with both ears rather than with only one. However, there are large individual differences in the amount of improvement they get from hearing aids (Nabalek and Robinson 1982). Those who obtain the least improvement probably introduce significant distortion during the transduction of the acoustic signal to neural signal in the cochlea and/or they abnormally process the signals from the two ears in the central auditory nervous system. Those who obtain substantial improve-

FIGURE 2.6. Speech spectrograms of the phrase "the beet again." In the left panel the words were spoken in an anechoic chamber in which the reverberation time was zero, and in the right panel they were spoken in a room with a reverberation time of 0.4 sec. From A. K. Nabelek 1982. "Temporal distortions and noise considerations." In *The Vanderbilt Hearing-Aid Report.* Ed. G. A. Studebaker and F. H. Bess. Reproduced with permission of the author and Monographs in Contemporary Audiology, Upper Darby, Pa.

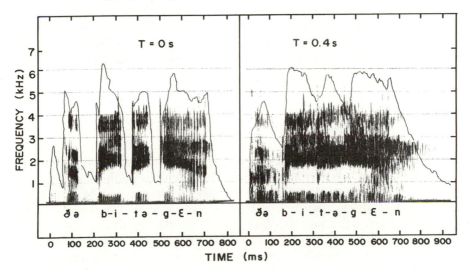

ment will probably benefit from binaural aids in moderately reverberant rooms (RT = less than 0.5 to approximately 1 sec.). In churches and large auditoriums that are very reverberant, hearing-impaired individuals need to avoid the adverse effects of reverberation by sitting as close to the source of speech as possible or by using FM, induction loop, or infrared transmission systems.

Speech Context

Adults who converse with one another have many years of experience with the language they are speaking and hearing. In most situations the words spoken are familiar and often predictable from the context of the conversation. However, occasionally words are unfamiliar or unpredictable from the context. In addition, some words may be unintelligible because they are masked by background noise or reverberation. In these adverse conditions normal-hearing individuals have to pay close attention both auditorily and visually to compensate for the cues that are not available. If the adverse conditions continue for a long time, people eventually become too tired to try to understand what is being said.

Hearing-impaired individuals who do not wear hearing aids have more difficulty understanding speech than normal-hearing individuals in the same listening conditions. For those with conductive hearing impairment, a hearing aid will compensate well for the loss of normal sound transmission to the inner ear. For those with cochlear or neural hearing impairment, presently available hearing aids cannot compensate for the lack of normal auditory processing in the inner ear or neural centers, but the aids can be adjusted to so that speech is maximally intelligible for the individual.

Normal-hearing children and those with hearing impairment need more acoustic cues than adults to perceive speech accurately. They are still in the process of learning language and cannot predict unfamiliar words or unclearly spoken words from the context of the conversation as easily as adults can. For this reason, it is just as important to adjust hearing aids to maximize speech intelligibility for children as it is for adults.

AUDITORY PROCESSING CAPABILITY

Normal-hearing adults understand speech accurately even under adverse circumstances, such as in noisy cafeterias, because their auditory processing capabilities are normal. In addition to audibility, these capabilities include the ability to (1) discriminate small changes in intensity, in frequency, and in the timing of successive sounds, (2) keep separate the frequency components that occur simultaneously in a complex sound, (3) hear speech at normal loudness levels, (4) integrate sound energy over time, and (5) localize the source of sounds accurately in space. Hearing-impaired individuals do not have normal auditory processing capabilities, and thus they have more difficulty discriminating speech under adverse conditions. Effects of conductive, cochlear, and neural hearing impairment on the processing of sound are described in the sections that follow.

Conductive Hearing Impairment

Individuals with a purely conductive hearing impairment have a lesion or malformation that blocks the normal transmission of sound to the inner ear. This blockage causes the sound at the inner ear to be less intense and often of different phase than if there had been normal transmission. Although the sound level is less intense at the inner ear, it is probably processed there and in the auditory nervous system in much the same way that it would be at that level in a normal-hearing person, except for small changes in phase. That is, the ability to detect changes in intensity and in frequency and to detect the time a sound begins and ends is similar to the normal ear at the same level above threshold (sensation level; SL). In everyday life the conductive hearing loss often causes speech and other sounds to be too soft to hear comfortably. Because of the phase shifts, such loss can make it a little more difficult to localize sounds in space (e.g. Nordlund 1964) and to detect signals in noise (at threshold) (Hall and Derlacki 1986). These listeners often obtain maximum benefit from hearing aids, since the aids compensate for the loss of intensity and many aspects of their auditory processing are essentially normal.

Cochlear Hearing Impairment (Hair-Cell Loss)

The most prevalent type of cochlear hearing impairment is caused by hair-cell dysfunction or loss. The degree of hearing loss is related to the number of hair cells that are dysfunctioning or have been lost in specific regions of the cochlea. Patterns of hair-cell loss are different at the base than at the apex and depend on the etiology of the loss. Some studies (Bredberg 1968; Clark and Bohne 1986) have shown a 30 to 50 percent loss of outer hair cells in the apical turn of the cochlea before there is an elevation of pure-tone thresholds in the low frequencies, whereas a smaller percentage of loss of hair cells in the basal turn is associated with threshold elevation in the high frequencies (Clark and Bohne 1978). Under some conditions there can be loss of outer hair cells with preservation of inner hair cells for hearing losses up to 50 dB HL in the frequencies at and above 1000 Hz. With hearing losses greater than 50 dB Hearing Level (HL), inner hair cells are lost in significant numbers (Bohne and Clark 1976). According to the knowledge presently available, the degeneration of primary auditory neurons is not significant until inner hair cells are lost (Morest and Bohne 1983). Thus, for mild or moderate hearing losses at and above 1000 Hz, there is generally a nearly normal population of neurons to encode the sound once its intensity is above threshold. However, the message these neurons carry is probably not normal. The current belief is that the outer hair cells exert some influence on the inner hair cells; if outer hair cells are missing, they cannot exert a normal influence on the inner hair cells (Kim 1984).

Frequency and timing resolution.   The lack of a normal population of hair cells can cause a decrease in the individual's ability to detect changes in frequency, to detect the time of onset and offset of sounds, to keep separate the frequency components that occur simultaneously in a complex sound, and to integrate intensity over time (Scharf and Florentine 1982; Tyler, Summerfield, Wood and Fernandes 1982). This decrease appears related to the number of hair cells missing (or nonfunctioning) and to the location in the cochlea. For example, if the hair cells are missing only in a small section of the basal turn of the cochlea, the decrease in ability will be specific to high-frequency sounds (for example, 3000 to 4000 Hz) that would normally be transduced by the hair cells that are missing. The greater the loss of cells, the poorer the ability to resolve frequency and timing information.

Unlike normal-hearing individuals, who are equally sensitive to small changes in the frequency and timing of a sound over a fairly large range of background intensities (for example, between 50 and 100 dB SPL), individuals with cochlear impairment have small ranges over which they are maximally sensitive (for example, 10 to 15 dB) (e.g., Jerger and Jerger 1967). The position of this maximally sensitive range re 0 dB SPL is dependent on the degree of hearing loss and often varies as a function of frequency. Commercially available hearing aids can be adjusted to amplify speech for the individual listener so that it falls in this maximally sensitive range in specific frequency regions. This enables individual listeners to take full advantage of the auditory processing capabilities they have.

Intensity resolution.   Individuals with mild or moderate cochlear hearing impairment are able to detect changes in intensity as well, or almost as well, as normal-hearing individuals can at the same background intensity. Only when sounds are very intense (for example, 110 dB SPL) does their ability become poorer than normal (Jerger and Jerger 1967). These individuals also have *loudness recruitment*, which can be defined as the abnormally rapid growth of loudness above threshold as the physical intensity of sound increases *or* a normal loudness sensation at moderate to high intensity levels (for example, 60 to 100 dB HL) despite loss of hearing sensitivity for softer sounds.

Individuals with severe and profound cochlear hearing impairment will have secondary degeneration of primary auditory neurons where inner hair cells are lost. This is associated with somewhat poorer ability to detect changes in intensity. However, as long as a few hair cells and some neurons are intact, these individuals will have loudness recruitment for sounds above threshold.

Frequency selectivity and masking.   Some individuals with mild or moderate cochlear hearing impairment appear to have normal (or nearly normal) ability to keep separate the frequency components of complex sounds that occur simultaneously (called *frequency selectivity*), though others do not (Wightman, McGee, and Kramer 1977). Unfortunately, one cannot predict frequency-selectivity ability from the pure-tone thresholds or dynamic range. Frequency-selectivity involves a filtering process that enables normal individuals to respond differently to sounds composed of frequencies within a certain bandwidth than to sounds outside this bandwidth. This bandwidth is called a *critical bandwidth*. When this filtering process is normal, the masking effect of irrelevant sound on speech is the same as it is for normal-hearing individuals. When this process is abnormal, the critical bandwidth is larger and it is more difficult for these individuals to perceive speech in the midst of noise than it is for normal-hearing individuals. This is particularly true for people with severe to profound cochlear impairment.

Frequency selectivity and loudness summation.   Another aspect of the filtering process is the perceived loudness of a complex sound as a function of its bandwidth. For example, if the bandwidth of a noise is increased and at the same time the sound-pressure level of the noise is kept constant, the loudness of the noise will remain constant for normal-hearing individuals as long as the noise is within a critical bandwidth. When the critical bandwidth is exceeded, the loudness will increase even though the sound-pressure level of the noise is kept constant. This is called *loudness summation*. Loudness summation for normal-hearing individuals is greatest at moderate intensities (55 to 65 dB HL) and is considerably less at intensities near uncomfortable listening levels (UCL), which are 90 to 100 dB HL. Some individuals with mild or moderate cochlear impairment appear to have normal loudness summation when compared with normal performance at the same sound level; others, particularly those with severe to profound hearing losses, do not summate the loudness of broad-band sounds in a normal fashion (e.g., Scharf and Hellman 1966). An example of loudness summation in a normal-hearing individual and a hypothetical example of no loudness summation are shown in figure 5.7.

An understanding of loudness summation is important in hearing aid fitting. For example, when an individual's UCL contour is obtained and the maximum output of the aid is set so that amplified sound does not surpass UCL in any specific frequency region (presuming that both the maximum output and the UCL are measured at the eardrum), a person with normal loudness summation will complain that intense sounds amplified by the hearing aid are too loud. These same sounds will not be too loud for someone with no loudness summation.

Cochlear Hearing Impairment (Strial Atrophy)

A rare type of cochlear hearing impairment is caused by degeneration of part of the stria vascularis; this has been called strial presbycusis. Individuals with this type of cochlear hearing impairment show no difference between their air-conduction and bone-conduction thresholds, and there is little or no loss of hair cells or primary auditory neurons. Since there is little loss of hair cells or neurons, these individuals seem to have nearly normal ability to resolve the frequency, intensity, and timing cues of speech; that is, they understand speech as well as normal-hearing listeners at the same sensation level (Schuknecht 1974). In addition, these individuals do not have loudness recruitment. The strial atrophy is thought to be associated with a lack of the normal amplification provided by the inner ear, which creates a loss similar to a conductive hearing loss.

Neural Hearing Impairment

Neural hearing impairment is caused by loss or dysfunction of auditory neurons. The loss or dysfunction may be localized at one site (such as that caused by an VIIIth cranial nerve neuroma), or it may be scattered throughout the central auditory pathways (such as that caused by multiple sclerosis). The pattern and extent of loss of neurons determines the effect on the individual's auditory processing capabilities. If the loss of neurons occurs only in the VIIIth cranial nerve or the lower brainstem, there is usually an elevation of pure-tone thresholds on the same side as the lesion. In addition, there is often a marked impairment of the ability to detect changes in intensity, frequency, and temporal order and to summate loudness (e.g., Jerger and Jerger 1967). This is associated with much poorer scores on word-identification tests than found with individuals with cochlear impairment who have the same pure-tone thresholds. The ability to understand speech in noise with the impaired ear is also much poorer than for individuals with the same degree of cochlear impairment. In addition, the defective neural input from the impaired ear also makes localization of a sound source inaccurate (Nordlund 1964).

Neural lesions in the upper brainstem, thalamus, or auditory cortex usually do not cause a hearing loss measured with pure tones, unless most of the auditory pathways are affected. Since there are many alternative routes for transmitting the neural signal to the cortex, the impairment of auditory processing often is not as marked as when the lesion occurs in the VIIIth cranial nerve. However, the impairment is often evident at both ears and not just at one ear. This impairment of binaural processing often makes it difficult for these individuals to understand speech in noisy or reverberant situations and to localize a sound source accurately. Individuals with neural impairment may not benefit from binaural amplification, unlike those with cochlear and conductive impairment.

Purely neural hearing impairments are rare. Most people with a neural impairment also have a cochlear impairment. This includes some people with presbycusis and those with tertiary syphilis and other diseases that affect both the cochlea and the central auditory nervous system. Individuals with both a cochlear and neural hearing impairment will have more difficulty understanding speech, particularly at poor speech-to-noise ratios (e.g., Olsen, Noffsinger, and Kurdziel 1975), and have MCL (most-comfortable listening level) and UCL contours at higher intensity levels than those with only cochlear hearing impairment. The MCL and UCL in specific frequency regions is probably elevated by the relative contribution of the neural dysfunction to the total hearing impairment.

RELATION OF SPEECH ENERGY TO DYNAMIC RANGE

Dynamic Range

The range of intensity levels between threshold and UCL is known as a hearing-impaired individual's *dynamic range* or *residual hearing*. This range is often determined as the person listens to speech. Specifically, it is calculated by subtracting the overall level associated with the speech-reception threshold (SRT) for spondaic words from the level of running speech that the person judges to be uncomfortably loud (UCL). Some clinicians also ask listeners to choose a level at which running speech is either most comfortable (MCL) or most intelligible (MIL); these two levels lie within the dynamic range. Listeners' judgments of UCL, MCL, and MIL are influenced by the instructions and by their own internal reference criteria. Although there is no generally accepted set of instructions, the ones used in clinical research at Central Institute for the Deaf are similar to those used by others (see Appendix 2).

The SRT, MCL, MIL, and UCL for speech are all affected by the spectral configuration of energy that reaches the inner ear. For example, the SRT for normal-hearing individuals is 4 dB lower when they listen in the sound field (at 0° azimuth) than when they listen under earphones. In the sound field the head diffraction and outer-ear resonances enhance the level of the high-frequency sound; this is the reason the SRT is 4 dB lower. The spectrum of speech amplified by hearing aids is often much different from that delivered by an audiometer through earphones or a loudspeaker. The

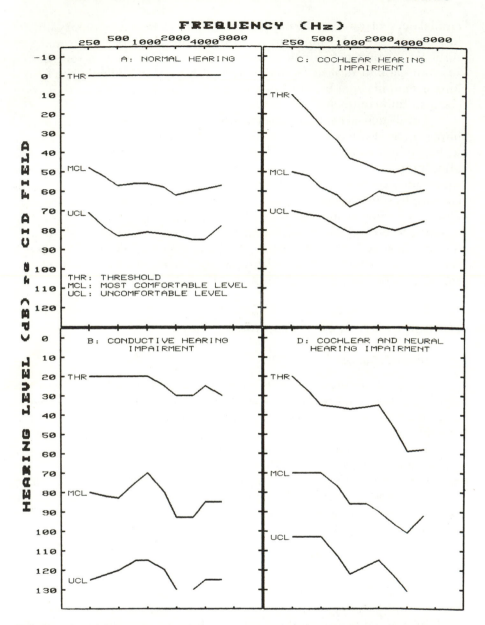

FIGURE 2.7. Examples of the dynamic range of normal-hearing individuals and three individuals with different kinds of hearing impairment. In these graphs the dynamic range is bounded by the threshold and UCL contour between 250 and 6000 Hz; the MCL contour falls within this range. **(A)** The average dynamic range for a group of normal-hearing young adults. **(B)** The normal dynamic range of a listener with normal bone conduction thresholds and a block in the external auditory canal. **(C)** The reduced dynamic range of a listener with a cochlear hearing impairment. **(D)** The nearly normal dynamic range of an elderly listener with both cochlear and neural hearing impairment.

aided SRT will reflect both the overall gain and the spectrum of the amplified speech.

The dynamic range can also be measured for frequency-specific signals such as pure tones or one-third-octave bands of noise. This is particularly useful with hearing-impaired individuals because the dynamic range often varies in ways that are not predictable from the audiogram. The dynamic range is also related to the anatomical site of dysfunction in the auditory system. The sound reaching the inner ear of an individual with conductive hearing impairment is lower by the amount of hearing loss. The UCL will usually be elevated by the amount of this conductive hearing loss except when the sound delivered to the eardrum is in excess of 120 to 140 dB SPL. When this occurs, the excessive movement of the eardrum and the middle-ear ossicles may cause discomfort. An example of the dynamic range of someone with a conductive impairment is shown in panel B of figure 2.7. Note that the dynamic range of the person with the conductive hearing impairment is approximately the same as that for the group of normal-hearing individuals shown in panel A.

Individuals with cochlear impairment (if it involves hair-cell loss and thresholds that do not exceed 50 dB HL) choose UCLs that are within the normal range, but since their thresholds are elevated they have reduced dynamic ranges. An example of the dynamic range of someone with this type of impairment is shown in panel C of figure 2.7. Note how much narrower this dynamic range is than that for the normal-hearing individuals.

Individuals with neural impairment choose UCLs that are higher than normal; they may have normal or expanded dynamic ranges depending on the degree of threshold and UCL elevation.

A number of older people with sensorineural hearing losses appear to have a combination of cochlear and neural dysfunction. A typical example of the dynamic range of someone with this type of loss is shown in panel D of figure 2.7. The dynamic range is approximately normal.

The dynamic range of a hearing-impaired individual probably reflects the composite effect of one or more sites of dysfunction in the auditory pathway and these effects vary as a function of frequency. Furthermore, the MCL contour probably approximates the range of intensity levels where this individual's frequency, intensity, and timing resolution is most sensitive.

Comparison of Speech Energy and Dynamic Range

The proportion of speech energy that falls within an individual's dynamic range can be determined, if the speech levels and the tones or noisebands (used for defining the dynamic range) are calibrated at the same reference point (for example, a microphone in the unobstructed field). An example of this comparison is shown in figure 2.8. The word-level contour is based on acoustical measurements of the Pascoe High-Frequency Word List

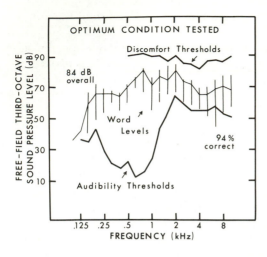

FIGURE 2.8.
Comparison of speech energy and dynamic range for a listener with a noise-induced hearing loss. The thresholds and UCLs were obtained with third-octave bands of noise presented in the field. The word-level contour represents the average of the range of levels that are approximately 12 dB above it and 18 dB below it in each frequency region (on this figure only the 10th to the 90th percentile of this range is shown by the vertical lines). The overall level is 84 dB SPL. Stimulus: Pascoe High-Frequency Word List spoken by a female. From M. W. Skinner 1979. "Audibility and intelligibility of speech for listeners with sensorineural hearing loss." In *Rehabilitative Strategies for Sensorineural Hearing Loss*. Ed. P. Yanick. Reprinted with permission of Grune & Stratton, Inc.

spoken by a female, and it is plotted on the same graph with a hearing-impaired listener's threshold and UCL contours. In an experiment in which there were nine variations in high-frequency gain and five intensity levels (9 × 5 conditions), this listener obtained the highest score with this particular configuration of the speech energy, for which the gain between 1600 and 6000 Hz was 22 dB greater than that between 100 and 800 Hz. Even if the 30-dB range of energy around the word-level contour is included, most of the speech energy between 250 and 6000 Hz falls within this listener's dynamic range; that is, it is audible and not uncomfortably loud. Note that the overall level is approximately 20 dB higher (84 dB SPL) than that of normal conversational speech (65 dB SPL).

Audibility

A crucial factor in the identification of speech sounds is the audibility of the speech. Clearly, the more of the relevant acoustic energy of the speech that is above threshold, the more likely it is that the listener will be able to detect and identify the phonemes. The greatest increases in score are associated with the increase in level of the speech until all of the signal is well above threshold. This finding is shown in figure 2.9. As shown for this listener in the left panel, the score increases from 38 to 94 percent correct as the overall level increases from 44 to 84 dB SPL.

The audibility of the speech energy in specific frequency regions can be associated with significant increases in score. As shown in figure 2.9, the amount of low-frequency energy is identical for the word-level contours with overall levels of 54 and 61 dB SPL in the left and right panels, respectively. As emphasized by the two dark arrows, the speech energy between

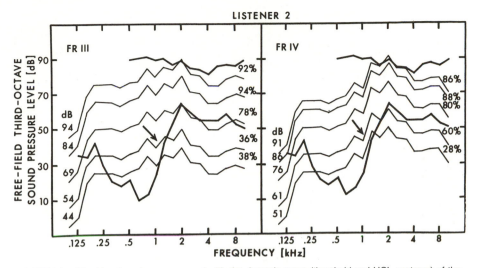

FIGURE 2.9. Word-level contours compared with the dynamic range (threshold and UCL contours) of the same listener whose data are shown in figure 2.8. The overall level of the speech is shown at the far left of each panel, and the word score in percent correct is shown at the far right. Stimulus: Pascoe High-Frequency Word List spoken by a female. From M. W. Skinner 1979. "Audibility and intelligibility of speech for listeners with sensorineural hearing loss." In *Rehabilitative Strategies for Sensorineural Hearing Loss*. Ed. P. Yanick. Reprinted with permission of Grune & Stratton, Inc.

approximately 1200 and 1600 Hz is audible in the right panel and not in the left panel. When this energy is audible, the score is 24 percent higher than when it is inaudible. Since the standard deviation of a single score for this investigation was 4 percent, this represents a significant difference.

Balance

The balance between low-frequency and high-frequency speech energy is important when much of it is above threshold. An example of this is shown in figure 2.10. The overall level in all three panels was associated with the highest word-identification score for that frequency response. These overall levels are approximately the same, and the word-level contours all fall within the listener's dynamic range. However, the balance between low- and high-frequency energy is different. For the uniform response there is more energy in the low-frequency than in the high-frequency region. The score associated with this balance is 10 percent lower than the balance shown in the middle panel, where there is approximately 22 dB more gain in the high frequencies. When there is too much high-frequency gain (see the bottom panel), the intelligibility of the speech decreases.

The importance of the appropriate balance between the low- and high-frequency speech energy for hearing-impaired listeners is also shown

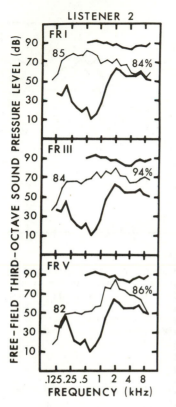

FIGURE 2.10.
Word-level contours associated with the highest word-identification scores for three frequency responses. Although the overall level (dB SPL) of the words (denoted by the number at the left of the speech contours) was approximately the same, the balance between low- and high-frequency energy is different. The highest score was associated with approximately 22 dB more gain in the high frequencies than in the low frequencies. Stimulus: Pascoe High-Frequency Word List spoken by a female. From M. W. Skinner 1979. "Audibility and intelligibility of speech for listeners with sensorineural hearing loss." In *Rehabilitative Strategies for Sensorineural Hearing Loss*. Ed. P. Yanick. Reprinted with permission of Grune & Stratton, Inc.

in figure 2.11. The two speech-level contours in each panel of this figure were achieved with specific settings of the amplification system; these settings were for a uniform response in the field and a response with high-frequency emphasis, the amount of which was determined by the hearing impairment and other criteria. The overall level for each speech level contour was chosen as MCL by each group of listeners. Although the overall levels associated with the two contours for each group are approximately the same, their shapes are different, particularly for the listeners with sharply sloping losses. Both groups obtained significantly higher phoneme-identification scores (standard deviation in this investigation: 2 percent) with the high-frequency emphasis than with the uniform response in the field. The improvement in mean score was 30 percent for the listeners with sharply sloping losses and 13 percent for the listeners with flat losses.

Uncomfortable Listening Level (UCL)

In experiments in which the overall level of speech has been varied below, at, and above the listeners's UCL, the scores for speech at and above the UCL are no higher and are sometimes lower than when the speech is

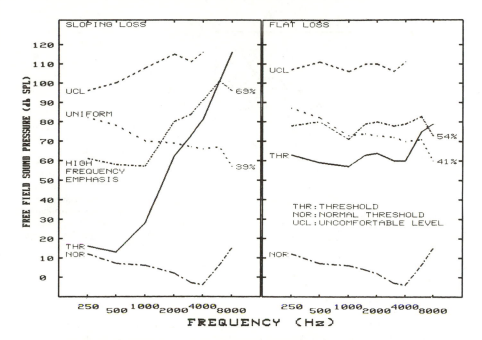

FIGURE 2.11.   Mean speech-level contours compared with the mean threshold and UCL contours in the field for three listeners with sharply sloping hearing losses and two listeners with flat losses. In the original experiment each listener chose the most comfortable listening level for three types of speech material (spoken by male and female talkers) presented with the amplification system set for four different frequency responses. In this figure only the speech-level contours associated with the highest and lowest mean scores are shown for each group, the high-frequency uniform response and a high-frequency response, respectively. Adapted from R. P. Lippman, L. D. Braida, and N. I. Durlach 1981. "Study of multichannel amplitude compression and linear amplification for persons with sensorineural hearing loss." *Journal of the Acoustical Society of America* 69:524−34. Reproduced with permission of the authors and the publisher.

presented below UCL. If the speech energy surpasses a listener's UCL in specific frequency regions, the score may be lower than when the speech energy is below the UCL (see figure 2.12). In this example the score associated with the word-level contour that is below the listener's UCL contour was 10 percent better than when the word-level contour surpassed the UCL contour.

There have been many anecdotal accounts of hearing-aid wearers who turn down the overall gain of their hearing aids when the maximum output is not limited at their UCL contour. They do this to prevent sudden environmental sounds from causing them discomfort. When they lower the gain, they do not receive speech at an overall level high enough for them to understand it maximally. Thus, it is very important to obtain an individual's UCL contour and limit the output of the hearing aid so that loud sounds cannot exceed UCL.

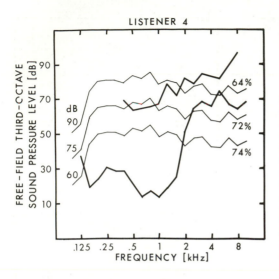

FIGURE 2.12.
Comparison of three word-level contours with the dynamic range of a listener with noise-induced hearing loss. The score is lower when the word-level contour surpasses the listener's UCL contour than when it does not. Stimulus: Pascoe High-Frequency Word List spoken by a female. From M. W. Skinner 1979. "Audibility and intelligibility of speech for listeners with sensorineural hearing loss." In *Rehabilitative Strategies for Sensorineural Hearing Loss.* Ed. P. Yanick. Reprinted with permission of Grune & Stratton, Inc.

Effective Bandwidth

The effective bandwidth of an amplification system is the bandwidth of amplified sound that is above threshold for the individual listener. For example, in figure 2.11, the effective bandwidth was 125 to 6000 Hz for those with flat losses, but for those with sloping losses the effective bandwidth was narrower (125 to 2000 Hz for the uniform response and 125 to 4000 Hz for the high-frequency-emphasis response).

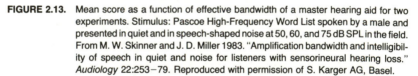

FIGURE 2.13.   Mean score as a function of effective bandwidth of a master hearing aid for two experiments. Stimulus: Pascoe High-Frequency Word List spoken by a male and presented in quiet and in speech-shaped noise at 50, 60, and 75 dB SPL in the field. From M. W. Skinner and J. D. Miller 1983. "Amplification bandwidth and intelligibility of speech in quiet and noise for listeners with sensorineural hearing loss." *Audiology* 22:253–79. Reproduced with permission of S. Karger AG, Basel.

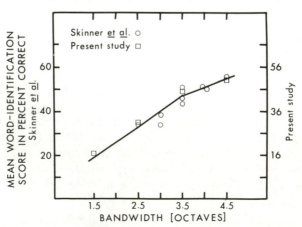

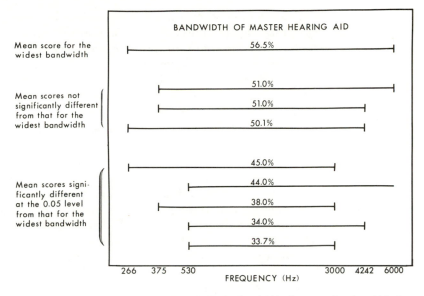

FIGURE 2.14.   Mean score as a function of effective bandwidth of a master hearing aid for two listeners with moderately severe sensorineural hearing losses. Stimuli: Pascoe High-Frequency Word List spoken by a male and presented in quiet at 50, 60, and 70 dB SPL in the field. From M. W. Skinner, M. M. Karstaedt, and J. D. Miller 1982. "Amplification bandwidth and speech intelligibility for two listeners with sensorineural hearing loss." *Audiology* 21:251–68. Reproduced with permission of S. Karger AG, Basel.

In two experiments in which the effective bandwidth of a master hearing aid was varied, all listeners obtained the highest scores with the widest bandwidth, as shown in figure 2.13. This aid was individually adjusted so the word-level contour (word list at 60 dB SPL overall) approximated each listener's MCL contour, and the maximum output was limited at each listener's UCL contour. In the first of these two experiments nine different combinations of low- and high-frequency cutoffs were tried. The mean scores were significantly lower for bandwidths that were an octave narrower at either the high or the low end of the spectrum (figure 2.14).

There is anecdotal evidence that hearing-impaired listeners accept hearing aids with wide effective bandwidths (250 to 6000 Hz) only when (1) the maximum output is limited below UCL, (2) the balance between low- and high-frequency gain is appropriate, and (3) there are no resonant peaks in the frequency response.

Articulation Index

Articulation Index theory was developed by engineers at Bell Telephone Laboratories to assist in the design of telephone communications systems (French and Steinberg 1947; Fletcher and Galt 1950). Through extensive experimentation with highly-trained, normal-hearing listeners and many conditions of filtering and noise, they found that speech recognition could be predicted from (1) the communicating proficiency of the talker and the listener, (2) measurements of the intensity and spectra of the speech and the noise, (3) the spread of masking, and (4) the auditory threshold of the listener. For each listening condition, an Articulation Index value (AI) was calculated from these quantities. Kryter (1962) modified the calculations slightly, and his method was adopted as the standard in calculating AI values (ANSI S3.5-1969).

The major elements of the formula for Kryter's calculation are (1) a *proficiency factor*, (2) an *importance function* that represents the contribution which speech energy makes to intelligibility in a specific frequency region, and (3) a *band efficiency function* that reflects the proportion of the speech signal that is above the listener's threshold (or masked threshold in noise) and below the discomfort level. The values for the importance function and the band efficiency function are multiplied for each of the frequency regions (e.g., third-octave bands between 200 and 5000 Hz), summed, and multiplied by the proficiency factor. The values for each of these factors and for the AI range between 0 and 1, 0 being associated with no contribution of information and 1 with perfect contribution of information. A graph of the actual speech recognition score in percent correct for AI values between 0 and 1 indicates that simpler materials, such as sentences, are recognized correctly 90 percent of the time at low AI values (such as 0.25), whereas materials that require accurate perception of the acoustic cues, such as nonsense syllables, are recognized 90 percent of the time at high AI values (such as 0.8).

In recent years there has been considerable interest in the application of Articulation Index theory to relate the residual hearing of hearing-impaired listeners to their ability to recognize speech (Dugal, Braida, and Durlach 1980; Kamm, Dirks, and Bell 1985; Pavlovic, Studebaker, and Sherbecoe 1985), and to select the frequency response of a hearing aid based on the one associated with the highest AI value (Byrne 1978). One application is to calculate an AI value for hearing-impaired adults listening to speech spoken at low- and normal-intensity levels without a hearing aid. Some clinicians suggest that AI values less than 0.8 for people listening under these conditions are supportive of the recommendation of a hearing aid, if this information is in agreement with the results of other tests and the individual's perception of hearing difficulty. Another application is to select the frequency response and gain of a hearing aid associated with the highest AI value for a particular individual. The major limitation of this application is that the formula for calculating the AI does not include an adjustment for the balance of the low- and high-frequency speech energy necessary for maximizing speech recognition, a concept described earlier in this chapter. Despite this limitation, calculation of the AI value using a proficiency factor of 1 will indicate the proportion of the speech spectrum that is audible, weighted by the contribution of specific frequency regions to intelligibility, for a hearing-impaired individual using a particular set of hearing aid characteristics and speech spectrum.

SUMMARY

Speech energy is constantly varying in frequency and intensity as a function of time and vocal effort of the person speaking. These fluctuations occur over at least a 55 dB range in specific frequency regions. For hearing-impaired individuals to function best with a hearing aid, they need to have a dynamic range between threshold and discomfort that is at least this large.

Speech is heard in a variety of contexts. High levels of background noise and room reverberation degrade the speech signal. The degrading effects of noise, room reverberation, and hearing impairment, if they are not excessive, can be minimized by adults who use the available auditory and visual cues to predict, on the basis of their long experience with the language, what someone is saying. Children, who are learning the language, need many more acoustic cues than do adults to accurately perceive speech.

Hearing-impaired individuals do not have normal auditory capabilities. Those with conductive hearing impairment have a blockage in the outer or middle ear that causes sound at the inner ear to be less intense and often of different phase than it would be if there had been normal transmission. The difficulties these individuals experience are that (1) speech is too soft, and is harder to detect in noise, and (2) sound sources may be harder for them to localize than they are for people with normal hearing. Individuals with cochlear hearing impairment from hair-cell dysfunction may have a decrease in the ability to (1) detect changes in frequency and temporal onset and offset, (2) keep separate the frequency components which occur simultaneously in a complex sound, and (3) integrate intensity over time, particularly with increasing magnitude of impairment. They can detect changes in intensity as well, or almost as well, as normal-hearing individuals at the same background intensity, and they have loudness recruitment. Individuals with cochlear hearing impairment due to strial atrophy have elevated thresholds, but speech recognition and other auditory processing capabilities appear normal. Individuals with neural hearing impairment often have greater difficulty detecting changes in intensity, frequency, and temporal order, separating signal from background noise, recognizing speech and localizing sounds in space than do individuals with cochlear impairment of the same magnitude.

The dynamic ranges of hearing-impaired individuals reflect dysfunction along the auditory pathway. The dynamic ranges for individuals with cochlear hearing impairment due to hair-cell dysfunction are smaller than those of individuals with conductive, neural, or cochlear hearing impairment due to strial atrophy.

The proportion of speech energy that falls within an individual's dynamic range can be determined if the speech and the sounds for dynamic range are calibrated at the same reference point. When the speech levels in specific frequency regions are compared with a listener's dynamic range for speech recognition tests, it is clear that hearing-impaired listeners can understand speech best if (1) it is audible between 250 and 6000 Hz (except for listeners who have no hearing in certain frequency regions), (2) the balance between the low- and high-frequency speech energy is appropriate, and (3) the amplified speech does not surpass the listener's UCL contour. The Articulation Index is a standard method for comparing speech levels with an individual's dynamic range. If it is used with a proficiency factor of 1, it is a measure of the audibility of speech weighted according to the contribution of specific frequency regions to speech intellibility, but it does not reflect the effect of the appropriate balance of low- and high-frequency speech energy on speech recognition by the hearing-impaired.

APPENDIX 2.   Instructions for obtaining the most comfortable listening level (MCL), most intelligible listening level (MIL), and uncomfortable listening level (UCL) for speech.

I will play a list of words at a certain loudness, and I want you to tell me which words describe the sound: Too loud, very loud, loud, comfortable but a little loud, comfortable (speech sounds clearest), comfortable but a little soft, soft, very soft, too soft, or nothing. I will change the loudness of the words several times. Each time tell me the words that best describe the sound.

Interpretation

With these instructions the MCL and MIL for speech are at the same level, the one consistently chosen as "comfortable." If comfortable is not defined as the level at which the speech sounds clearest, the MIL is often associated with a higher level (comfortable but a little loud) than that of the MCL (comfortable). The UCL is the level consistently chosen as too loud.

Chapter Three
ROOM, STIMULI, AND EQUIPMENT

The room, sound stimuli, and equipment used to present sound must be considered in evaluating the effect of a hearing aid on a hearing-impaired listener's ability to hear. The interaction of the effects of the room, stimuli, and equipment on the signal at the listener's ear or the hearing aid microphone is complex. At present there is no calibration standard (such as from the American National Standards Institute or the International Standards Organization) for sound-field testing except for the ambient noise levels (ANSI S3.1-1977) at which normal sound-field thresholds can be obtained. Consequently, the clinical testing situations in use today are very diverse.

A number of compromises must be made in choosing rooms, stimuli, and equipment for hearing aid evaluations. Important issues for making these choices and taking appropriate precautions when doing sound-field testing will be described in the following sections.

ROOM

In the United States many hearing aid evaluations are done in sound booths (for example, those manufactured by Industrial Acoustics Company or Tracoustics, Inc.) or in sound-treated rooms, most of which were individually designed and built prior to 1960. Both types of rooms are intended to isolate listeners from environmental noise outside the room that would interfere with the listeners' response to sounds. The amount of sound isolation, the acoustic reverberation, and the size of these rooms are important factors affecting the sound used for testing.

Ambient Noise Level

The ambient noise level in the room depends on the noise level outside the room and the attenuation provided by the walls, floor, ceiling, window, doors, and ventilating ducts of the room. The amount of attenuation provided by sound booths is much greater at high frequencies than at low frequencies, as shown in figure 3.1; double-walled booths provide 20 to 30 dB greater attenuation than single-walled booths. Since the attenuation in double-walled booths is only 40 to 55 dB between 100 and 200 Hz and the low-frequency components of environmental noise are often the most intense, sound booths and sound-treated rooms should be situated in quiet areas in a building.

The ambient noise level inside the room needs to be at a lower level for obtaining bone-conduction or sound-field thresholds than earphone thresholds; when earphones are used, they attenuate the noise. Unless the noise is at a low enough level, it will mask the test sound at threshold, and the measured threshold will be higher than the true hearing threshold. To obtain accurate thresholds at 1 dB HL with the ears uncovered, the maxi-

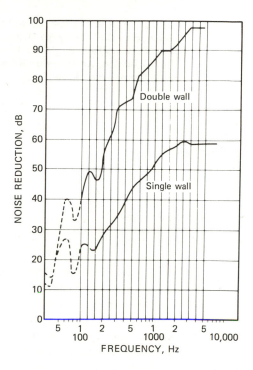

FIGURE 3.1.
The noise reduction provided by standard single- and double-walled audiometric sound booths. Reproduced with permission of Tracoustics Co.

mum allowable sound-pressure levels for octave and one-third-octave bands centered at the audiometric frequencies should be those shown in table 3.1. When the measured noise levels are higher than the maximum allowable levels, it may be possible to reduce the noise by eliminating one or more sources of noise (for example, turn off the fan of a forced-air ventilating system during testing). If the noise level cannot be reduced, then the lowest level at which an accurate threshold can be obtained can be calculated by subtracting the maximum allowable levels shown in table 3.1 from the measured levels, an example of which is shown in table 3.2. In this example

TABLE 3.1.   Maximum Allowable Sound-Pressure Levels in dB re 20 μPa for One-Ear Listening (with the Ear Uncovered) for No More Than 1-dB Threshold Elevation re the Reference Hearing Threshold Levels Given in ANSI S3.6-1969. From ANSI S 3.1-1977, Criteria for Permissible Ambient Noise During Audiometric Testing.

	FREQUENCY (Hz)						
	125	250	500	1000	2000	4000	8000
Octave band levels	28	18.5	14.5	14	8.5	9	20.5
One-third-octave band levels	23	13.5	9.5	9	3.5	4	15.5

TABLE 3.2. **Calculation of the Lowest Level at Which an Accurate Threshold Can Be Obtained by Comparing the Measured Levels with the Maximum Allowable Level Shown in Table 3.1 (Minus 1 dB Since the Criteria Are Based on 1 dB HL). The Calculations Are Based on Measurements Made with Octave-Band Filters in the Sound-Level Meter.**

	FREQUENCY (Hz)					
	250	500	1000	2000	4000	8000
Level measured in room (dB SPL)	23.0	19.0	8.5	7.8	9.5	11.5
Maximum allowable level (dB SPL) minus 1 dB	17.5	13.5	13.0	7.5	8.0	19.5
Lowest hearing threshold levels that can be measured (dB HL)	5.5	5.5	−4.5	0.3	1.5	−8.0

one cannot obtain accurate thresholds below 6 dB HL at 250 and 500 Hz. This limitation will not cause a problem unless a hearing-impaired listener's *unaided* or *aided* threshold at these frequencies is 6 dB HL. In this case the 6 dB HL threshold may be a masked threshold and not indicative of the actual, more sensitive threshold. This principle also applies to rooms with higher ambient noise levels; the major concern with hearing-impaired listeners is that the aided thresholds may be limited by the masking noise in the room.

Acoustic Reverberation

Anechoic chambers have very low levels of reverberant sound. However, these chambers cost so much that they are not economically feasible for the clinical evaluation of hearing aids. Consequently, sound booths or sound-treated rooms are generally used. Although these booths and rooms have much shorter reverberation times than most other untreated rooms (see figure 3.2), the reflected sound causes regions of high and low sound levels (resonances and antiresonances, respectively) within the room. The exact pattern of sound levels within the room depends on the frequency spectrum of the sound stimulus, the frequency response, directivity and placement of the loudspeaker, the dimensions and absorptivity of the room, and furniture or people within the room.

The effect of room reverberation on the sound level of a signal is shown in the three-dimensional graphs in the left and right panels of figure 3.3. When the reverberation time (RT) of the room is 0.52 seconds (see the top panel), 30-dB variations in level often occur as the frequency and/or distance from the loudspeaker is changed. Although there is a 30-dB change in level around 1125 Hz in the sound booth (RT = 0.05 seconds) as shown in the bottom panel of figure 3.3, there is much less variation in level with frequency and distance from the loudspeaker than in the more rever-

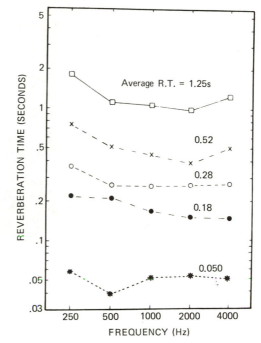

FIGURE 3.2.
The reverberation time (RT) measured as a function of the center frequency of a frequency-modulated tone used to excite the room. The top four curves were measured in a room (4.22 m long × 3.22 m wide × 2.73 m high) in which the absorptivity was changed. The bottom curve is for a standard sound booth (IAC Model 404A). From H. Dillon and G. Walker 1981. "The effect of acoustic environment on the reliability of sound field audiometry." *Australian Journal of Audiology* 3:67−72. Reproduced with permission of the authors and publisher.

berant room. Since listeners often move their heads and torsos during testing, the level in the sound field should vary as little as possible as a function of frequency and position in the room. Therefore, the room should have as much absorption and as little reverberation as possible.

The sound-pressure level at a particular point in the room may depend predominantly on the sound that comes directly from the loudspeaker (*direct sound field*) or predominantly on the sound that is reflected from the room surfaces (*reverberant sound field*). The difference between direct and reflected sound is illustrated in figure 3.4. In figure 3.5 the direct sound field extends from about 0.1 to about 0.7 m in front of the loudspeaker. In this region the sound level decreases 6 dB for each doubling of the distance from the sound source. The sound field very close to the loudspeaker (less than 0.1 m away at this frequency) is called the *near field*. In the near field the sound-pressure level changes rapidly with increasing distance from the loudspeaker; the size of this region depends on the stimulus frequency and the radiation characteristics of the loudspeaker. The reverberant sound field in figure 3.5 extends from about 0.8 to about 2.0 m in front of the loudspeaker. In this region the mean sound level remains approximately the same, but there are variations in level, particularly for the pure tone (see the dashed line). These variations are caused by the interaction between direct and reflected sound, which produce standing-wave patterns. These variations can be reduced by

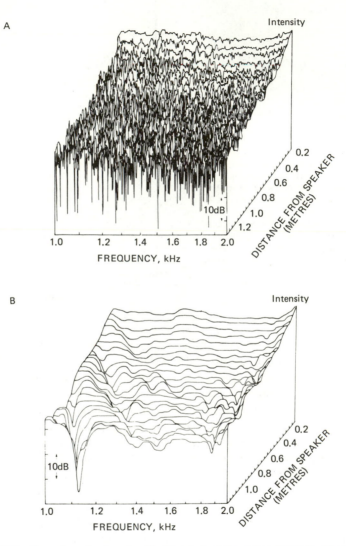

FIGURE 3.3.   Three-dimensional graphs of the intensity level of pure-tone signals (1–2 kHz) as a function of the distance of the microphone from the loudspeaker (0.2 to 1.3 m). The microphone was placed at the same height as the cone of the loudspeaker and moved along the axis of the cone. The graph for the room with the 0.52-sec RT is shown in the top panel, and the graph for the sound booth with the 0.05 sec RT is shown in the bottom panel. From H. Dillon and G. Walker 1981. "The effect of acoustic environment on the reliability of sound field audiometry." *Australian Journal of Audiology* 3:67–72. Reproduced with permission of the authors and publisher.

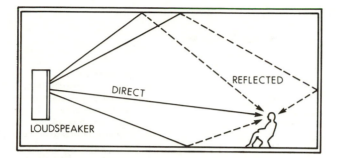

FIGURE 3.4. Diagram of direct and reflected sound within a room. The sound reaching the listener at this distance from the loudspeaker is mainly reflected sound. Adapted from A. F. Niemoeller 1981. "Physical concepts of speech communication in classrooms for the deaf." In *Amplification in Education*. Ed. F. H. Bess, B. A. Freeman, and J. J. Sinclair, 164–179, figure 10-3. Reproduced with permission of the author and the Alexander Graham Bell Association for the Deaf, Washington, DC.

using a frequency-modulated (FM) tone (see the solid curve in figure 3.5) or a narrow band of noise.

An FM tone has a broader bandwidth than a pure tone. This spread of spectral energy reduces the effects of resonances and antiresonances in the room. As the bandwidth of the FM tone (1350 Hz) is increased from 1 percent to 20 percent of the center frequency, the variability of the sound

FIGURE 3.5. The relative sound level (dB) of a pure tone (dashed line) and an FM tone (solid line) centered at 1350 Hz as a function of distance from a loudspeaker in the standard sound booth described in the legend for figure 3.2. From H. Dillon and G. Walker 1982. "Comparison of stimuli used in sound field audiometric testing." *Journal of the Acoustical Society of America* 71:161–72. Reproduced with permission of the authors and the publisher.

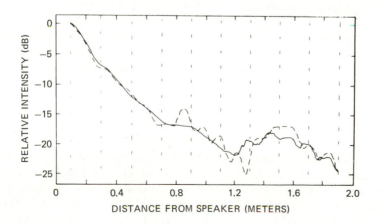

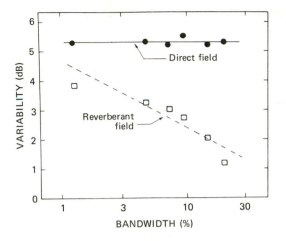

FIGURE 3.6.
Average variability of the SPL (dB) within the direct and reverberant sound fields as a function of stimulus bandwidth for an FM tone with a center frequency of 1350 Hz. The values shown in this graph are based on measurements made under the same conditions noted in figure 3.5. From H. Dillon and G. Walker 1982. "Comparison of stimuli used in sound field audiometric testing." *Journal of the Acoustical Society of America* 71:161–72. Reproduced with permission of the authors and the publisher.

level decreases from 4 dB to 1 dB (see figure 3.6). It is important to note that this increase in bandwidth does not affect the variability in sound level in the direct sound field; in this region reverberant sound makes little contribution to the overall sound level.

To obtain reliable thresholds in the sound field, there needs to be as little variation in the sound-pressure level as possible so that small changes in head position will not cause relatively large changes in the actual sound level at the listener's ear or at the microphone of the hearing aid. The sound field in existing test rooms will be most uniform (least variable) if the listener is placed in the reverberant sound field and the sounds have sufficient spread of spectral energy to minimize the effects of the resonances and anti-resonances of the room. Although the exact position of the reverberant field that is most uniform may be determined for each room, loudspeaker, and test-stimulus combination, a position 1 m in front of the loudspeaker is often appropriate.

In addition to being in the reverberant field, the listener needs to be as far away as possible from the reflecting surfaces in the room, particularly the walls. This will avoid the greater variation in the sound level near these reflecting surfaces. Although compromises may need to be made, the listener should be at least 1 m from each wall.

Room Size

The room chosen for sound-field testing needs to have sufficient space for the loudspeaker, and for the listener to be at least 1 m from the loudspeaker and from each surrounding wall. Loudspeakers, including their enclosures, vary in size. An estimated volume of 2 ft. × 2 ft. × 2 ft. (0.6 m × 0.6 m × 0.6 m) should accommodate most loudspeakers used in clinical testing. If there is sufficient space, the loudspeaker should be located from 1 ft. to 3 ft. (0.3 m to 1 m) from the wall to reduce the level of reflected sound energy that may result from radiation to the back and sides of the loudspeaker.

The smallest room feasible for sound-field testing is one that is: (1) approximately 7½ ft. (2.3 m) long to accommodate the loudspeaker, the listener, and the distance between them and the walls, (2) 7 ft. (2.1 m) wide to allow sufficient room between the listener and the two walls, and (3) approximately 6½ ft. (2 m) high to allow most adults to stand up without bumping their heads. Larger rooms are more likely to have larger areas in which the sound field is relatively uniform; this is particularly desirable when testing small children, who move more than adults and for whom other equipment, such as toys and a table, is placed in the room.

STIMULI

A number of sounds are used for different purposes during a hearing aid evaluation. The purposes include determination of (1) the dynamic range of hearing, (2) the listener's unaided and aided thresholds in the field, and (3) the listener's response to speech stimuli in quiet and in the presence of competing sounds. The stimuli include pure tones, frequency-specific complex sounds, speech, and competing sounds.

Pure Tones

Pure tones presented through an earphone are recommended for determining the dynamic range of hearing-impaired individuals for the following reasons. A number of these individuals have uncomfortable listening levels (UCLs) that occur at high sound-pressure levels (greater than 100 dB SPL). Many loudspeakers cannot deliver these sound levels without undue harmonic distortion, whereas TDH, Telex and ER-3A earphones can deliver pure tones up to 130 dB SPL between 750 and 2000 Hz. Pure tones, which have a lower peak factor than narrow bands of noise, can be delivered at root-mean-squared (rms) sound levels about 5 dB higher than the rms levels of narrow bands of noise for the same amount of harmonic and intermodulation distortion. If the signal used to measure UCLs is distorted by the loudspeaker, the listener may be responding to the distortion products rather than to the test stimulus. For accurate testing the distortion products should be at least 40 dB below the level of the test stimulus.

Frequency-Specific Complex Sounds

The stimuli chosen for determining threshold in the sound field should be *frequency specific* and provide *sound-field uniformity*. A sound can be considered frequency specific when its energy is limited to a narrow band of frequencies centered at the test frequency and sound energy outside of this band is 50 to 80 dB below the energy within the band. A sound field is uniform if the SPL of the test stimulus does not vary more than ±2 dB within the region that the listener's head could occupy during testing. As shown in figure 3.3 the sound field for pure tones varies more than ±2 dB in clinical sound rooms; consequently complex sounds must be used to achieve the necessary sound-field uniformity. Four types of stimuli have been used clinically: FM tones (often called warble tones), narrow bands of noise, damped wave trains, and amplitude-modulated tones. The subsequent discussion will be confined to FM tones and narrow bands of noise, since they are generated by many clinical audiometers in use today. The suitability of either of these signals depends on the manner in which they are generated and the equipment with which they are amplified and transduced into sound energy. The following sections will focus on what parameters of FM tones and narrow bands of noise will provide sufficient frequency specificity and sound-field uniformity.

FM tones. Frequency-modulated tones are generated by changing the frequency of a tone over a given range at a stated rate. The frequency deviation is often expressed in terms of the percentage of the center frequency, such as ±5% of 1000 Hz, which would be ±50 Hz, or 950 to 1050 Hz. The number of times per second the tone changes from the lowest to the highest and back to the lowest frequency within this range or bandwidth is called the *modulation rate* (Hz). The manner in which the tone changes affects the spread of spectral energy. Sinusoidal, triangular, sawtooth, and square-wave modulation of FM tones have been or are available on clinical audiometers. In sinusoidal modulation the frequency of the tone changes sinusoidally in time. When the frequency changes sinusoidally, more energy occurs near the upper and lower extremes of the total frequency range because more time elapses while the signal is there than at the center frequencies. In triangular modulation the energy is more evenly distributed across the frequency range because the change in frequency is constant as a function of time. In sawtooth modulation the change in frequency is constant from the lowest to the highest frequency; this is followed by an instantaneous change back to the lowest frequency. In square-wave modulation the tone remains for equal lengths of time at the lowest and highest frequency of the range and changes instantaneously between them. Examples of the change in frequency as a function of time for sinusoidal, triangular, sawtooth, and square-wave modulation are shown in the top panel of figure 3.7. Three-dimensional graphs of the spectral energy (frequency versus intensity) as a function of time for these four types of FM tones are shown in figure 3.7. Note that the sinusoidally modulated tone has steep stimulus skirts and the spectral energy is confined to the nominal frequency range or bandwidth of the signal. The stimulus skirts are not quite as steep for the triangularly

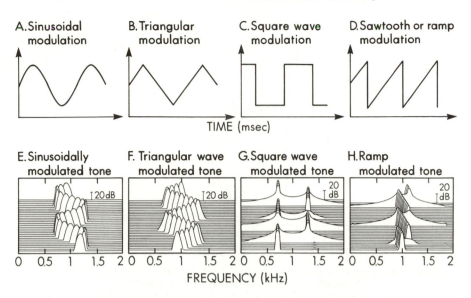

FIGURE 3.7.   The change in frequency as a function of time for FM tones is shown in the top four graphs for **(A)** sinusoidal, **(B)** triangular, **(C)** square-wave, and **(D)** sawtooth or ramp modulation. The change in frequency and intensity as a function of time is shown in the bottom four graphs **(E, F, G,** and **H)** for these four types of modulation. From H. Dillon and G. Walker 1981. "The selection of modulation waveform for frequency modulated sound field stimuli." *Australian Journal of Audiology* 4(2):56−61. Reproduced with permission of the authors and the publisher.

modulated tone as for the sinusoidally modulated one. In the sawtooth- and square-wave-modulated tones, a spread of spectral energy at frequencies above and below the nominal bandwidth is caused by the instantaneous change in frequency. The spread of spectral energy is too large to allow accurate, frequency-specific thresholds. For audiometric testing the FM tones should be sinusoidally or triangularly modulated.

It is interesting to note that the harmonics of a pure tone produced by an oscillator are also modulated during FM signal generation. Harmonics are tones occurring at integral multiples of the test-signal frequency. The SPL of the harmonics is almost always lower than that of the test signal, as shown in figure 3.8. The test signal is a 250 Hz FM tone, and the harmonics occur at 500, 750, and 1000 Hz. It is important for the SPL of the harmonics to be below threshold when obtaining a listener's threshold for the test signal. This may be difficult to achieve for people who have thresholds that are 50 to 60 dB better at high frequencies than at low frequencies.

The modulation rate and bandwidth of FM tones affect the uniformity of the sound field. For an FM tone centered at 1350 Hz, the average variation in sound level in a sound booth is least (and the uniformity of the field is greatest) at a modulation rate between 10 and 90 Hz and with a

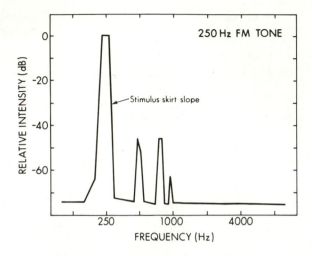

FIGURE 3.8.   Spectrum of an FM tone (250 Hz) that was sinusoidally modulated and measured electrically at the output of an audiometer. The stimulus skirt slopes are greater than 300 dB per octave. The oscillator generated harmonics at 500, 750, and 1000 Hz; the test tone and harmonics are both modulated.

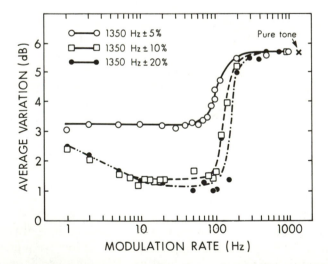

FIGURE 3.9.   The average variation in field SPL (dB) for a 1350-Hz FM tone as a function of modulation rate, for each of three bandwidths. From G. Walker and H. Dillon 1983. "The selection of modulation rates for frequency modulated sound field stimuli." *Scandinavian Audiology* 12:151–56. Reproduced with permission of the authors and the publisher.

frequency range of $\pm10\%$ to 20% (±135 to 270 Hz) as shown in figure 3.9. With a $\pm5\%$ range, the variation of the sound level in the field is larger than if a larger frequency range is used.

It is obvious that the SPL in the field is more uniform with wider stimulus bandwidths, but then the signals are less frequency specific for determining thresholds for individuals with steeply sloping hearing losses. Consequently, a compromise has to be made between field uniformity and frequency specificity of the sound. The standard bandwidths shown in table 3.3 are an example of such a compromise. They were chosen to obtain the greatest field uniformity for signals that were sufficiently frequency specific to get reasonably close agreement between pure-tone and FM-tone thresholds for people with gently sloping audiograms. The narrow bandwidths are for individuals with steeply sloping audiograms, and the wide bandwidths are for individuals, such as small children, who move in the test space. The wider the bandwidth, the more sound-field uniformity and less frequency specificity there is. An FM tone generator that produces these sounds is used in the clinics of the National Acoustic Laboratories in Australia. The bandwidth of FM tones (with $\pm5\%$ frequency deviation) that are available on audiometers in the United States are less than the standard bandwidths at all frequencies, as shown in table 3.3. Between 250 and 1500 Hz the sound-field uniformity for $\pm5\%$ frequency deviation is approximately 2 dB less than for the deviations recommended in table 3.3. For hearing losses that have extremely steep slopes, the $\pm5\%$ frequency deviation is too wide above 1000 Hz to provide sufficient frequency specificity. Consequently, their thresholds for FM tones between 1500 and 8000 Hz may be at less intense levels than for pure tones presented with earphones.

TABLE 3.3.   Recommended Bandwidths of Stimuli for Use in the Sound Field.

FREQUENCY (Hz)	NARROW		STANDARD		WIDE	
	DEVIATION % OF CENTER FREQUENCY	BAND-WIDTH Hz	DEVIATION % OF CENTER FREQUENCY	BAND-WIDTH Hz	DEVIATION % OF CENTER FREQUENCY	BAND-WIDTH Hz
250	9.7	24	29	72	58	145
500	8.0	40	24	120	48	240
1000	5.7	58	17	170	34	340
1500	4.3	64	13	195	26	390
2000	3.7	74	11	220	22	440
3000	3.0	90	9	270	18	540
4000	2.7	108	8	320	16	640
6000	2.7	162	8	480	16	960
8000	2.7	216	8	740	16	1280

From G. Walker, H. Dillon, and D. Byrne. 1984. "Sound field audiometry: Recommended stimuli and procedures." *Ear and Hearing* 5(1):13–21. Copyright Williams & Wilkins, 1984. Reprinted with permission of the authors and publisher.

If the modulation rate of FM tones is too slow, the normal-hearing person will respond only to the peak sound intensity and not integrate fluctuations in intensity as the frequency changes. A modulation rate of 5 to 10 Hz is sufficient for normal-hearing listeners to integrate these fluctuations. A higher modulation rate is needed for some individuals with a sensorineural hearing loss who have smaller integration times than normal. Although the optimum rate increases with the center frequency of the FM tone, a modulation rate of 20 Hz is a feasible choice for these individuals. At the present time the modulation rate of FM tones on a number of clinical audiometers is 10 Hz. Although this rate is low, it is clinically usable.

Narrow bands of noise. These stimuli have been available on clinical audiometers for a number of years to provide contralateral masking for pure-tone testing. Although the bandwidth is often approximately one-third-octave wide, the stimulus skirt slopes may vary between approximately 10 and 60 dB per octave, and the energy outside the noise band may only be 35 dB lower than the level within it. Thus, even if the stimulus skirt slope is relatively steep, sufficient frequency specificity is not obtained unless this slope is maintained down to a level between 50 and 80 dB below the test-signal level. An example of the electrical output from a recent-model audiometer is shown in figure 3.10. If hearing-impaired individuals with hearing losses that are 40 dB worse at 4000 Hz than at any frequency between 125 and 2000 Hz are tested with this 4000-Hz narrow band of noise, the thresholds obtained would be based on the sound heard at the other frequencies instead of that at 4000 Hz. To obtain an accurate threshold for sound energy around 4000 Hz, you need a narrow band of noise with stimulus skirt slopes that continue to fall off so that the level at 2000 Hz and below is more than 50 dB lower than the level at 4000 Hz.

The one-third-octave bands of noise used at Central Institute for the Deaf are produced with a locally built white-noise generator and filters; the stimulus skirt slopes of these noise bands are shown in figure 3.11. With these noise bands accurate thresholds can be obtained for the listeners

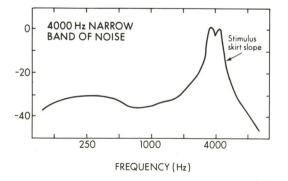

FIGURE 3.10.
Spectrum of a narrow band of noise measured electrically at the output of a clinical audiometer. This noise is intended for use in masking the nontest ear during pure-tone audiometry. Although the steepest portion of the stimulus skirt slope is approximately 115 dB per octave, the low-frequency energy between 125 and 1000 Hz is only 30 to 35 dB lower than that at the 4000-Hz test frequency. This does not provide sufficient frequency specificity if these narrow bands are used in threshold testing.

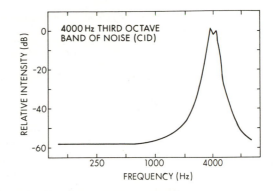

FIGURE 3.11.
Spectrum of a third-octave band of noise produced by a narrow-band-noise generator built at CID. The signal from the generator was fed to the auxillary input of a clinical audiometer and measured electrically at the output to the earphones (prior to the power amplifier). The steepest portion of the stimulus skirt slopes is approximately 115 dB per octave, and the energy between 125 and 1000 Hz is at least 55 dB less than that at the test frequency.

described above. However, the stimulus skirt slope would not be steep enough to get an accurate threshold if there was a 60 dB difference between the threshold at 2000 Hz and that at 4000 Hz. Some audiometers now have narrow bands of noise that are digitally filtered so that the stimulus skirt slopes are more than 100 dB per octave (see figure 3.12). More accurate thresholds can be obtained with these digitally filtered stimuli with very steep stimulus skirt slopes, if the level outside the noise band is more than 70 dB lower than the level within the noise band.

If we compare the bandwidth of one-third-octave bands of noise (see table 3.4) with the standard frequency deviations of FM tones recommended as a good clinical compromise in table 3.3, they are fairly close at low frequencies but the bandwidths of bands of noise are much wider at the high frequencies. For example, the bandwidth at 500 Hz is 116 Hz for the narrow

FIGURE 3.12.   Spectrum of a digitally filtered narrow band of noise measured electrically at the output of a clinical audiometer. This noise is intended for use in masking the nontest ear for pure-tone audiometry and for obtaining sound-field thresholds. Although the steepest portion of the stimulus skirt slopes is approximately 125 dB/per octave, the slope decreases so that the low-frequency energy is not more than 50 dB below that of the test frequency. This noise band is suitable for sound-field testing if the threshold at 250 and 500 Hz is not 50 dB better than that at 1000 Hz. Data from Tracoustics 1982.

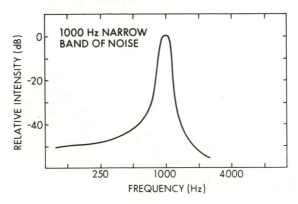

TABLE 3.4. Bandwidth (Hz) of One-Third-Octave Bands of Noise at the Audiometric Frequencies.

	FREQUENCY (Hz)							
	250	500	1000	1500	2000	3000	4000	6000
Bandwidth (Hz)	58	116	230	348	460	694	920	1390

band of noise and 120 Hz for the FM tone, whereas the bandwidth at 4000 Hz is 920 Hz for the narrow band of noise and 320 Hz for the FM tone. The third-octave bands of noise may not provide sufficient frequency specificity for those with steeply sloping losses to obtain thresholds that compare closely with pure-tone thresholds. If, however, a stimulus that more closely approximates speech energy in a normal critical band is desired, then the third-octave bandwidth is an appropriate choice for obtaining unaided and aided thresholds.

Narrow bands of noise having a bandwidth that is 20 percent of the center frequency or greater (this includes third-octave bands of noise at the audiometric frequencies) provide essentially the same field uniformity as FM tones (see figure 3.13). As the bandwidth of both stimuli is narrowed, the sound-field uniformity of the narrow band noise is significantly less than that of the FM tone for the same bandwidth because of the random amplitude fluctuations characteristic of the noise. It appears that FM tones with frequency deviations less than ±10% (that is, 20%) are a better choice than narrow bands of noise (of the same bandwidth), if frequency specificity is needed to test individuals with steeply sloping hearing losses.

Speech

Speech is used in hearing aid evaluations for determining the unaided and aided (1) speech-reception threshold, (2) ability to identify words, (3)

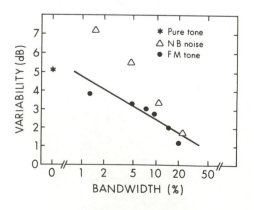

FIGURE 3.13.
The average variation in SPL (dB) in the reverberant field as a function of bandwidth (percent of center frequency) for FM tones and narrow bands of noise. Adapted from H. Dillon and G. Walker 1982. "Comparison of stimuli used in sound field audiometric testing." *Journal of the Acoustical Society of America* 71:161–72. Reproduced with permission of the authors and the publisher.

MCL, and (4) UCL. Speech is also presented at a conversational level for listeners to adjust the gain of their hearing aids so that the output is at their MCL or MIL.

Speech can be spoken "live voice" or presented with recordings. The test-retest variability in performance is lower when recordings rather than live voice are used. With recordings the utterance of each word is the same each time it is presented, whereas for live voice, the word is different each time it is spoken, even if the same person says it. Although recordings are used whenever possible, live-voice testing is appropriate in the following situations. First, in testing small children or some elderly people, the word set may need to be reduced to include only words they understand, and each word may need to be enunciated carefully at just the right time for them to respond optimally. Second, with children and adults it may be important to compare the ability to understand speech with and without speech-reading cues when no videotape recordings are available. Finally, in some clinical situations, it is important to quickly estimate the listener's aided response to speech. In all these situations the level and spectral content of speech presented live voice is more variable than that on recordings, and consequently the results should be interpreted cautiously.

Two-syllable words with equal stress on each syllable (spondees) are used for obtaining the lowest level at which the listener can identify 50 percent of the words correctly. This is called the speech-reception threshold (SRT). The CID W-1 list of 36 spondees is used most widely in the United States for obtaining the SRT for adults and older children. Recordings of this list by two different talkers are commercially available. A recording of a children's list of twelve spondees is also commercially available.

One-syllable words are used by most clinics to evaluate the ability of hearing-impaired listeners to identify speech at SPLs above the SRT. The most widely used clinical tests are the CID W-22 tests, the NU-6 lists, and the PB-50 lists; the PBK-50, WIPI, and NU-CHIPS lists are designed for children. Commercial recordings are available for all these tests. Except for the WIPI and NU-CHIPS tests, these word lists are phonetically balanced to reflect the relative rate of occurrence of speech sounds in spoken American English. Since vowels and consonants with predominantly low-frequency energy occur much more often than consonants with predominantly high-frequency energy, this is reflected in the spectral content of these phonetically balanced word lists. In addition, the original recordings of the CID lists (spoken by Ira Hirsh) and the PB-50 lists (spoken by Rush Hughes) do not have significant energy beyond 3500 Hz. For both reasons these lists are appropriate for evaluating changes in amplification below approximately 2500 Hz; they are not appropriate for evaluating changes above 2500 Hz.

The California Consonant Test (Owens and Schubert 1977) is a four-alternative forced-choice test in which the consonants to be identified are predominantly those with high-frequency energy. This commercially available recording is particularly appropriate for determining the effect of changes in amplification between 2500 Hz and 6000 Hz on hearing-impaired listeners' ability to identify these speech sounds. Other word lists have a high percentage of consonants with high-frequency energy, but recordings of them are not commercially available.

The Nonsense Syllable Test developed by Resnick, Dubno, Hoffnung, and Levitt (1975) and the Pascoe High-Frequency Word List include more speech sounds with high-frequency energy than the phonetically balanced word lists described above. These lists are appropriate for evaluating the effect of changes in low- as well as high-frequency amplification on the listeners' identification of speech sounds. Commercial recordings of these lists are not available at present.

Several sentence tests have been designed for clinical use. These include the CID Everyday Sentences test (and its revision to sentences of equal word length), the Synthetic Sentence Identification test, and the Speech Perception Test in Noise (SPIN). In sentence tests the SPL of the phonemes varies over a larger range than in tests of single words; this variation in level makes it a good test for evaluating the value of linear versus compression amplification of hearing-impaired listeners with narrow dynamic ranges. Sentence tests also can provide a measure of everyday listening skills.

Recordings of three different talkers reading passages from a book (often called "connected discourse") are available commercially. These recordings can be used for obtaining listeners' MCL and UCL for speech, and for setting the volume control of their hearing aids so that the amplified speech is at their MCL or MIL.

Speech tests for which commercial recordings are available are listed in Appendix 3A under the name of the company from which they can be obtained. References for speech tests that are not commercially available are also given.

Competing Sounds

To simulate some listening conditions in everyday life, competing sounds are presented simultaneously with speech in the evaluation of hearing aids. The competing sounds include cafeteria noise, multitalker babble, white noise, white noise shaped to the long-term spectrum of speech (speech-shaped noise), and a person reading a passage from a book. When the competing sound is a person reading aloud, it is spoken by the same person who made the speech recording. In this case the sentences and competing sounds are recorded simultaneously on separate channels of the same magnetic tape; an example of this is the Synthetic Sentence Identification test, which is available commercially. Recordings of cafeteria noise and multitalker babble are also commercially available with the CID W-22 or NU-6 lists. The spectral content and the level of the person reading, the cafeteria noise, and the multitalker babble all vary widely. However, these competing sounds are more similar to the speech the listener is trying to identify (and consequently cause the listener more difficulty) than white noise or speech-shaped noise. Clinically, the white or speech-shaped noise is generated by most audiometers and can be used with any speech test, whereas the other competing sounds are available on the second channel of specific speech recordings. A list of these is included in Appendix 3A.

EQUIPMENT

Audiometer

An audiometer is an essential piece of equipment for the clinical evaluation of hearing aids. This audiometer must be capable of:

1. generating FM tones (sinusoidal or triangular modulation) or narrow bands of noise that are no more than one-third-octave wide, have stimulus skirt slopes that are sufficiently steep (approximately 45 dB per octave), and sound energy beyond one octave that is 50 to 60 dB lower than that at the center of the narrow bands of noise, *or* accepting one of these inputs from a separate stimulus generator,
2. accepting input from two channels of a reel-to-reel recorder, cassette recorder, or phonograph,
3. pulsing the narrow bands of noise with an on-time between 200 and 500 msec. and an off-time equal to the on-time,
4. generating white noise or speech-shaped noise,
5. delivering two signals simultaneously on two separate channels,
6. amplifying signals over a range from 0 to 120 dB HL in each channel,
7. attenuating sound linearly over this range in 2- or 2.5-dB steps (5-dB steps can be used if no other is available) in each channel,
8. switching the signal delivery to the right or the left earphone or to one or both loudspeakers, and
9. communicating with the listener with a talk-back system.

The audiometer should comply with the "Specifications for Audiometers" of the ANSI S3.6-1969 standard.

Earphones

Earphones are used for obtaining estimates of an individual's thresholds, contour of MCLs, and contour of UCLs for pure tones or narrow bands of noise. They also are used to deliver speech stimuli to assess the threshold (SRT), MCL, and UCL for speech, and to obtain a speech recognition score. In the United States, most audiological testing is done with TDH series or Telex 1470 earphones mounted in MX-41/AR or P/N 510C017-1 cushions that are held against the pinna by a spring headband. These are called *supra-aural earphones* because of their placement in relation to the ear. The nominal acoustic immittance of these earphones is either 10 or 50 ohms, and the frequency response for the TDH-49, TDH-50P, and Telex 1470 earphones in MX-41/AR cushions is uniform (±3.5 dB) between 100 and 6000 Hz; this is also true for the TDH-39 earphones except for a 7 dB resonant peak at around 5800 Hz. The output of the TDH series earphones falls off rapidly above 6000 Hz whereas that of the Telex 1470 earphones is maintained out to 10,000 Hz. The maximum output for the TDH series and Telex 1470 earphones is about 130 dB SPL between 750 and 2000 Hz.

There are several disadvantages in using supra-aural earphones for testing hearing. First, the cushion does not fit tightly against the ear, which allows (1) room noise to reach the listener's eardrum (necessitating quiet test conditions to obtain accurate thresholds), and (2) a leak of low-frequency sound energy (particularly at 125 and 250 Hz) that varies from one individual to the next and from one placement of the earphone to the next. Second, sounds delivered to the test ear at approximately 40 dB or more above the bone-conduction threshold at the nontest ear are heard at the latter, making it necessary to use masking noise at the nontest ear. Third, the pressure of the earphones against the ear causes collapse of the earcanal in some patients, causing the air-conduction thresholds to appear elevated when, in fact, they are not. Fourth, a listener's thresholds, MCLs, and UCLs obtained with supra-aural earphones (a low acoustic immittance source) are difficult to relate to the same measurements obtained with a hearing-aid receiver (a high acoustic immittance source). An *insert earphone* can be used to eliminate these disadvantages.

Commercially available hearing-aid receivers are used as insert earphones. In figure 3.14, the insert earphone in the top panel is a button-type receiver from a body hearing aid, and the insert earphone in the bottom panel is a small receiver from a behind-the-ear hearing aid which is enclosed in the box. The components for using the insert earphone in the top panel are relatively inexpensive to purchase and assemble. This earphone can be used for frequency-specific testing. Although it can be plugged into the earphone jack of an audiometer, there is no provision for matching the low acoustic immittance of the output of the audiometer to the high acoustic immittance of the insert earphone. In addition, its frequency response is not uniform; for this reason, it is not recommended for speech testing. The insert earphone in the bottom panel of figure 3.14 has been designed to closely approximate the overall output and frequency response of the TDH-39 earphone, and to provide the appropriate immittance matching between the

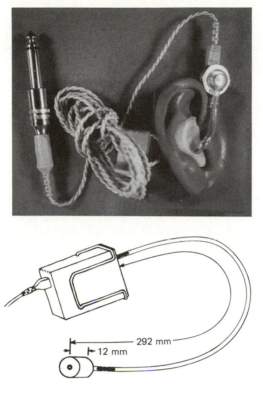

FIGURE 3.14. Insert earphones for audiological testing. Top: example of an insert earphone which is a button-type receiver used with a body hearing aid. If a Danavox SMW 100-ohm receiver is used, the 2-cc coupler calibration should be corrected by subtracting 2 dB at 1000 Hz and adding 5 dB at 2500 Hz. From R. M. Cox 1983. "Using ULCL measures to find frequency/gain and SSPL 90." *Hearing Instruments* 34(7):17–21. Reproduced with permission of the author and publisher. Bottom: diagram of an ER-3A insert earphone that has the same output as a TDH-series supra-aural earphone. The foam tip can be replaced with the person's own earmold. From M. C. Killion, L. A. Wilber, and G. I. Gudmundsen 1985. "Insert earphones for more interaural attenuation." *Hearing Instruments* 36(2):34–36. Reproduced with permission of the authors and publisher.

output of the audiometer (10 or 50 ohms) and the insert earphone. For these reasons, this earphone can be used for testing with speech as well as with frequency-specific sounds. Although it is more expensive than the insert earphone shown in the top panel, it can be used for all types of audiological testing. The sound from both types of insert earphones is delivered through a plastic tube held in the external earcanal by a custom earmold or an EAR™ foamtip.

If supra-aural or insert earphones are dropped or driven with signals that are too high in level, they will produce excessive distortion. This distortion can be heard as a crackling or rattling sound as the SPL of either narrow bands of noise or speech is increased. If this distortion occurs, the earphone must be replaced to get accurate results.

Amplifier

A power amplifier, in addition to the amplifier in the audiometer, is needed to provide the necessary gain to drive the loudspeaker at the desired sound levels. This amplifier should have a dynamic range of about 100 dB (unweighted). The amplifier should have a bandwidth greater than 20 to 20,000 Hz and a uniform frequency response (±0.01 dB). It should introduce less than 0.1% distortion at full power. To achieve this, the maximum output of the amplifier should be 10 dB greater than the highest signal to be generated. This will allow signals that have high crest factors, such as random noise or speech, to be amplified without peak clipping. If the amplifier is capable of producing more power than the rating of the loudspeaker, a suitably rated, fast-responding fuse should be placed between the amplifier and the loudspeaker.

Loudspeaker

A loudspeaker should be chosen based on the following qualities:

1. bandwidth at least 100 to 10,000 Hz
2. smooth frequency response
3. enclosure for direct radiation of sound to the listener
4. low distortion
5. high efficiency
6. capacity for handling large amounts of power for long periods
7. reliability

These qualities are described in greater detail below.

Bandwidth. Few single-cone loudspeakers manufactured today are capable of reproducing a sound with a bandwidth from 100 to 10,000 Hz. To provide this bandwidth, two or three loudspeakers, each of which exhibits a uniform frequency response over a limited frequency range, are combined with electrical crossover networks designed to provide a minimum of overlap in the sounds transduced by each speaker. A common positioning of two loudspeakers is a coaxial array as shown in the top panel of figure 3.15. In this array the high-frequency speaker is on the axis of the low-frequency speaker so that there is only one apparent source of sound for both frequency regions. The crossover point for these two speakers is clearly shown

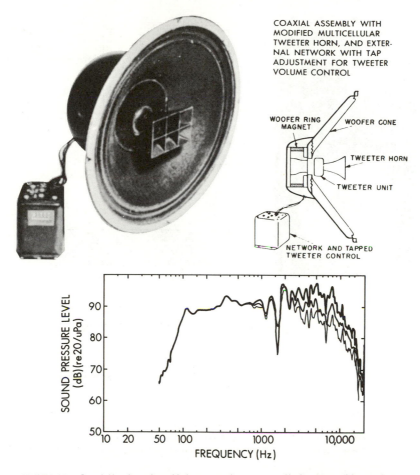

COAXIAL ASSEMBLY WITH
MODIFIED MULTICELLULAR
TWEETER HORN, AND EXTER-
NAL NETWORK WITH TAP
ADJUSTMENT FOR TWEETER
VOLUME CONTROL

WOOFER RING
MAGNET

WOOFER CONE

TWEETER HORN

TWEETER UNIT

NETWORK AND TAPPED
TWEETER CONTROL

FIGURE 3.15.   Coaxial loudspeaker with the tweeter horn mounted in the center of the woofer cone (top panel). The frequency response of this loudspeaker was measured at 0° azimuth at the same height as the cone and at a distance of 2 m in an anechoic chamber. The notch at 1600 Hz is associated with the crossover between the woofer and the tweeter; there are three settings for the high-frequency response (bottom panel). Top panel from A. B. Cohen 1968. *Hi-Fi Loudspeakers and Enclosures*, 2nd ed., based on loudspeaker manufactured by Altec Lansing Corporation. Reproduced with permission of Altec Lansing Corp., and A. B. Cohen's son.

by the dip in the frequency response at approximately 1600 Hz (lower panel of figure 3.15). Another common positioning is the three-speaker array shown in the top panel of figure 3.16. The sound source for each frequency region is slightly different, and although this can be detected by the normal-hearing listener for narrow-band sounds, this should not cause difficulty in

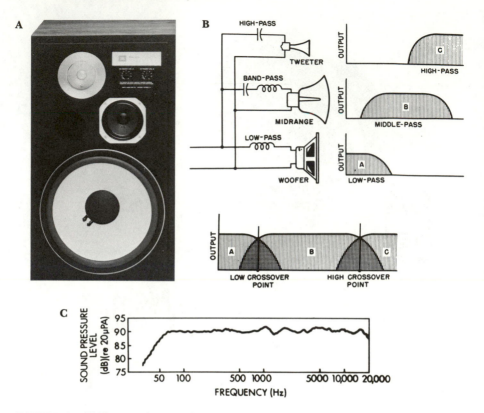

FIGURE 3.16. **(A)** Three-speaker array. Reproduced with the permission of James B. Lansing Sound, Inc. **(B)** The diagram of the cross-over network with the frequency range carried by each speaker. From A. B. Cohen 1968. *Hi-Fi Loudspeakers and Enclosures*, 2nd ed. Reproduced with permission of A. B. Cohen's son. **(C)** The frequency response of one of these loudspeakers.

clinical testing. The two crossover points are not discernible in the frequency response shown in the lower panel of figure 3.16.

Frequency response.   The frequency response of a loudspeaker is measured by delivering pure tones of equal electrical intensity (for example, between 100 and 10,000 Hz) to the terminals and monitoring its output (in dB SPL) with a microphone placed a given distance on a given axis in front of it in an anechoic chamber. If there is little variation in the SPL as a function of frequency, as shown in the lower panel of figure 3.16, this is considered a smooth frequency response. A loudspeaker with a smooth frequency response will give a more faithful reproduction of the original sound than one that is not smooth. This is highly desirable in providing a uniform sound

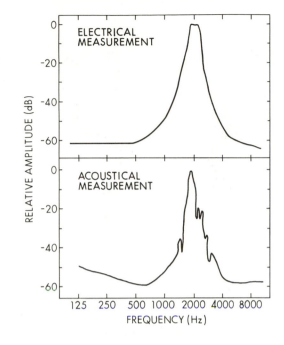

FIGURE 3.17.
Spectra for a third-octave band of noise (centered at 2000 Hz) measured electrically at the output of the audiometer (top panel) and acoustically (bottom panel) in a sound-treated room 2 m from the loudspeaker at the center of where the listener's head would be. The SPL between 125 and 500 Hz is higher in the acoustical measurement because of ambient noise in the room. The significant difference between the two spectra in the region of 2000 Hz is largely caused by the filtering effect of the frequency response of the coaxial loudspeaker (see the bottom panel of figure 3.15) in which the crossover frequency is approximately 1600 Hz. To a far smaller extent the spectrum measured acoustically also reflects the effects of the amplifier noise floor and the variability in the SPL in this reverberant field.

field for narrow-band sounds and in delivering an undistorted speech signal for clinical testing.

A coaxial loudspeaker with a crossover frequency at 1600 Hz (see figure 3.15) is used in many clinics. When a third-octave band of noise centered at 2000 Hz was measured electrically (top panel of figure 3.17) and acoustically (bottom panel of figure 3.17) and the two spectra compared, it was clear that the acoustic stimulus reflects the resonances and antiresonances of the loudspeaker in this frequency region. Similar measurements at 250 and 500 Hz showed close correspondence between the electrical and acoustic stimuli because the frequency response of the loudspeaker was relatively uniform at these frequencies. This loudspeaker is often chosen instead of one with a smoother frequency response because it produces 10 to 15 dB higher SPLs.

Enclosure. Loudspeakers can be housed in two major types of enclosures: a direct radiator or a horn enclosure. Most enclosures are of the direct-radiator type because direct-radiator enclosures are simple to construct, require less space, and provide a relatively uniform frequency response. At Central Institute for the Deaf a direct-radiator, a closed-baffle, or a bass-reflex-baffle enclosure (see figure 3.18) with glass wool lining the closed space at the back of the loudspeaker is used. These enclosures were chosen not only for the reasons noted above but to have an apparent sound

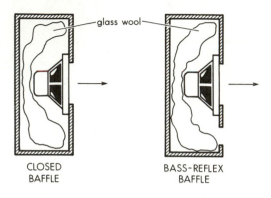

CLOSED
BAFFLE

BASS-REFLEX
BAFFLE

FIGURE 3.18.
Closed-baffle and bass-reflex-baffle enclosures for loudspeakers. These are direct-radiator enclosures. The baffle is formed by the enclosure surface that extends in the same plane as the edge around the loudspeaker cone and helps to prevent the sound radiating in front of the loudspeaker from interacting with sound radiating in back. The bass reflex is a small hole in the enclosure that creates an acoustic enhancement of the low-frequency response of the loudspeaker. Modified from A. B. Cohen 1968. *Hi-Fi Loudspeakers and Enclosures*, 2nd ed. Reproduced with permission of A. B. Cohen's son.

source similar to that of the human voice for testing with speech stimuli. The enclosures were built so that the panels vibrate as little as possible. This was accomplished by building the enclosure with ¾-in. plywood, cross-bracing and fastening with screws, and gluing all the connections.

Low distortion. Loudspeakers for use in audiometry should be capable of transducing narrow-band sounds (such as FM tones or narrow bands of noise) so that harmonic distortion and intermodulation distortion (sound energy at sum and difference frequencies of the test signal) are at least 50 to 80 dB below the test signal. When loudspeakers are driven with high SPLs, harmonic and intermodulation distortion will increase. Some loudspeakers will begin to distort with output levels of 80 dB SPL (measured 1 m in front of the speaker); for others this occurs at 90 to 110 dB SPL. Since some hearing-impaired listeners have severe or profound hearing losses, it is desirable to choose the loudspeaker that will give the highest output with the least distortion.

Efficiency. Loudspeakers that give high output with little distortion must also be efficient. For 1 watt electrical input the most efficient loudspeakers commercially available will produce about 105 dB SPL (measured at 1 m) and the least efficient will produce about 75 dB SPL. For clinical testing a loudspeaker with the highest undistorted output *and* a uniform frequency response should be chosen.

Power-handling capacity. Professional loudspeakers, such as those used in auditoriums, are designed to handle large amounts of power for long periods with no damage to the cones. Home-entertainment loudspeakers typically are designed for lower power levels and will burn out when they are driven over long durations by high-level signals. In testing people with severe hearing losses unaided in the field, it is necessary to deliver narrow-band sounds of at least 80 to 100 dB SPL. For this reason, a professional loudspeaker is usually more suitable for clinical testing than a home-entertainment speaker.

Reliability.   The frequency-response and distortion characteristics of home-entertainment loudspeakers are more likely to change with age than those of professional loudspeakers. Since these characteristics should re-main constant, this is another reason for choosing a professional loud-speaker.

Summary.   An efficient professional loudspeaker is more likely to have the qualities that are best for clinical, sound-field testing than a home-entertainment loudspeaker. It costs more, but with it more accurate thresh-olds can be obtained over a wider range of levels, and speech can be presented that is a more faithful reproduction of the original recording.

Reel-to-Reel Recorder or Cassette Player

Most reel-to-reel recorders or cassette players used in audiological testing have two channels, and the output of each can be fed to the two channels of an audiometer. The test stimulus, such as a phonetically bal-anced word list, is recorded on one channel, and a competing signal, such as cafeteria noise, may be recorded on the other. In hearing aid evaluations the test words and the competing signal can be fed to two different loudspeakers separated in space by 90° or 180° to simulate everyday listening situations; the test words can also be presented to one loudspeaker and no signal presented to the other.

Good reel-to-reel recorders and cassette players should comply with the standards of the National Association of Broadcasters (1771 N Street, N.W., Washington, D.C. 20036). The performance characteristics that are particularly important for audiometry are as follows:

1. uniform frequency response between 100 and 10,000 Hz,
2. "crosstalk" from one channel to the other is 50 dB or more down at 20,000 Hz,
3. wow and flutter below 0.1%, and
4. signal-to-noise ratio (for recordings made at 0 VU) that is 50 dB or greater (unweighted) without a noise-reduction system being activated (e.g., Dolby).

For the same cost the performance characteristics for a reel-to-reel recorder are better than for a cassette player. The major advantage of the cassette player is that it takes much less time to change a cassette than to change a reel-to-reel tape.

A variety of polyester tapes with ferromagnetic coating are available.

Recordings should be made on tape that provides the best signal-to-noise ratio according to the guidelines of the National Association of Broadcasters.

All reel-to-reel recorders and cassette players need to have the tape heads cleaned after every 20 to 30 hours of use to remove material that rubs off the tape. In addition, the tape heads should be demagnetized every 50 to 100 hours. The manufacturer's instructions should be followed for cleaning and demagnetization. Unless this cleaning is done regularly, the high-frequency sound may not be reproduced accurately.

Earmuff and Earplug

In hearing evaluations it is important to determine the response to sound by each ear separately. For sound-field testing the sound reaching the nontest ear can be reduced by inserting an earplug and placing an earmuff over that ear. An example of the attenuation provided by the earplug and earmuff is shown in figure 3.19. The attenuation of the two is greater than that provided by either one but much lower than the sum of the attenuation associated with each.

To achieve 35 to 55 dB attenuation, the earplug must fit tightly in the earcanal, and the earmuff must fit snugly against the head and surround the pinna. If the coupling of either the earplug or the earmuff is loose, the attenuation will be lower at all frequencies but particularly at 125 to 500 Hz. With hearing losses that are the same at both ears at all frequencies, it is not critical that there be 35 to 40 dB attenuation. However, when the nontest ear has substantially better thresholds than the test ear, less than 35 to 40 dB attenuation will result in the individual's responding to sound at the nontest ear.

A number of earplugs and earmuffs are available commercially, and some provide more attenuation than others. A listing of some of the companies that sell them is included in Appendix 3B.

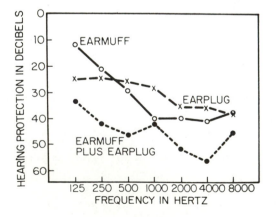

FIGURE 3.19.
The hearing protection or attenuation (dB) provided by earmuffs, earplugs, and a combination of both. From C. W. Nixon 1979. "Hearing protective devices: Ear protectors." In *Handbook of Noise Control*, 2nd ed. Ed. C. M. Harris, figure 12.3. Copyright 1979, McGraw-Hill Book Co., New York. Reproduced with permission of the author and the publisher.

Chair

The chair in which the listeners sit should not extend above their shoulders; if it does, it may cause sound reflections that interfere with the uniformity of the sound field. If possible, the chair should be equipped with a headrest that is only as large as the back of a person's head to prevent it from interfering with the sound field. For testing, the listeners can position their heads on the headrest; this will reduce the variation in sound level at the ear resulting from small head movements when unaided and aided thresholds are obtained.

Table

For testing small children, toys or pictures are often placed on a low table in front of the loudspeaker. The sound reflected from the hard surfaces of the table can cause the level in the sound field to be less uniform than if it were not there. If the table is padded with absorbent material, this will decrease the sound reflections. Even with the padding, the table may still affect the sound field. For this reason, calibration of sound levels for the test signals should be made with the table, chairs, toys, and people who will be assisting with the testing in the room in the same place as when the child is tested.

Sound-Level Meter

A sound-level meter is an instrument designed for measurement of SPL. Two types of sound-level meters are used in calibrating or measuring sound for hearing aid evaluations. The first type is used for the daily acoustic calibration of the overall level of stimuli in the sound field. This meter with a 2-cc coupler can also be used to measure the approximate output of hearing aids in response to speech, warble tones, or narrow-band-noise inputs. With a phone jack and a pair of earphones one can also listen to the output of the hearing aid in response to these inputs. This sound-level meter can be set to measure the rms sound-pressure level of a sound on the A-, B-, or C-weighted scale with a fast or slow speed of the needle-deflection response. Although there are several qualities of meters available with these features, it is important to get an ANSI standard (S l.4-1971) Type 2 meter because it gives more accurate measurements of the sound than a Type 3 meter. A picture of a Type 2 meter coupled to a hearing aid is shown in figure 3.20.

The second type of sound-level meter is used for measuring the sound level of test signals as well as the level at frequency regions an octave or more away from the test signals (that is, the stimulus skirt slopes, the noise floor, and the distortion products). It is also used for measuring the ambient-noise

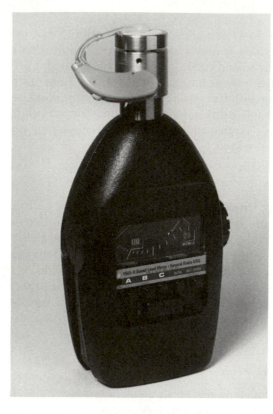

FIGURE 3.20.   Sound-level meter (Type 2) with a 2-cc coupler to which a hearing aid is coupled. The gain and the saturation SPL of a hearing aid can be estimated with speech stimuli or FM tones by measuring the SPL of the input sound (without the coupler) and the output sound from the hearing aid and comparing the two.

levels in the test room. This sound-level meter should be capable of measuring the overall level of sounds, and it must have octave or third-octave filters so that the sound can be measured in discrete frequency regions. It should be capable of measuring on the peak or rms scales with either a slow or fast speed of the needle-deflection response. An ANSI standard (S1.4-1971) Type 1 precision sound-level meter is required for these measurements. Although it would be advantageous to own one of these meters, they are very expensive. Consequently, many clinicians pay a company that has the meter and expertise to calibrate their equipment and sound field at regular intervals. If a company does the calibration, each clinician should understand what is being done and monitor the results, since s/he is legally responsible for the accuracy of the calibration.

Hearing Aid Test System

Hearing aid test systems are designed to measure the electroacoustic performance of hearing aids. Commercially available test systems comply with the equipment described in the ANSI standard (ANSI S3.22-1982), "Specifications of Hearing Aid Characteristics." These systems include a test enclosure in which a loudspeaker (driven by a sound source), a monitor microphone, and a coupler (with microphone) are situated; an amplifier, a sound-level meter, and an X-Y plotter, graphic level recorder, or printer are also included.

The test enclosure is like an anechoic chamber. Its walls are highly absorbent to minimize reflected and standing waves, and they are constructed to reduce the ambient noise level inside the chamber. The sound level of the tones can be varied between 50 and 90 dB SPL at the hearing aid microphone. The output of the speaker is monitored with a microphone and an automatic-gain-control system that ensures that the signal delivered to the hearing aid does not differ from the nominal input intensity by more than ± 1.5 dB between 200 and 2000 Hz and ± 2.5 dB between 2000 and 5000 Hz. The output of the hearing aid is delivered to a standard 2-cc coupler (an HA-2 coupler for body, behind-the-ear, and eyeglass aids and an HA-1 coupler for in-the-ear aids and other aids attached to the listener's own earmold). The hearing aid output is transduced by the coupler microphone, and the SPL of the amplified signal is measured with a sound-level meter. In some systems there is a digital printout, in others there is a graphic printout of the output as a function of input SPL, and some have both.

With the hearing aid test system the gain, the frequency response, the frequency range, the saturation SPL (often called the maximum power output), and the harmonic distortion of a hearing aid can be measured. Some systems are also designed to measure the input noise level, the attack and release times of compression hearing aids, the battery current, and the frequency response and gain of the induction (telephone) coil.

A hearing aid test system is an essential piece of equipment for the clinical evaluation of hearing aids. With it new, used, or repaired aids can be evaluated to determine whether they perform according to the manufacturer's specifications using standard procedures and equipment (ANSI S3.22-1982). The output of the aid can be measured before and after making changes in its electroacoustic characteristics when fitting it to an individual client.

If a hearing aid test system is not available, a Type 2 sound-level meter can be used to first measure speech and warble tones (or narrow bands of noise) in the field (use the C-weighted scale), and then to measure the output of the hearing aid in a 2-cc coupler to get a rough estimate of the gain, frequency response and saturation sound pressure level of the hearing aid.

Since more accurate and more complete measurements are specified by the ANSI standard than is possible with the Type 2 sound-level meter, the purchase of a hearing aid test system should be a high-priority item.

Probe and Probe-Tube Microphone Systems

In the last few years probe and probe-tube microphone systems have been developed commercially to clinically measure the unaided and aided SPL in an individual's external earcanal. One company sells a probe microphone system in which the miniature, silicone-covered microphone is inserted in the space between an earmold tip and the eardrum. A block diagram of this system, which is shown in figure 3.21, includes coupling to a commercially available hearing aid test system. The SPL output of the control microphone is part of a feedback system which produces a sweep-frequency, pure-tone stimulus through a loudspeaker at a constant SPL at the port of this microphone. In this figure the control microphone is shown in the left earcanal (nontest ear); it can also be placed at the top of the superior helix of the test ear. The major reasons this probe microphone system has not received widespread acceptance are (1) the microphone is too large to fit easily into the earcanal of a number of adults, as well as children,

FIGURE 3.21. Block diagram of a probe microphone system for measuring the unaided and aided SPL in the earcanal. From E. R. Harford 1981. "A new clinical technique for verification of hearing aid response." *Archives of Otolaryngology* 107:461–68. Copyright 1981, American Medical Association. Reproduced with permission of the author and the publisher.

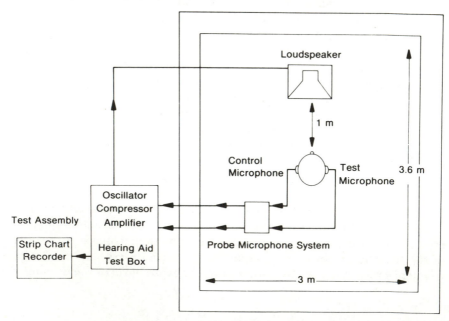

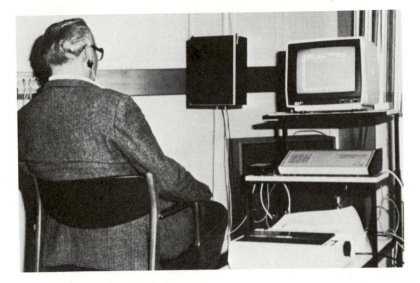

FIGURE 3.22.   Probe-tube microphone system (Rastronics CCI-10 Computer System) for measuring the
unaided and aided SPL in the earcanal. The equipment is placed in a sound room with the client
seated approximately 30 to 50 cm from the loudspeaker, which is mounted at ear level at 0°
azimuth. From H. Birk-Nielsen 1985. "Hearing aid fitting based on insertion gain measurements." *Audecibel* 34(1):16—19. Reproduced with permission of the author and the publisher.

and (2) there is a slight risk of injuring the canal wall or eardrum if placed by
inexperienced clinicians.

Probe-tube microphone systems avoid these drawbacks, because a very
thin, flexible tube, attached to the port of the probe microphone, is placed in
the earcanal instead of the microphone. One of these systems is shown in
figure 3.22. The equipment includes a loudspeaker, reference and probe
microphone, preamplifier, dedicated computer, computer controlled pure-
tone stimuli (FM modulated and constant), acoustic monitoring earphone
for the clinician, display screen, and printer. This system, as well as most of
the other systems, has options for measuring the electroacoustic characteristics of hearing aids with a coupler in a hearing aid test box. Manufacturers of
hearing aid test systems are now offering options for probe-tube microphone measurements.

The computer for some of these probe-tube microphone systems is
dedicated so that the individual clinician cannot expand the applicability of
the system by calculating the real-ear gain for a specific prescriptive procedure or by making other modifications that may be helpful in the clinical
dispensing of hearing aids. It is advantageous to have the capacity for this
expansion. Some systems have the option of presenting a click through the
loudspeaker, and the spectrum of this click, measured with the probe-tube
microphone, is analyzed using the Fast Fourier Transform (Schweitzer
1986). It takes a much shorter time to present a click than sweeping a tone

from low to high frequencies, and the click gives a more realistic analysis of the output of a hearing aid with a compression circuit than the pure-tone sweep. In addition, an aid's temporal response to a transient stimulus can be analyzed.

SUMMARY

An understanding of the effect of the room, sound stimuli, and equipment on the reliability and validity of the test results is important in evaluating the effect of a hearing aid on a hearing-impaired individual's ability to hear. The room size, its reverberation patterns, the ambient noise level, and the individual's position in the room affect the sound reaching the ear and the hearing aid microphone. A number of sound stimuli are used to evaluate the person's hearing with and without a hearing aid. These should include speech and frequency-specific stimuli, such as tones and narrow bands of noise. For sound-field-threshold testing, it is essential to choose frequency-specific stimuli so that if the person moves his or her head, the level will not change more than ± 2 dB. In addition, the sound should be centered in the small range around the test frequency; sound more than one octave from the test frequency should be 45 to 60 dB lower than that at the test frequency. Many of these same considerations are applicable to measurements of unaided and aided SPL in the earcanal using probe and probe-tube microphone systems. Equipment for presenting and measuring sound should be chosen after considering the criteria described in this chapter.

APPENDIX 3A. Speech materials and competing sounds for the clinical evaluation of hearing aids.

A. Reel-to-reel and cassette recordings commercially available from Auditec of St. Louis, 330 Selma Avenue, St. Louis, Missouri 63119

  1. Adult spondee word lists
  2. Children's spondee word lists
  3. Children's pictured spondee words (12)
  4. W-22 word lists
  5. NU-6 word lists
  6. California Consonant Test
  7. Synthetic Sentence Identification Test
  8. Children's PBK-50 word lists
  9. Children's Word Intelligibility by Picture Index (WIPI)
  10. Northwestern University—Children's Perception of Speech Test (NU-CHIPS)
  11. Bell Telephone sentences

12.   Connected Discourse, male and female talkers
13.   Multitalker complex
14.   Four-talker complex
15.   Cafeteria noise

B.   Phonograph or cassette recordings available from Technisonic Studios, 1201 South Brentwood Boulevard, St. Louis, Missouri 63117

1.   CID W-1 and W-2 spondee word lists (Ira Hirsh recording)
2.   CID W-22 word lists (Ira Hirsh recording)
3.   CID PB-50 word lists (Rush Hughes recording)
4.   Connected Discourse (Fulton Lewis, Jr., recording).

C.   References to speech materials, recordings of which are not commercially available.

1.   CID Everyday Sentences: Davis, H., and S. R. Silverman. 1978. *Hearing and deafness.* 4th ed. New York: Holt, Rinehart, and Winston, 536–38.

2.   Revised CID Everyday Sentences: Elkins, E., G.D. Causey, L.B. Beck, D. Brewer, and J. B. de Moll. 1975. Normal and impaired listener performance on the University of Maryland Revised CID Sentence Lists. Unpublished report, University of Maryland.

3.   Nonsense Syllable Test: Resnick, S. B., J. R. Dubno, S. Hoffnung, and H. Levitt. 1975. Phoneme errors on a nonsense syllable test, *Journal of the Acoustical Society of America* 58:114.

4.   Speech Perception in Noise Test (SPIN): Kalikow, D. N., K. N. Stevens, and L. L. Elliott. 1977. *Journal of the Acoustical Society of America* 61:1337–51. Also, Bilger, R. C., J. M. Nuetzel, W. M. Rabinowitz, and C. Rzeczkowski. 1984. "Standardization of a test of speech perception in noise." *Journal of Speech and Hearing Research* 27:32–48.

APPENDIX 3B.   Alphabetical list of some companies that manufacture earmuffs (M) and earplugs (P).

(P)   American Optical Corporation
14 Mechanic Street
Southbridge, Massachusetts 01550

(P)   E A R Division of Cabot Corporation
7911 Zionsville Road
Indianapolis, Indiana 46268

(M)   M S A (Mine Safety Appliances)
600 Penn Center Boulevard
Pittsburgh, Pennsylvania 15235

(P)   Norton Company Safety Products
2000 Plainfield Pike
Providence, Rhode Island 02920

(M)   Racal Airstream, Incorporated
      7309-A Grove Road
      Frederick, Maryland 21701

(M)   Sellstrom Manufacturing Company
      213 South Hicks Road
      Palatine, Illinois 60067

(M)   U.S. Safety Service Company
(P)   1535 Walnut, Box 1237
      Kansas City, Missouri 64141

(M)   Willson Safety Products
(P)   Box 622
      Reading, Pennsylvania 19603

Chapter Four
MEASURING SOUND FOR HEARING AID EVALUATIONS

SUPRA-AURAL EARPHONE
Sound-Pressure-Level Measurements
6-cc Coupler versus Eardrum Sound-Pressure Level
Zwislocki Coupler versus Eardrum Sound-Pressure Level

INSERT EARPHONE
Sound-Pressure-Level Measurements
2-cc, Zwislocki Coupler, and Eardrum Sound-Pressure Level

SOUND FIELD
Location of Loudspeaker and Listener
Sound-Pressure-Level Measurements
Microphone Position
Ambient Noise
Frequency-Specific Sounds
Speech and Competing Sounds
Sound Field versus Eardrum Sound-Pressure Level
Loudspeaker Azimuth
Effect of Listener on the Sound Field
Normal Sound-Field Thresholds
Estimates of Sound Field versus
Eardrum Sound-Pressure Level

HEARING AID
Coupler Measurements
Test-Box Calibration
Couplers
Placement of Hearing Aid in Test Box
Standard Tests of Hearing Aid Performance
Acoustic Characteristics of an Earmold
Listening to Hearing Aid Output
Factors That Affect the Actual Frequency Response
for the Listener
Differences in the Sound Field at the Hearing Aid Input
Differences in Sound at the Hearing Aid Output
Measurements with KEMAR and Zwislocki Coupler
Probe and Probe-Tube Microphone Measurements

COMPARISON OF SUPRA-AURAL-EARPHONE, SOUND-FIELD, AND INSERT-EARPHONE MEASURES OF AN INDIVIDUAL'S AUDITORY AREA WITH HEARING AID OUTPUT
SUMMARY

One of the major challenges in hearing aid evaluations is to select and adjust the frequency response, gain, and SSPL90 of a hearing aid so that amplified speech and other sounds will be comfortably loud between 250 and 6000 Hz, and no amplified sound will be uncomfortable. An important aspect in selecting these hearing aid characteristics is to make the appropriate comparison between an individual's thresholds, MCLs and UCLs (auditory area) and the hearing aid output between 250 and 6000 Hz. A direct comparison of these data cannot be made, unless the SPL measurement is made at the same reference point, such as the microphone in a 2-cc coupler. For example, when an insert earphone is used to obtain an individual's auditory area, a direct comparison (in dB SPL) can be made with the hearing aid output because both are measured with a 2-cc coupler. However, when the auditory area is obtained with a supra-aural earphone (or in the sound field), the SPL for the auditory area is measured in a 6-cc coupler (or in the center of the place where the listener's head would be for testing), whereas the SPL for the hearing aid is measured in the 2-cc coupler. The SPL for these two sets of data can be compared only when both are referred to the SPL at the eardrum.

The purpose of this chapter is to describe procedures for measuring sound from earphones and hearing aids in couplers, from loudspeakers in the sound field, and from all these sources with probe and probe-tube microphone systems. Also described is the relation of the SPL measured by these procedures to (1) the average, normal-hearing threshold (to convert the levels to dB HL) and (2) the SPL at the listener's eardrum.

SUPRA-AURAL EARPHONE

Sound-Pressure-Level Measurements

The standard procedure (ANSI S3.6-1969) for measuring sound from supra-aural earphones is with a microphone in an NBS 9-A coupler (see figure 4.1). In this procedure the earphone cushion is fitted tightly against the lip of the coupler by the pressure of a 500 gram force applied to the top of the earphone. The 6-cc cavity bounded by the microphone, the earphone and the coupler approximates the acoustic transfer immittance of the average human ear between about 400 and 3000 Hz but not at higher and lower frequencies.

Although a description of the procedure for calibrating the earphone output of an audiometer is beyond the scope of this book, there are several aspects that are particularly important for a hearing aid evaluation. The standard (ANSI S3.6-1969) specifies the SPLs associated with the mean threshold for pure tones and speech for normal-hearing listeners. These are shown in table 4.1. The SPL for recorded speech is measured with a 1000 Hz

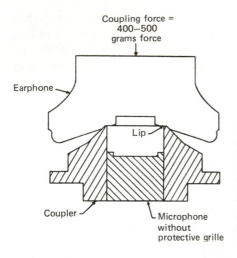

Coupling force =
400—500
grams force

Earphone

Lip

Coupler

Microphone
without
protective grille

FIGURE 4.1.
A schematic drawing of the NBS 9-A coupler showing
the method of placing a TDH-series earphone mounted
in a MX-41/AR cushion on the coupler with a 500-g force
on top of the earphone. This figure is reproduced with
permission from American National Standard Specifications for Audiometers, ANSI S3.6-1969. Copyright 1969,
American National Standards Institute. Copies of this
standard may be purchased from the American National
Standards Institute, 1430 Broadway, New York, NY 10018.

calibration tone set at 0 VU on the audiometer; this calibration tone should
be recorded so that "the average peak VU meter deflection produced by the
speech signal" (ANSI S3.6-1969) is equal to the deflection caused by the
calibration tone. To compare the output of the earphone with the standard
values, subtract the standard value for the signal being measured (pure
tones or speech) from the reading on the sound level meter. In a properly
operating audiometer, this should equal the attenuator dial reading within
the acceptable range (± 3 dB at $250-3000$ Hz, ± 4 dB at 4000 Hz, ± 5 dB at
125, 6000, and 8000 Hz, and ± 3 dB for speech). The relation between the
audiometer dial readings and the earphone output should be linear (i.e.,
within 0.3 of the interval step or 1.5 dB, whichever is smaller) over the entire
range of attenuator settings. In addition, the pure tones should be within ± 3
percent of the indicated frequency, and any harmonics should be at least 30
dB below the fundamental at the highest level output of the audiometer. For

TABLE 4.1.   Reference Threshold Values in dB SPL at 0 dB HL for TDH Series Supra-Aural
Earphones (ANSI S3.6-1969) and Provisional Values for ER-3A Insert Ear-
phones (Libby 1985b). The SPL Output of the Supra-Aural Earphones Is
Measured in a 6-cc Coupler and That of the Insert Earphone (Attached to
Tubing Used for Testing) Is Measured in a 2-cc, HA-1 Coupler.

	FREQUENCY (Hz)								
	250	500	1000	1500	2000	3000	4000	6000	SPONDEE WORDS
TDH-39	25.5	11.5	7.0	6.5	9.0	10.0	9.5	15.5	19.5
TDH-49 and TDH-50P	26.5	13.5	7.5	7.5	11.0	9.5	10.5	13.5	20.0
ER-3A	15.5	8.5	3.5	2.5	6.5	5.5	1.5	−1.5	—

speech there should be no audible distortion at the highest levels of output. If the audiometer is not functioning within the above limits, it should be adjusted or repaired.

6-cc Coupler versus Eardrum Sound-Pressure Level

One way to determine the relation between the SPL output of a supra-aural earphone measured in a 6-cc coupler and at the eardrum is to compare the SPLs associated with average, normal-hearing thresholds in the coupler and at the eardrum. The coupler threshold values for the TDH-39 earphones are shown in table 4.1. The eardrum threshold values were derived by Killion (1978a) from (1) coupler data (NBS 9-A; ANSI S3.6-1969) corrected for physiological noise, (2) free-field data (ISO R266-1961), and (3) SPL measurements made by Shaw (1966b, 1974a) using a supra-aural earphone and a free-field sound source. The eardrum threshold values, called Minimum Audible Pressure (MAP), and the coupler threshold values for the TDH-39 earphone with MX-41/AR cushion are plotted in the bottom panel of figure 4.2. When the coupler values are subtracted from the eardrum values, the resulting difference (dB) is the ratio of the *average* eardrum SPL to the *average* 6-cc coupler pressure for this earphone/cushion. This difference (dB) is plotted in the top panel of figure 4.2, and the values are given in table 4.2. The levels at the eardrum are higher than those in the coupler at all frequencies except 250 Hz, where there is a loss of low-frequency energy due to the fit of the earphone cushion against the pinna. The values in table 4.2 should be corrected if a supra-aural earphone other than the TDH-39 with an MX-41/AR cushion is used.

The SPL reaching the earcanal from a supra-aural earphone varies among individuals and from one placement to the next on the same individual. This variability can be seen in measurements Shaw (1966a) made of the SPL output of a TDH-39 earphone in the 6-cc coupler and at the entrance of the earcanal. A drawing of the probe tube placement for the earcanal

FIGURE 4.2.
Top panel: calculated average difference between the SPL at the eardrum and that in an NBS 9-A coupler for a TDH-39 earphone in an MX-41/AR cushion. Bottom panel: SPL associated with normal hearing threshold for TDH-39 earphones in MX-41/AR cushions measured in the coupler and at the eardrum. Drawn from calculations by Killion 1978, based on data from Shaw 1966b and Shaw 1974a.

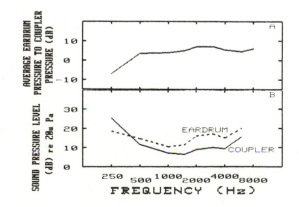

TABLE 4.2.   The Difference (dB) Between the Average SPL at the Eardrum and That Measured in a Coupler. This Difference Is Shown for a Supra-Aural Earphone (TDH-39 in a MX-41/AR Cushion) Measured in a 6-cc Coupler and for an Insert Earphone (Hearing Aid Receiver) Measured in a 2-cc Coupler.

	FREQUENCY (Hz)						
	250	500	1000	2000	3000	4000	6000
6-cc Coupler/ Eardrum[1]	−7	0.5	2	6	5	3.5	−2.5
2-cc Coupler/ Eardrum[2]	4	4	5	8	10	12	14

[1]These values were calculated by subtracting the SPLs associated with the normal reference thresholds for this earphone/cushion from the SPLs associated with normal hearing threshold at the eardrum (Killion 1978).
[2]Sachs and Burkhard 1972, in Levitt et al. 1980.

FIGURE 4.3.   (A) Drawing of the left ear showing placement of the probe tube. The broken lines indicate the boundaries of the concha and the meatus. **(B)** Cross-section of the auricle looking toward the front of the head and showing the position of the probe-tube orifice. **(C)** The critical dimensions of the tube. From E. A. G. Shaw 1966. "Earcanal pressure generated by a free sound field." *Journal of the Acoustical Society of America* 39:465-70. Reproduced with permission of the author and the publisher.

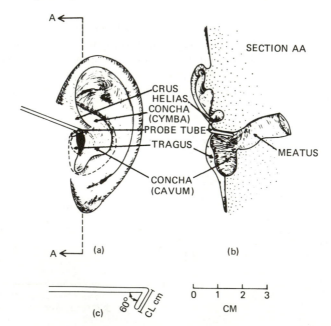

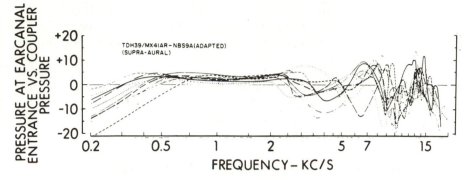

FIGURE 4.4. Ratio of the SPL at the earcanal entrance to coupler pressure (normalized response) from 10 adult male subjects. From E. A. G. Shaw 1966b. "Earcanal pressure generated by circumaural and supra-aural earphones." *Journal of the Acoustical Society of America* 39:471-79. Reproduced with permission of the author and the publisher.

measurements is shown in figure 4.3, and the data from ten subjects is shown in figure 4.4. The difference (dB) between the SPL at the earcanal entrance and the SPL in the coupler varies across subjects only 5dB between 750 and 2500 Hz, but it varies 20 dB at 250 Hz, and 10 dB or more at 3000 Hz and above. The large variation at 250 Hz reflects the differences in the amount of low-frequency sound in the earcanal caused by how well the earphone fits against the pinna. The variation above 3000 Hz is due to earcanal resonances and antiresonances that are not present in the coupler.

The amount of sound reaching the earcanal also varies throughout repeated placements of the earphone on a single person. The ranges for three fittings averaged over nine adult males are shown in figure 4.5.

Similar studies for children between 6 and 11 years and for adult females indicate that the ratio of SPL at the earcanal entrance to that in the

FIGURE 4.5. Ranges (dB) of SPL at the earcanal entrance occurring with three successive fittings of an earphone (single sitting), averaged over nine adult male subjects. From E. A. G. Shaw 1966. "Earcanal pressure generated by circumaural and supra-aural earphone." *Journal of the Acoustical Society of America* 39:471-79. Reproduced with permission of the author and the publisher.

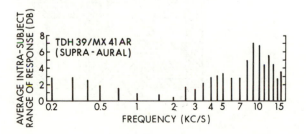

6-cc coupler is 1 dB higher from 500 to 2000 Hz and 2 to 4 dB higher at 250 and 4000 Hz than it is for adult males (e.g., Erber 1968). Consequently, the values in table 4.2 for the 6-cc coupler/eardrum difference should be corrected by these amounts for females and children.

The variability in the level of sound reaching the earcanal is directly related to the sound level at the eardrum. Based on the data shown in figures 4.4 and 4.5, it appears that the values in table 4.2 can be used to predict the SPL at the eardrum from the 6-cc coupler SPL with reasonable accuracy between 750 and 2000 Hz, but not at higher and lower frequencies.

Zwislocki Coupler versus Eardrum Sound-Pressure Level

An ear simulator, originally designed by Zwislocki (1970) and usually called a Zwislocki coupler, provides the same acoustic immittance and standing-wave sound field as a median adult human ear does, including the pinna, concha, earcanal, and eardrum (see figure 4.6). This coupler can be adapted to accommodate supra-aural, circumaural, and insert (hearing-

FIGURE 4.6. A simplified cross-section of an ear simulator, originally designed by Zwislocki (1970), for measurement of earphone responses. Z_1, Z_2, Z_3, Z_4, and Z_c are acoustic networks simulating components of acoustic immittance of the human ear. Construction of the simulator should permit separation of the portion below the line X-X' for measuring hearing aid or insert-earphone outputs. This portion, called an occluded-ear simulator, is described in the American National Standard for an Occluded Ear Simulator, ANSI S3.25-1979, that can be obtained from the Standards Secretariat, Acoustical Society of America, 335 East 45th Street, New York, NY 10017.

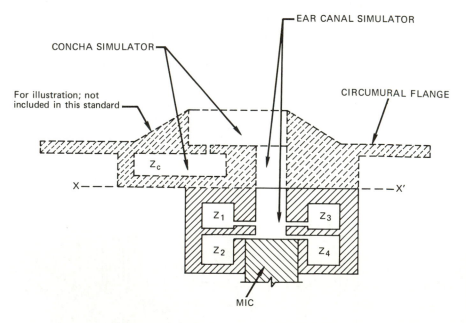

aid type) earphones. The SPL measured in the Zwislocki coupler is essentially the same as the SPL measured at the eardrum for the *median* adult between 100 and 8000 Hz.

INSERT EARPHONE

Sound-Pressure-Level Measurements

The SPL output of insert earphones can be measured with a microphone in a 2-cc or Zwislocki coupler (occluded ear simulator). Since insert earphones are coupled to the ear with tubing in an earmold or canal-occluding tip, the output is measured by placing the earcanal end of the tubing flush with the cavity in the coupler (this would be the HA-1 version of the 2-cc coupler shown in fig. 4.19). Fun-Tak™ is used to make a tight seal between the earmold and coupler; care should be taken to eliminate any air leaks or air pockets that would be contiguous with the tubing opening, because these will create unwanted acoustic pathways and cause inaccurate measurement of the output. After sealing the tubing to the coupler, the SPL output for the audiometric frequencies can be measured with a SPL meter or hearing aid test system. The SPL measured with the 2-cc coupler will be lower than that with the Zwislocki coupler; this difference will be described below in "2-cc Coupler, Zwislocki Coupler, and Eardrum Sound-Pressure Level."

The provisional reference SPLs associated with the mean normal thresholds for the ER-3A insert earphone are shown in table 4.1. If these insert earphones are used for all audiological testing, the potentiometer or digital memory of the audiometer should be set so that the SPL output at each frequency is greater than the dial reading in dB HL by these amounts. If the insert earphones are only used for hearing aid evaluations, then correction factors need to be calculated by (1) adding the values in table 4.1 for the ER-3A to the dial readings used during sound measurement, and (2) subtracting the actual SPL measured at each frequency. The resulting values should be added to the dial readings to obtain the level in dB HL at each frequency. For comparison with the 2-cc coupler output of hearing aids, the output should be expressed in dB SPL. In this case, the dial reading should be subtracted from the actual SPL measured at each frequency, and the resulting value should be added to the dial readings for auditory area data for an individual.

Although insert earphones and supra-aural earphones both may be calibrated in dB HL using mean normal-hearing thresholds, the insert earphone thresholds at 250 and 500 Hz may be 10 to 15 dB higher than the supra-aural-earphone thresholds for individuals with unusually low acoustic immittance at the eardrum. For example, this could occur in someone with a disarticulated ossicular chain or someone who did not have an eardrum. The reason for this difference in SPL needed to reach threshold is that the acoustic immittance of the supra-aural earphone is low, whereas the acoustic immittance of the insert earphone is high. The acoustic immittance mismatch between the high immittance of the insert earphone and the abnormally low immittance of the middle ear requires additional sound energy to reach threshold. The additional SPL needed with the insert earphone closely approximates the SPL needed with a hearing aid receiver. Consequently, the use of an insert earphone is desirable. However, it is important to note that for these individuals the insert earphone thresholds (dB HL) will *not* be a good approximation of the unaided sound-field thresholds at these frequencies, because the sound field is a low-immittance source which is reasonably well matched to the abnormally low immittance of the middle ear. In this case, the supra-aural earphone thresholds will be closer to the sound-field thresholds.

2-cc Coupler, Zwislocki Coupler, and Eardrum Sound-Pressure Level

The relation between the SPL measured in a 2-cc coupler, in a Zwislocki coupler, and in the SPL at the eardrum is shown in the top panel of figure 4.7. Sachs and Burkhard (1972) obtained this data with an insert earphone that was driven by a constant voltage for all three measurement sites: the two couplers and the earcanals of eleven adults. The real-ear SPLs were measured with a probe tube that extended 5 mm beyond the earmold; these SPLs were corrected to give the SPL at the eardrum based on data from Zwislocki (1970). The median, real-ear SPLs at the eardrum differ no more than 3 dB from the Zwislocki coupler SPLs between 200 and 7500 Hz. For this reason, the Zwislocki coupler SPLs can be considered essentially the same as the median, real-ear SPLs at the eardrum. In contrast, the 2-cc coupler SPLs are less than the Zwislocki coupler SPLs, and these values, which represent the *average* difference (dB) between SPL at the eardrum and SPL in a 2-cc coupler are given in table 4.2. The variation in individual differences between 2-cc coupler and eardrum SPLs are substantial above 1500 Hz, as shown by the vertical bars representing ± one standard deviation in the top panel of figure 4.7.

The residual volume between the insert earphone tubing (including earmold or foamtip) and the eardrum has a significant effect on the SPL at the eardrum. As shown in the bottom panel of figure 4.7, the SPL at the eardrum is approximately 5 dB higher in female than in male ears between approximately 1600 and 8000 Hz for the same SPL in the 2-cc coupler. This frequency-specific effect is associated with the smaller residual volume in female ears compared to male ears. An even higher SPL would be expected in infants and small children who have an even smaller residual volume.

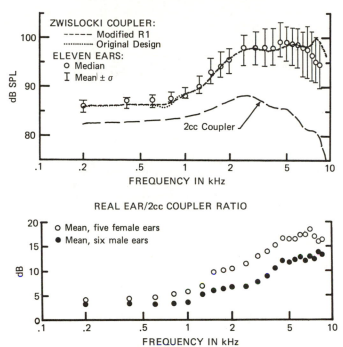

REAL EAR AND COUPLER RESPONSE

REAL EAR/2cc COUPLER RATIO

FIGURE 4.7. Top panel: The SPL output of an insert earphone measured in a 2-cc coupler, a Zwislocki coupler and in eleven adult ears. The median data for the real ears has been corrected to give the SPL at the eardrum. Bottom panel: The difference between the SPL output of an insert receiver in a 2-cc coupler and the mean SPL at the eardrum of 5 females and 6 males. Both panels from R. M. Sachs and M. D. Burkhard 1972. "Earphone pressure response in ears and couplers." Project 20021 for Knowles Electronics, Franklin Park, Ill. Reprinted in *Sensory Aids for the Hearing Impaired*. Ed. H. Levitt, J. M. Pickett, and R. A. Houde 1980. New York: IEEE Press. Reproduced with permission of the authors and Knowles Electronics.

SOUND FIELD

Location of Loudspeaker and Listener

The first step in setting up for sound-field audiometry is to find a position for the loudspeaker and listener where the levels of frequency-specific stimuli between 250 and 6000 Hz are least variable. There are two reasons to have listeners face the loudspeaker at 0° azimuth as shown in the left panel of figure 4.8. First, it simulates the typical position in which one listens to another person talk, and second, the level reaching each ear is

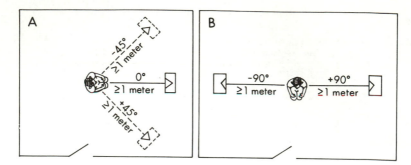

FIGURE 4.8. Three possible arrangements of loudspeakers in relation to a listener in a sound booth. Left panel: In one arrangement the listener is facing the loudspeaker at 0° azimuth, and in a second arrangement the listener is at +45° and -45° to two loudspeakers. Right panel: In the third arrangement the listener is at +90° and -90° azimuth to two loudspeakers. Adapted from W. Melnick 1979. "Instrument calibration." In *Hearing Assessment*. Ed. W. F. Rintelmann. Reproduced with permission of the author and PRO-ED, Inc., Austin, TX.

approximately the same. Another arrangement that is often used is that of two equidistant loudspeakers at 45-degree angles to the right and left of the listener. In some clinics two loudspeakers are placed at either end of the room, and the listener is placed in the position shown in the right panel of figure 4.8.

To find the best position for the loudspeaker and listener, start by placing the loudspeaker about 1 ft. (0.3 m) away from a wall (if there is sufficient space in the room) with the cone facing the center of the room. Mount the loudspeaker on a sturdy base so that the cone is at the same height as the listener's external earcanals. Then present an FM tone or narrow band of noise centered at 250 or 500 Hz at an SPL of approximately 75 dB and adjust a hand-held sound-level meter so that the needle is on scale (rms, slow, linear or C-weighted). Hold the meter at the same level as the central axis of the loudspeaker and extend it at arm's length so your body influences the sound field as little as possible.

Start with the microphone approximately 0.5 m in front of the loud-speaker and slowly move backward noting at what points the SPL is lower than at adjacent points. These low points, or dips, are places of antireson-ances in the room and should be avoided in choosing a position for the center of the listener's head. The position chosen should be in the reverber-ant field, and the SPL level should be uniform (about ± 2 dB) in the space in which listeners may move their heads during testing. For adults a spherical space with a 6-in. (15 cm) radius will allow for forward, backward, and side-to-side movements as well as for variations in height. For children the radius needs to be about 12 in. (30 cm).

To test the uniformity of the field, measure the SPL for signals cen-tered at 250, 1000, and 4000 Hz at six points in this spherical space (that is, in front, in back, above, below, and to each side of the position of the center of the head). These levels should be compared with that for the center position. If most of the values fall within a ±2 dB range, this is a good position for the listener. If many of the values fall outside this range, explore other positions for the listener and/or loudspeaker to find one with the least variability in level.

Sound-Pressure-Level Measurements

Microphone position. A field microphone mounted on a stand and attached to a Type I sound-level meter by a long cable should be placed facing the loudspeaker at the center position described above.[1] It is useful to have a plumb bob (such as surveyors or carpenters use) that marks this position in space to place the microphone accurately.

Ambient noise. The ambient noise should be measured with the field microphone at the center position at a time when the noise levels during testing hours are highest. The sound-level meter should be set for octave or third-octave analysis (rms, slow scale), and an average level (the level will fluctuate) for the frequency bands between 250 and 6000 Hz should be entered in a table (see table 3.1 in chapter 3). Compare these values with the maximum permissible levels for uncovered ears from the ANSI standard (ANSI S3.1-1977) to determine whether the measured levels are higher. If they are, then calculate the lowest level at which an accurate threshold can be obtained as shown in table 3.2 in chapter 3. It is important to have this information to evaluate whether the thresholds are accurate or are masked thesholds.

If a sound-level meter with octave or third-octave filters is not available, a meter set on the A-weighted scale can be used to estimate whether the ambient noise levels meet the standard criteria (Killion and Studebaker 1978). Ambient noises with no prominent tonal components (such as hums or whistles) that are 15 dBA or less probably meet the standard criteria. If the noise level is higher than 15 dBA, estimate the maximum threshold elevation by subtracting 15 dB from the measured level. If the ambient noise does have tonal components, obtain sound-field thresholds from normal-hearing listeners to determine the lowest obtainable thresholds for frequency-specific sounds.

Frequency-specific sounds. The first step in calibrating frequency-specific sounds is to determine the difference between the level of the test signal and that at frequency regions distant from the test signal. To do this, the microphone should be in the center position and the sound level meter

---

[1]If a sound-pressure microphone is used, it should be perpendicular to, instead of facing, the loudspeaker.

TABLE 4.3. Calibration Worksheet for Measurements (dB SPL) Made in the Sound Field at the Center of Where the Listener's Head Would Be and at Six Positions 15 cm from that Point. After H. Dillon 1982, with Permission.

SIGNAL	DIAL READING	MEASUREMENT POSITIONS						MAXIMUM DEVIATION FROM CENTER
		CENTER	LEFT	RIGHT	FRONT	BACK	UP	DOWN
250 Hz								
500 Hz								
1000 Hz								
1500 Hz								
2000 Hz								
3000 Hz								
4000 Hz								
6000 Hz								
Speech (calibration tone)								
Competing sound								

should be set for third-octave or octave analysis (rms, fast scale for FM tones; rms, slow scale for narrow bands of noise). The level of the test signal should be 30 dB higher than sound an octave above or below it, and 45 to 60 dB higher than sound energy two or more octaves above and below it. To measure this accurately, the test signal needs to be about 60 dB higher than the ambient noise floor (this usually will not be possible at 250 Hz). If the test signals do not meet these criteria for frequency specificity, one or more components in the sound system may be causing this problem. These may need to be repaired or replaced.

When the criteria for frequency specificity are met, determine the level of the test stimuli at the center position and at the other six points described above and noted in table 4.3. For these seven measurements the dial reading at each audiometric frequency should be held constant and recorded in the table. After all the measurements are made at each frequency, note the value that deviates most from that for the center position. For the stimuli and room, this is the possible difference between the measured level and the actual level that could be caused by head movement.

To calculate the correction from dial reading to SPL for determining a listener's thresholds (dB SPL), insert the values obtained for the center position shown in table 4.3 into the first line of table 4.4. Insert the dial readings in the second line of table 4.4 and then subtract line 2 from line 1 to obtain line 3. These will be the SPL at 0 dB on the dial, and they are added to the dial reading associated with a listener's thresholds to determine the thresholds in dB SPL. In most clinics listener's sound-field thresholds are expressed in dB HL. The conversion from dB SPL to dB HL is described later in the chapter.

TABLE 4.4. **An Example of the Calculation of the Sound-Field SPL at 0 dB on the Audiometer Dial by Subtracting the Dial Reading from the Measured Levels Obtained for the Center Head Position in Table 4.3. When Calculations Such as These Are Made for a Specific Audiometer and Sound-Field System, the Values in Line 3 Are Subtracted from the Dial Readings Associated with an Individual's Thresholds To Express Them in dB SPL.**

	FREQUENCY (Hz)								
	250	500	1000	1500	2000	3000	4000	6000	SPONDEES (0° AZIMUTH)
1. SPL (dB) center position	103	104	105	104	103	104	104	102	75
2. Dial reading	85	85	85	85	85	85	85	85	83
3. SPL (dB) at 0 dB on the dial	18	19	20	19	18	19	19	17	−8

The next step is to determine the linearity of the signal output, and the highest level that can be used without undue distortion. As described above for earphones, the low- and high-level portions of the range should be checked to see whether a 10-dB change in dial reading results in a 10-dB change in SPL. As the highest levels are approached, a 10-dB increase in dial reading may produce less than a 10-dB increase in the SPL of the signal.

At some point in this high range the level of the harmonic and inter-modulation distortion of the signal may grow more rapidly than the level of the signal, and this distortion can be heard. To measure this distortion, present sound at a moderate intensity level, such as 65 dB SPL, and with third-octave-band filters measure the SPL at the test frequency and at one and two octaves above and below the test frequency. Note the difference between the SPL at the test frequency and those levels above (harmonic distortion) and below (intermodulation distortion). Then present the sound at a high level, such as 90 dB SPL, and measure with the same filter settings. If the difference in SPL between the test frequency and harmonic and intermodulation distortion is lower than with the test frequency at 65 dB SPL, then there is undue distortion. Lower the test frequency in 5-dB steps until you find a level at which the difference is the same as that for the 65-dB-SPL test frequency. Testing should be limited to levels at and below this point.

Speech and competing sounds.   Since the instantaneous levels of speech and competing sounds are always changing as a function of time, a 1000-Hz calibration tone recorded with the speech or competing sounds is

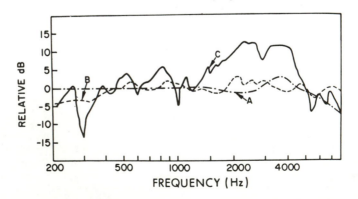

FIGURE 4.9.   Frequency response characteristics from **(A)** TDH-39 earphones in MX-41/AR cushions, **(B)** loudspeaker 1, and **(C)** loudspeaker 2. From D. D. Dirks, D. E. Morgan, and R. H. Wilson 1976. "Experimental Audiology." In *Handbook of Auditory and Vestibular Research.* Ed. C. A. Smith and J. A. Vernon. Reproduced with permission of the authors and Charles C. Thomas, Springfield, Ill.

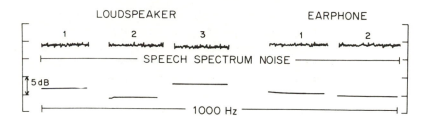

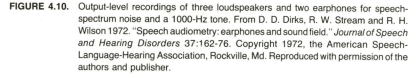

FIGURE 4.10. Output-level recordings of three loudspeakers and two earphones for speech-spectrum noise and a 1000-Hz tone. From D. D. Dirks, R. W. Stream and R. H. Wilson 1972. "Speech audiometry: earphones and sound field." *Journal of Speech and Hearing Disorders* 37:162-76. Copyright 1972, the American Speech-Language-Hearing Association, Rockville, Md. Reproduced with permission of the authors and publisher.

used to represent the average SPL. This method gives an accurate estimate of the level of these broad-band sounds for a TDH-series earphone because the frequency response is essentially uniform in the coupler (as shown by curve *A* in figure 4.9). This method for estimating the level of these sounds may not be accurate for loudspeakers in sound booths because the frequency response can vary markedly as a function of the loudspeaker characteristics and the room reverberation (as described in chapter 3). For example, look at the frequency response of two different loudspeakers shown by curves *B* and *C* in figure 4.9. Although the frequency responses intertwine between 200 and 1250 Hz and between 5000 and 7000 Hz, there is about 10 dB more gain in the region between 2000 and 4000 Hz for loudspeaker 2 than for loudspeaker 1. If a 1000-Hz calibration tone was set at 0 VU for loudspeaker 2 (curve *C*), the overall level would be at least 6 dB higher than for loudspeaker 1 (curve *B*). Furthermore, the overall level in loudspeaker 2 might be even higher, because the frequency response between 1500 and 4000 Hz is about 10 dB higher than that for loudspeaker 1. As shown in figure 4.10, speech-spectrum noise would give a more accurate estimate of the overall level of speech or competing sounds than the 1000-Hz tone. However, at present this calibration noise is not generally available on recordings.

The SPL for the calibration signal for speech and competing sound recordings should be measured at all the positions shown in table 4.3, and the dial readings and values should be entered in the table. The SPL associated with 0 dB on the dial should be calculated and entered in a table like table 4.4. The conversion from dB SPL to dB HL is described later in this chapter.

The highest level at which the speech and competing signals should be used can be determined by listening to them (not the calibration tone) and finding the point at which they sound distorted. Since these are broad-band sounds, the harmonic and intermodulation distortion cannot be measured with a sound-level meter; however, with an oscilloscope the level at which the waveform peaks become clipped can be determined.

If white noise or speech-shaped noise is used for a competing signal, the overall SPL of each of these signals can be measured in the same way that the recorded calibration tone was measured for speech. These values can be entered in table 4.3, and the SPL associated with 0 dB on the dial should be calculated and entered in a table like table 4.4.

Sound Field versus Eardrum Sound-Pressure Level

Loudspeaker azimuth. The common notation for the placement of the loudspeaker in relation to the listener is in degrees azimuth. (As mentioned earlier, at 0° azimuth the listener is facing the loudspeaker as shown in the left panel of Figure 4.8.) The loudspeaker can be placed anywhere in a circle of 360° around the listener as shown in Figure 4.11. Those angles to the right of the listener's face may be denoted with a positive sign, and those to the left with a negative sign or with a positive sign with 180° to 359° rotation (see the loudspeaker positioned at 300°).

Effect of listener on the sound field. When the SPL of signals are measured in the field, the listener is not present (undisturbed field). When an individual is seated so that the center of the head is at the former position of the microphone, the torso, head, and pinna diffract the sound and cause resonances and antiresonances to occur in the concha and outer earcanal. When the listener faces the loudspeaker at 0° azimuth, the change in SPL from the measured levels obtained in the undisturbed field to the level at the eardrum is approximately equal at the two ears.

For 0° azimuth the average difference in level between the undisturbed field and the sound field at the eardrum as a function of frequency is shown by the dotted curve in figure 4.12. The SPL at the eardrum is no more than

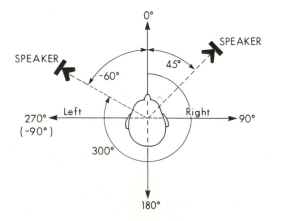

FIGURE 4.11.
Azimuth angles around the head. The loudspeaker toward the right is at an azimuth of 45°; the one at the left is at an azimuth of -60° (or 300°).

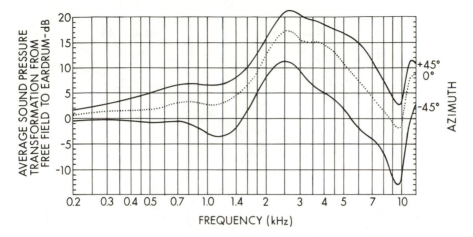

FIGURE 4.12.   Average sound-pressure transformation from free field to the eardrum in the horizontal plane as a function of frequency for 0°, +45°, and -45° azimuth. Free-field SPL was measured at the position to be occupied by the center of the head. Functions are based on a synthesis of data from twelve studies. From E. A. G. Shaw 1974. "The external ear." In *Handbook of Sensory Physiology* 5(1). Ed. W. D. Keidel and W. D. Neff. Reproduced with permission of the author and Springer-Verlag, Heidelberg.

3 dB higher than that in the undisturbed field between 200 and 1200 Hz, but between 2000 and 5000 Hz the level is 10 to 17 dB higher at the eardrum. When the listener turns so that the loudspeaker is at +45° azimuth, the level at the eardrum increases 3 to 7 dB at most frequencies over that for 0° azimuth. In this position the sound reaches the earcanal more efficiently than at 0° azimuth. At −45° azimuth the head causes a sound shadow for tones higher than about 700 Hz. This shadow causes the sound to be 5 to 10 dB lower at the eardrum than in the field in this frequency region (as shown in figure 4.12). The average difference in level at the eardrum can be plotted as a function of loudspeaker azimuth (this is shown in figure 4.13 for 500, 1000, and 4000 Hz). The marked effect of the head shadow on the SPL at the eardrum begins at 1500 Hz and is shown on this graph at 4000 Hz for the −60° and −90° azimuths.

The data plotted in figures 4.12 and 4.13 are an average across many listeners. Although it is important to remember the average transformation of sound from the undisturbed field to the eardrum, it is also important to know that the variability across subjects is large for frequencies above 2000 Hz (as shown for that part of the sound-pressure transformation from the free field to the earcanal entrance in figure 4.14). This variability is caused by individual differences in sound diffraction (caused by the torso, head, and pinna), and in resonances and antiresonances (caused by the concha and outer earcanal).

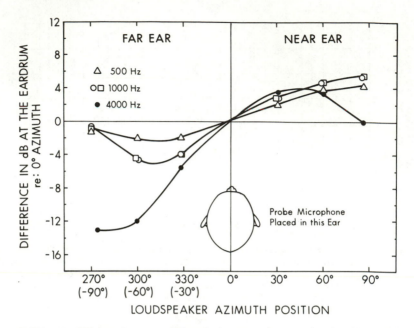

FIGURE 4.13.   Difference in average SPL at the human eardrum as a function of loudspeaker azimuth. Functions based on a synthesis of data from twelve studies. Based on data from E. A. G. Shaw 1974. "The external ear." In *Handbook of Sensory Physiology* 5(1). Ed. W. D. Keidel and W. D. Neff. Reproduced with permission of the author and Springer-Verlag, Heidelberg.

FIGURE 4.14.   Ratio of SPL at the earcanal entrance to the free-field SPL as a function of frequency for ten subjects facing the loudspeaker at 0° azimuth. Free-field SPL was measured at the position to be occupied by the center of the listener's head. From E. A. G. Shaw 1966. "Earcanal pressure generated by a free sound field." *Journal of the Acoustical Society of America* 39:471-79. Reproduced with permission of the author and the publisher.

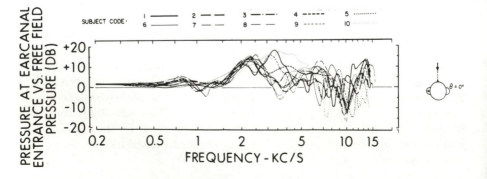

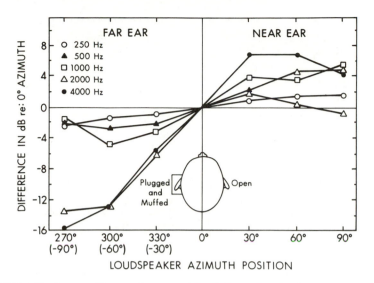

FIGURE 4.15. Average differences in monaural, free-field, pure-tone thresholds as a function of loudspeaker location. From D. D. Dirks, D. E. Morgan, and R. H. Wilson 1976. "Experimental audiology." In *Handbook of Auditory and Vestibular Research Methods*. Ed. C. A. Smith and J. A. Vernon. Reproduced with permission of the authors and Charles C. Thomas, Springfield, Ill. Based on data from D. Dirks, R. Stream and R. Wilson 1972.

Normal sound-field thresholds. Normal sound-field thresholds for one ear (monaural) must be defined in terms of the azimuth of the listener in relation to the loudspeaker. If the average differences in monaural pure-tone thresholds (shown in Figure 4.15) obtained in an anechoic chamber are compared with the differences in SPL at the earcanal entrance (shown in figure 4.13), it is obvious that the differences in threshold are a result of the differences in SPL reaching the eardrum. A graph of the relation between monaural, spondaic-word thresholds and loudspeaker azimuth (see figure 4.16) is almost the same as the 1000-Hz curve in figure 4.15.

The 0°-azimuth position was chosen by the International Organization for Standardization for the ISO R226-1961 standard for the binaural human auditory threshold in a free field (obtained in an anechoic chamber); this is often called the Minimum Audible Field (MAF). The ISO values for pure-tone stimuli are shown in figure 4.17. These values are very close to the binaural thresholds (also shown in Figure 4.17) for third-octave bands of noise obtained in a sound-treated room. The thresholds for noise bands below 630 Hz are probably masked by ambient noise in the test room and thus are higher than the ISO values for tones. This close correspondence between pure-tone thresholds and noise-band thresholds is expected since the energy in both signals falls within a single critical band. The monaural

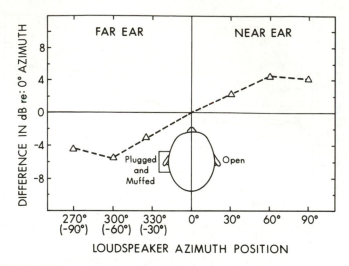

FIGURE 4.16.   Average difference in spondaic word thresholds as a function of loudspeaker location obtained with the right ear (open ear) of twelve listeners seated in an anechoic chamber. Adapted from R. H. Wilson and R. H. Margolis 1983. "Measurements of auditory thresholds for speech stimuli." In *Principles of Speech Audiometry*. Ed. D. F. Konkle and W. F. Rintlemann. Reproduced with permission of the authors and PRO-ED, Inc., Austin, TX.

thresholds for FM tones (also shown in figure 4.17) are adequately close to the binaural thresholds for pure tones and narrow bands of noise; it is generally accepted that the monaural thresholds are about 3 dB higher than the binaural thresholds as shown in figure 4.18.

The curves shown in figures 4.17 and 4.18 are based on average data. The variation in thresholds across normal-hearing listeners at any one frequency is between 13 and 18 dB (± 2 standard deviations as shown in figure 4.18).

Since there is no American National Standard for sound-field testing, and the stimuli, loudspeaker, and room vary widely from one clinic to

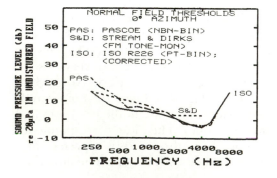

FIGURE 4.17.
Normal field thresholds at 0° azimuth for pure tones (ISO R226-1961 standard; corrected by Killion 1978), narrow bands of noise (Pascoe 1975), and FM tones (Stream and Dirks 1974). The SPL was measured at the position to be occupied by the center of the listener's head. The pure-tone and narrow-band-noise thresholds were obtained binaurally, and the FM tone thresholds were obtained monaurally.

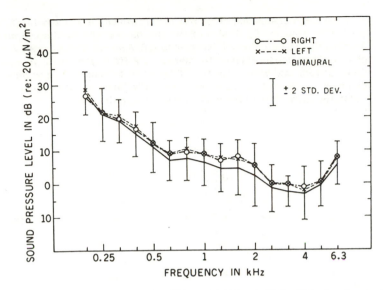

FIGURE 4.18. Average monaural and binaural field thresholds for third-octave bands of noise presented at 0° azimuth to twenty normal-hearing listeners. (The SPL reference of 20 μN/m² is the same as 20 μPa.) From D. P. Pascoe 1975. "Frequency responses of hearing aids and their effects on the speech perception of hearing-impaired subjects." *Annals of Otology, Rhinology and Laryngology* 84 supp. 23:1-40. Reproduced with permission of the author and the publisher.

another, it is important to obtain sound-field thresholds from at least ten young normal-hearing listeners to determine the average threshold at each audiometric frequency at the azimuth chosen for testing. Thresholds for spondaic words should also be obtained at the same azimuth since the loudspeaker-room combination may cause normal-hearing listeners to have different thresholds than the suggested 16-dB SPL threshold for 0° to 30° azimuths and 13-dB SPL thresholds for 30° to 60° azimuths (Dirks, Stream, and Wilson 1972; also see Konkle and Townsend 1983).

If an audiometer has potentiometers or digital memory for setting the level at each audiometric frequency, then a calculation such as the one shown in table 4.5 will give the SPL to which the audiometer should be adjusted. In this example, the audiometer dial reading is set at 70 dB, the listener faces the loudspeaker at 0° azimuth, the average normal sound-field thresholds are from Pascoe (1975; corrected for masked threshold at 250 Hz), and the average normal spondee thresholds are from Dirks, Stream, and Wilson (1972). With other dial readings, azimuths, or average normal sound-field thresholds (such as those obtained from normal listeners with a specific audiometer, loudspeaker, and sound field), these values should be entered in a table such as table 4.5.

If an audiometer does not have potentiometers or digital memory for

TABLE 4.5. Example of the Calculation of the SPL (dB) to Which the Audiometer Output Should Be Adjusted So That 0 dB HL on the Dial Will Be the Output for Average Normal Sound-Field Thresholds at 0° Azimuth (Third-Octave Bands of Noise Corrected for Masked Threshold at 250 Hz: Pascoe 1975; Spondees: Dirks, Stream, and Wilson 1972). If Different Dial Readings and/or Different Estimates of Normal Sound-Field Thresholds (Such as Stream and Dirks 1974) Are Used, These Should Be Substituted in the Table.

	Frequency (Hz)								
	250	500	1000	1500	2000	3000	4000	6000	SPONDEES (0° AZIMUTH)
Audiometer Dial Reading	70	70	70	70	70	70	70	70	70
Average Normal Threshold (dB SPL)	15	11	7	5	3	−2	−3	6	16
SPL (dB) to which audiometer should be adjusted	85	81	77	75	73	68	67	76	86

TABLE 4.6. An Example of the Calculation of the Sound-Field HL (dB) at 0 dB on the Audiometer Dial by Subtracting the Average Normal Sound-Field Thresholds (Third-Octave Bands of Noise Corrected for Masked Threshold at 250 Hz: Pascoe 1975) from the Values from Table 4.4 for the Sound-Field SPL at 0 dB on the Audiometer Dial. When Calculations Such as These are Made for a Specific Audiometer and Sound-Field System, the Values in the Third Line are Subtracted from the Dial Readings Associated with an Individual's Thresholds to Express Them in dB HL.

	Frequency (Hz)								
	250	500	1000	1500	2000	3000	4000	6000	SPONDEES (0° AZIMUTH)
SPL (dB) at 0 dB on the dial	18	19	20	19	18	19	19	17	17
Average Normal Threshold (dB SPL) (0° Azimuth)	15	11	7	5	3	−2	−3	6	16
HL (dB) at 0 dB on the dial	3	8	13	14	15	21	22	11	1

setting the SPLs in the sound field, then a set of correction factors needs to be calculated to convert the dial readings to dB HL. The measured SPLs can be entered in a table like table 4.4, and the SPL (dB) at 0 dB on the dial can be calculated. Then these values can be entered in a table like table 4.6 to calculate the HL (dB) in the sound field for 0 dB on the audiometer dial. These values are then subtracted from the dial readings obtained with a specific individual.

Estimates of Sound-Field versus Eardrum Sound-Pressure Level

There are two ways to estimate the difference (dB) between the SPL measured in the undisturbed sound field and the SPL measured at the eardrum. One way is to compare the SPLs associated with the average, normal-hearing threshold at each of these two reference points. This difference can be calculated by subtracting the average, normal thresholds at 0° azimuth (Pascoe 1975, corrected at 250 Hz) from the eardrum threshold values (MAP; Killion 1978), as shown in table 4.7. These values can then be compared with an estimation of the difference between the physical measurements of SPL in the undisturbed sound field and at the eardrum for 0° azimuth, as shown in figure 4.12 and in table 4.7. The threshold and physical measurement estimates are within 1.5 dB at all frequencies except 250 Hz, which is considered good agreement.

TABLE 4.7. The Difference (dB) Between the Average SPL at the Eardrum and That Measured in the Undisturbed Sound Field When the Individual Faces a Loudspeaker at 0° Azimuth. This Difference Is Estimated from Average Normal Thresholds and from Physical Measurements of the SPL at These Two Reference Points.

	Frequency (Hz)							
	250	500	1000	1500	2000	3000	4000	6000
Threshold								
MAP (Eardrum) (dB SPL)[1]	19	12	9	11	15	15	13	13
Average Normal Threshold (dB SPL)[2]	15	11	7	5	3	−2	−3	6
Sound-Field/ Eardrum	4	1	2	6	12	17	16	7
Physical Measurement Sound-Field/ Eardrum[3]	1	2	3	5.5	13	15.5	14.5	7.5

[1]Killion 1978.
[2]Pascoe 1975 corrected at 250 Hz.
[3]Shaw 1974b.

HEARING AID

Coupler Measurements

The electroacoustic performance of a hearing aid can be evaluated (1) by presenting sounds that are picked up by the hearing aid microphone, (2) by measuring the sound energy at the output of the hearing aid, and (3) by comparing the input and output signals to determine the transformation that has occurred in the hearing aid. The standard procedure for making these measurements is with a microphone in a 2-cc coupler in an anechoic-like chamber (ANSI S3.22-1982), such as the test-box system described in chapter 3. The purpose of this standard procedure is to measure hearing aid performance accurately in a manner that can be easily replicated in other settings to determine whether a hearing aid meets the manufacturer's specifications. It is not intended to simulate the input-output function of the hearing aid as worn by a hearing-impaired individual.

Test-box calibration.   To be certain that the measurements of a hearing aid in the test box are accurate, the output of the measurement system needs to be adjusted so that the sound-level meter gives the same reading as the output level of the calibrator. The SPL of the loudspeaker output in the test box also needs to be measured with a microphone at the point where the hearing aid microphone will be placed, and adjusted so that it is the same as the nominal input on the text box.

Couplers.   There are two standard couplers for measuring the output of hearing aids: the HA-1 and the HA-2 couplers (see figure 4.19). The HA-1 coupler is used for measuring the output from in-the-ear hearing aids and from other hearing aids attached to an earmold. With this coupler the tip of the earmold should be placed even with the top of the 2-cc cavity wall and centered over the access hole into it. As described in the section on SPL measurements of the output of insert earphones, Fun-tak^{TM} is used to make a tight seal between the earmold and the coupler, taking care to avoid any air leaks or air pockets around the earmold opening.

The amplified sound from in-the-ear aids with vents (or other aids with vented earmolds) can cause feedback when amplified sound escapes through the vent and combines with the sound in the vicinity of the hearing aid microphone. Although this feedback can also occur when the person wears the hearing aid, the feedback in the test box, because of the confined enclosure, may not be the same as when the hearing aid is worn. For this reason, the standard recommends that coupler measurements be made with the vents plugged. These vents should be plugged at the earmold tip to eliminate the possible resonance of the hearing aid output in the vent cavity.

The HA-2 coupler is used to measure the output from an external

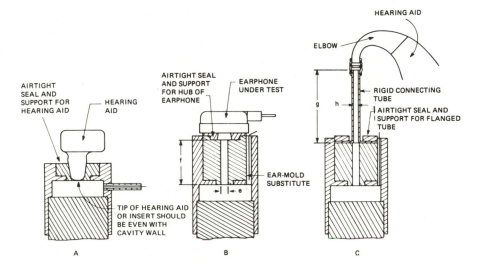

FIGURE 4.19.   Standard couplers for measuring the output of hearing aids. The HA-I coupler is shown in the left panel, and two configurations of the HA-2 coupler are shown in the middle and right panels. In both couplers the microphone diaphragm is shown as the lower boundary of the 2-cc cavity that is intended to roughly approximate the acoustic load of the listener's ear. The long, narrow cavity (length denoted *f* and diameter denoted *e*) in the HA-2 coupler simulates the bore of an earmold with a *3-cm* diameter. The HA-2 coupler in the middle panel is used with receivers for body aids. The HA-2 coupler in the right panel is attached to behind-the-ear or eyeglass aids with standard tubing that is 2.5 cm ±4% long and has a diameter of 0.193 cm ±2%. From W. R. Hodgson 1986. *Hearing Aid Assessment and Use in Audiologic Habilitation*, 3rd ed. Figure 3.1 in "Electroacoustic characteristics of hearing aids" by R. N. Kasten and J. R. Franks. Copyright 1986, Williams and Wilkins Co., Baltimore. Reproduced with permission of the authors and publisher.

receiver (for a body aid) by snapping the earphone port into the coupler as shown in the middle panel of figure 4.19. The HA-2 coupler is also used with behind-the-ear and eyeglass hearing aids, as shown in the right panel of figure 4.19.

The Zwislocki coupler can be configured to measure the output of hearing aids, as described in the section on insert earphones. When identical settings are used, the hearing aid output (dB SPL) will be higher than that in the 2-cc coupler by the amount shown in figure 4.7 (Sachs and Burkhard 1972).

Placement of hearing aid in test box.   For accurate measurements the hearing aid microphone must be placed within the designated space in the test box (preferably on a marked test point) at a position close to the reference microphone that monitors the input level to the hearing aid. The hearing aid microphone, particularly a directional microphone, should face the sound source. The actual level at the hearing aid microphone of in-the-ear and behind-the-ear hearing aids closely approximates that at the reference microphone; the frames and lenses for eyeglass hearing aids can cause acoustic perturbations in the sound field so that the level at the hearing aid microphone for certain frequencies may be as much as 17 dB different from the level at the reference microphone.

Standard tests of hearing aid performance. Table 4.8 is a summary of the tests recommended in the ANSI standard for hearing aid specifications (ANSI S3.22-1982). These tests are used to evaluate the electroacoustic performance of a hearing aid and then compare its performance with the manufacturer's specification. This procedure is important for evaluating new aids, for determining whether the performance of the aid has changed since it was purchased, and for determining whether an aid has been properly repaired. Since a number of internal adjustments can be made on many hearing aids, the settings and battery used when the aid is measured should be carefully recorded. In comparing the performance of an aid with the manufacturer's specifications or with its prior performance, the standard makes allowance for a small amount of variation in the hearing aid as well as in test-equipment performance. The range of predicted and measured variation in hearing aid output for one commercially available test system is shown in table 4.9. The observed measurement variation listed in this table is probably significantly lower than in the usual clinical setting.

Although a complete description of the standard measurements is not intended in this book, it is important to understand the meaning of *frequency response, gain,* and *saturation sound-pressure level.* The frequency response of an aid is the output SPL variation as a function of frequency for a known, constant input level at the sampled frequencies. A typical graph of the frequency response of a hearing aid measured in a test box is shown in the top panel of figure 4.20. The frequency response is obtained with the input sound set at 60 dB SPL (or at 50 dB SPL for Automatic Gain Control aids) and the hearing aid volume wheel set to the *reference test gain* position (for a definition see table 4.8) or to the volume-wheel setting the individual uses in everyday life. This use-gain setting, or the reference test-gain setting, is usually below full-on gain except for mild-gain hearing aids. The frequency response of an aid measured in the test box is often very different from that measured at the eardrum; variables that cause these differences will be described in the next section of this chapter.

The gain of a hearing aid is the difference between the input and output SPL levels as a function of frequency. The gain can be calculated from the frequency response (see top panel of figure 4.20) by subtracting the input level (60 dB SPL) from the output. This gain is shown in the middle panel of figure 4.20.

TABLE 4.8.   Summary of Tests Recommended in the ANSI Standard for Hearing Aid Specifications (ANSI S3.22-1982). Modified from Kasten and Franks 1986b, with Permission of Williams and Wilkins Co., Baltimore.

CHARACTERISTIC	INPUT SPL (dB) re 20µPa	FREQUENCY (Hz)	GAIN CONTROL SETTING	PRESENTATION	TOLERANCE REQUIREMENTS
SSPL90 (Saturation)	90	200–5000	Full on	Curve	Basic test equipment tolerance
Maximum SSPL90	90	Any frequency between 200 & 5000	Full on	Number (dB)	Mfr. to state max. value for model
Average SSPL90	90	1000, 1600, 2500	Full on	Number (dB) (3 freq. average)	±4 dB
Average full-on gain	60 or 50 (State which) 50 for AGC	1000, 1600, 2500	Full on	Number (dB) (3 freq. average)	±5 dB
Reference test gain control position*	60	1000, 1600, 2500	Set gain control back to give output SPL 17 dB less than averge SSPL90, or full on for low gain aids.		17 ± 1 dB
Frequency response	60 (linear) 50 (AGC)	200–5000 or to 20 dB below 3 freq. avg.	Reference test position	Curve	Low band ± 4 dB High band ± 6 dB
Total harmonic distortion	70 65	500, 800, 1600	Reference test position	Number (%)	Mfr. to state max. value for model
Equivalent input noise level, L_n	60 (linear) 50 (AGC)	1000, 1600, 2500 (Avg. to get L_{av})	Reference test position	Number (dB) $L_n=L_2(L_{av}60)$**	Mfr. to state max. value for model
Telephone pickup (Induction coil)	10 mA/m rms magnetic field	1000	Full on	Number (dB)	Within ±6 dB of mfr's. specified value

(continued)

* Reference test gain control position for AGC aids is full on.
** L_2 is the noise reading in the coupler with the input signal turned off.

TABLE 4.8. (*Continued*)

CHARACTERISTIC	INPUT SPL (dB) re 20μPa	FREQUENCY (Hz)	GAIN CONTROL SETTING	PRESENTATION	TOLERANCE REQUIREMENTS
Battery current	65	1000	Reference test	Number (mA)	Not to exceed mfr's. specified maximum for the model
Input-output curves (AGC only)	50 to 90	2000	Full on	Curve Input-abscissa Output-ordinate	Match at 70 dB input then to be within ±5 dB of specified
Attack and release times (AGC only)	Abrupt 55 to 80 80 to 55	2000	Full on	Numbers (ms)	To be within ±5 msec. or ±50% of values specified by mfr.

TABLE 4.9. Range of Predicted and Measured Variation in Hearing Aid Output for One Commercially Available Test System. From T.H. Townsend 1982. "Revised Estimates of Hearing Aid Test System Accuracy." *Journal of Speech and Hearing Research* 25:166-70. Copyright 1982, American Speech-Language-Hearing Association, Rockville, Md. Reproduced with permission of the Author and Publisher.

MEASUREMENT	1 SD (TOLERANCE)	2 SD*
Predicted[a]	.4 dB	.8 dB
Observed[b]		
Required measures[c]		
Maximum SSPL90	.1 dB	.2 dB
HF-avg. SSPL90	.1 dB	.2 dB
HF-avg. gain	.3 dB	.6 dB
THD (800 Hz)	.6 dB	1.2 dB
THD (1600 Hz)	.3 dB	.6 dB
L_n	.4 dB	.8 dB
AGC (50–70 dB)	.1 dB	.2 dB
AGC (70–90 dB)	.1 dB	.2 dB
Measures for information purposes		
f_1	5.0 Hz	10.0 Hz
f_2	12.0 Hz	24.0 Hz

[a]Presented in Townsend (1980).
[b]All measurements on a linear aid except AGC measures on an AGC aid.
[c]Derivation of frequency response variability explained in text; value for $p < .10$ is 1.0 dB.
*$p < .05$.

The saturation sound-pressure level (SSPL) is an estimate of the maximum acoustic output of the hearing aid as a function of frequency. The standard input level is 90 dB SPL, and the standard hearing aid setting is at full-on gain. An example of the SSPL90 of this hearing aid is shown in the bottom panel of figure 4.20.

Measurements of the frequency response, gain, SSPL90, distortion, and equivalent input-noise level can be made at hearing aid settings recommended by the standard and compared with the manufacturer's specifications. In addition, electroacoustic measurements can be made at the same internal and volume-wheel settings at which aided field thresholds were obtained, so the coupler gain can be compared directly with the real-ear gain, which is the actual gain provided by the hearing aid to the individual. If changes are needed in the frequency response, compression circuit, or SSPL90, the hearing aid output is remeasured in the coupler to see whether the desired changes have been achieved.

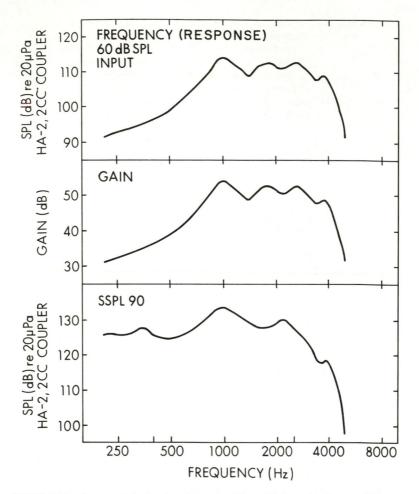

FIGURE 4.20.   The output of a hearing aid measured in an HA-2 coupler. Top panel: The SPL measured with the aid set at the reference test gain position. Middle panel: Corresponding gain of this hearing aid calculated from the output measurement in the top panel. Bottom panel: Saturation sound-pressure level (SSPL) of this hearing aid for input sound of 90 dB SPL and the volume wheel set at full-on. From W. R. Hodgson 1986. *Hearing Aid Assessment and Use in Audiologic Habilitation,* 3rd ed. Adapted from figure 3.5 in "Electroacoustic characteristics of hearing aids" by R. N. Kasten and J. R. Franks. Copyright 1986, Williams and Wilkins Co., Baltimore. Reproduced with permission of the authors and publisher.

Acoustic characteristics of an earmold.   An approximation of the acoustic characteristics of an earmold for behind-the-ear aids can also be estimated. When an individual is first fitted with a hearing aid and earmold, the ouptut of the hearing aid is measured first with the standard tubing and an HA-2 coupler and then with the individual's earmold and an HA-1 coupler.

The hearing aid settings must be exactly the same for these two measurements, so that when the HA-2 values are subtracted from the HA-1 values, the difference will be an accurate estimate of the acoustic characteristics of the earmold, but they may not be the same when the earmold is worn by the individual. These values are useful to compare with subsequent measurements in case this person returns complaining that the hearing aid is not working as well as it once did. If the two sets of values are different, changes in the earmold acoustics are a contributing factor. The most common changes are caused by cerumen, moisture, or split tubing.

Listening to hearing aid output. Although a hearing aid may meet the manufacturer's specifications according to the standard measurements, it may produce distortion that can be heard by listening to the hearing aid output. This distortion can be monitored in the following manner. Set the volume wheel of the aid at the use-gain or reference-test-gain setting and attach the aid to a 2-cc coupler on a Type 2 sound-level meter in the test room (see figure 3.19). Then present FM tones or narrow bands of noise, speech, and music at 60 to 80 dB SPL at the hearing aid microphone and listen to the amplified sound with a pair of high-quality circumaural or insert earphones coupled to the sound-level meter.

Factors That Affect the Actual Frequency Response for the Listener

The frequency response of a hearing aid measured in a coupler is not the same as that at the individual's eardrum. Some of the factors that cause this difference in frequency response are related to differences in the sound field at the hearing aid input (microphone), and other factors are related to differences in the acoustic load at the output of the hearing aid.

Differences in sound field at the hearing aid input. Factors that cause differences in the sound field at the hearing aid input (microphone) include the position of the microphone on the head or body, the relation of the microphone to the location of the sound source, and the effect of acoustic feedback that is not audible.

The head and body cause reflection and absorption of sound in the field that differs according to frequency. Therefore, the SPL in the undisturbed field is different from that measured at the microphone of the hearing aid as it is worn by an individual. For behind-the-ear aids the mean level in the undisturbed field and that at the hearing aid microphone facing forward at the top of the individual's pinna are almost the same between 250 and 4000 Hz, as shown in the top panel of figure 4.21. For directional sounds such as those used for this set of measurements, the across listener range is 7 to 10 dB between 1000 and 6300 Hz. For in-the-ear aids there is an average

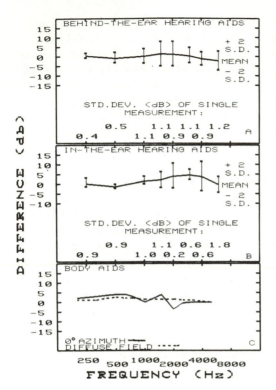

FIGURE 4.21.
Effect of microphone position (on a listener's head or body when facing the loudspeaker at 0° azimuth) on the SPL at the input to a hearing aid. Top panel: Level at the port of the microphone minus the level in the undisturbed field for behind-the-ear hearing aids. The function shown is based on data obtained from fourteen listeners, and the vertical lines show the across listener range (±2 standard deviations). The standard deviation of a single measurement (based on measurements made on two different days on the fourteen listeners) is also shown (Skinner, Miller, DeFilippo, Dawson, and Popelka 1986). Middle panel: Level at the port of the microphone in the listener's ear minus the level in the undisturbed field for in-the-ear aids. The function shown is based on data obtained from four listeners (Skinner, Miller, DeFilippo, Dawson, and Popelka 1986). Bottom panel: Level at the hearing-aid microphone of a body-type aid minus the level in the undisturbed sound field. The data for the directional sound source at 0° azimuth is the average of measurements with 6 males and 6 females (Lybarger 1983 in Kuhn and Guernsey 1983), and the data for the diffuse sound field is the average of measurements from a number of studies summarized in Kuhn and Guernsey (1983).

of 2 to 5 dB enhancement of the sound between 1000 and 4000 Hz, related to the microphone being placed in the center of the pinna (see the middle panel of figure 4.21). The across listener range between 1600 and 6300 Hz is between 5 and 15 dB. This large across listener range shown for the hearing aids in this figure makes it difficult to predict exactly the individual difference in level between the undisturbed field and the field at the hearing aid microphone for testing with a directional sound source. However, in many real-world listening situations there is a diffuse sound field, in which these differences across individuals are probably less than 1 dB.

Behind-the-ear aids with microphones that are on the bottom of the case behind the pinna provide 6 to 10 dB less sound in the frequency region between 1500 and 3000 Hz than aids with front-facing microphones on top of the pinna.

Body aids are usually worn under clothing on the chest. The body-baffle effect of this placement causes the level at the hearing aid microphone to be about 3 dB higher between 250 and 750 Hz and about 4 dB lower between 1000 and 2500 Hz than the level in the undisturbed sound field (see figure 4.21, bottom panel).

The SPL at the hearing aid input is affected by the position of the

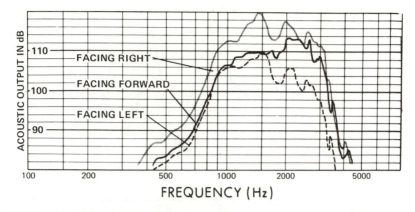

FIGURE 4.22.   Effect of head turning on the frequency response of an ear-level aid. From Zenith Corporation in M. C. Pollack 1980. "Electroacoustic characteristics." In *Amplification for the Hearing Impaired*, 2nd ed. Ed. M. C. Pollack. Tampa, Fla.: Grune & Stratton. Reproduced with permission of Zenetron, Inc., Grune & Stratton, Inc., and the author.

microphone on the head (or chest) in relation to the sound source. As an individual faces the sound source (0° azimuth), the sound at the microphone will be at a lower level for frequencies up to 2500 Hz than when the person faces right (90° azimuth; see figure 4.22). When the person turns left (−90° azimuth), the sound shadow of the head lowers the level of frequencies above 1500 Hz. This is essentially the same effect as shown in figure 4.14.

The blatant squeal of acoustic feedback is caused by the sound from the output of a hearing aid reaching the hearing aid microphone via unintentional leaks around the outside of the earmold or via vents in the earmold intended to change the frequency response of the aid. When the amplified sound combines with the unamplified sound and the appropriate relations between level and phase occur, resonances result in certain frequency regions causing feedback that may be audible (see figure 4.23). The effects of acoustic feedback increase as the volume-wheel setting is increased, as shown in figure 4.24. It is clear that the input sound to the microphone is affected by acoustic feedback even though the aid may not be in sustained oscillation and it is inaudible to a person listening nearby.

Differences in sound at the hearing aid output.   The factors that affect the hearing aid output at the individual's eardrum include internal dimensions of the earhook, tubing length, diameter and configuration of the earmold, acoustic dampers, vents, the residual volume between the tip of the earmold and the eardrum, and the acoustic immittance of the individual's eardrum and middle-ear system.

The tubing length, and especially its diameter, affect the frequency

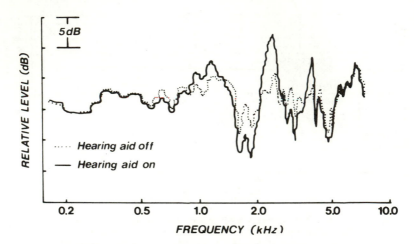

FIGURE 4.23.   The spectra of a broad-band white noise measured at the hearing-aid microphone with the hearing aid turned off and with the hearing aid turned on and set to a gain level slightly below audible oscillation. The differences between the two curves are due to the effects of acoustic feedback. R. M. Cox 1981. "Combined effects of earmold vents and suboscillatory feedback on hearing aid frequency response." *Ear and Hearing* 3(1): 12-17. Copyright 1981, Williams and Wilkins Co. Reproduced with permission of the author and the publisher.

FIGURE 4.24.   Effects of acoustic feedback portrayed using the differences between hearing-aid-on and hearing-aid-off spectra as shown in figure 4.23. The dotted, solid, and dashed curves were obtained at successively higher volume wheel settings on the hearing aid. The external signal remained constant. Oscillation was barely audible in a quiet room in the dashed-curve condition. R. M. Cox 1981. "Combined effects of earmold vents and suboscillatory feedback on hearing aid frequency response." *Ear and Hearing* 3(1): 12-17. Copyright 1981, Williams and Wilkins Co. Reproduced with permission of the author and the publisher.

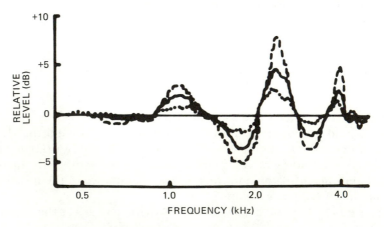

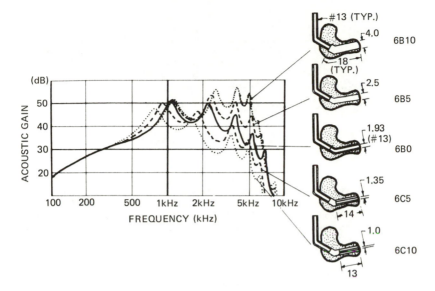

FIGURE 4.25. Frequency responses of a wideband hearing aid using Killion 6BC earmolds without acoustic damping measured with a 2-cc coupler (HA-1 configuration). The earmold with the largest-diameter opening is associated with the most high-frequency energy, and the one with the smallest with the least high-frequency energy. From M. C. Killion 1981. "Earmold options for wideband hearing aids." *Journal of Speech and Hearing Disorders* 46: 10-20. Copyright 1981, American Speech-Language-Hearing Association, Rockville, Md. Reproduced with permission of the author and publisher.

response of the amplified sound at the eardrum. The ratio of the diameter at the receiver to the diameter at the earmold tip affects the amount of high-frequency energy that reaches the eardrum. When the tubing forms a horn so that the diameter at the tip of the earmold is larger than that at the receiver, the high-frequency energy is greater (see 6B10 in figure 4.25) than when the tubing diameter stays constant (see 6B0). When the diameter is smaller at the earmold tip (see 6C10) than at the receiver, the high-frequency energy is even lower. Note that as the diameter of the earmold tip becomes smaller the frequency at which resonant peaks and antiresonant valleys occur in the frequency response becomes lower.

The resonances and antiresonances in the frequency response caused by the earhook and tubing can be reduced or eliminated with acoustic dampers placed at the appropriate locations in the tubing (see figure 4.26). A pair of 680-ohm dampers (placed as shown in the figure) eliminate most of the irregularity in the frequency response without substantially changing the overall gain; greater damping also reduces irregularity but further lowers the output. In clinical practice, when an acoustic damper is placed near the earmold tip, it often becomes blocked with earcanal moisture, causing a reduction in sound reaching the eardrum. For this reason, one

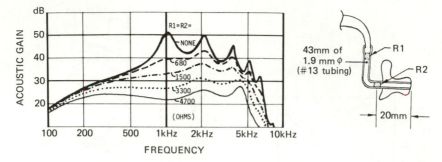

FIGURE 4.26. Frequency response of a wide-band aid showing the effect of a pair of 680, 1500, 3300, and 4700 ohms of acoustic damping compared to no damping. From M. C. Killion 1981. "Earmold options for wideband hearing aids." *Journal of Speech and Hearing Disorders* 46: 10-20. Copyright 1981, American Speech-Language-Hearing Association, Rockville, Md. Reproduced with permission of the author and publisher.

FIGURE 4.27. Frequency response of a hearing aid measured in a person's earcanal with a custom-made, unvented earmold (upper curves) and a vented earmold (lower curves). The dotted curves were obtained when the earmold was seated normally in the earcanal, and the solid curves were obtained when considerable effort was made to seal all acoustic leaks. From R. M. Cox and G. A. Studebaker 1980. "Problems in the recording and reproduction of hearing-aid processed signals." In *Acoustical Factors Affecting Hearing Aid Performance*. Ed. G. A. Studebaker and I. Hochberg. Baltimore: University Park Press. Reproduced with permission of the authors and PRO-ED, Inc., Austin, TX.

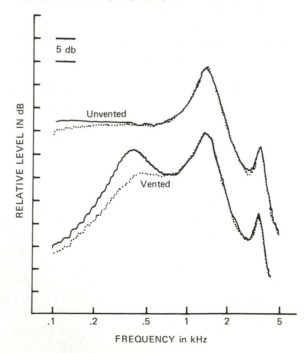

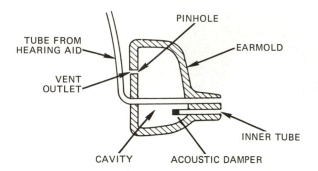

FIGURE 4.28.   Diagram of a damped cavity vent in an earmold to be used with a high-powered hearing aid to prevent acoustic feedback from the vent. From J. Macrae 1983. "Vents for high-powered hearing aids." *The Hearing Journal* 36: 13-16. Reproduced with permission of the author and publisher.

damper is usually placed in the earhook of behind-the-ear aids, *or* no dampers are used and the electronic circuitry of the aid is designed to compensate for the tubing resonances and antiresonances.

Vents in the earmold and unintentional leaks around the perimeter of the earmold cause loss of low-frequency energy (as shown in figure 4.27). The larger the diameter of the vent, the more loss of low-frequency energy there will be (see chapter 8 for a more detailed description of vents). The major drawback of using vents to control the amount of low-frequency energy is that inaudible acoustic feedback occurs at reasonably low-gain settings, and audible feedback prevents high-gain settings. A new method for venting that is designed to eliminate acoustic feedback associated with vents is shown in figure 4.28.

The residual volume between the tip of the earmold and the eardrum, and the acoustic immittance of an individual's eardrum and middle-ear system affect the hearing aid output. The smaller the volume of air in this space and the stiffer the middle-ear system, the higher the SPL will be. The larger the volume of air and the more flaccid the middle-ear system, the lower the SPL. The resultant SPL of the amplified sound depends on the complex interaction of these factors and the acoustic immittance of the hearing aid receiver. In addition, there is a frequency-specific effect due to the magnitude of the residual volume of the earcanal, as shown for female and male ears in the bottom panel of figure 4.8.

Measurements with KEMAR and Zwislocki Coupler

The manikin, KEMAR (Knowles Electronics Manikin for Auditory Research; see figure 4.29), was designed to represent the median dimensions of the adult human head and torso. The diffraction effects of the head and torso on the sound field and the resonance properties of the pinna and earcanal closely approximate those of an average person. KEMAR is used

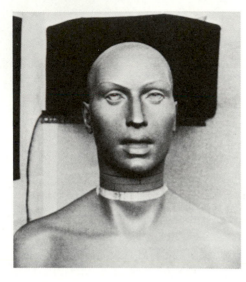

FIGURE 4.29.
The manikin KEMAR (Knowles Electronics Manikin for Auditory Research). From W. R. Hodgson 1986. *Hearing Aid Assessment and Use in Audiologic Habilitation*, 3rd ed. Figure 3.10 in "Electroacoustic characteristics of hearing aids" by R. N. Kasten and J. R. Franks. Copyright 1986, Williams and Wilkins Co., Baltimore. Reproduced with permission of the authors and publisher.

with a Zwislocki coupler, positioned so that the simulated earcanal of the coupler forms part of KEMAR's earcanal. The half-inch pressure microphone of the coupler is located in the position of KEMAR's eardrum.

Earmolds are available for KEMAR's earcanal, and measurements of the *in situ* (on the head or body) frequency response and SSPL90 at the output of a hearing aid can be made in an anechoic chamber. The results are a closer approximation of the effective sound for an individual than are the results of 2-cc coupler measurements, but they represent those for the *median* adult. The effect of a person's own earmold coupling system, the configuration of the body, head, pinna and earcanal, the acoustic leaks around the earmold, the residual volume of air between the earmold tip and the eardrum, and the acoustic immittance of the eardrum and middle-ear system are not reflected in the *in situ* measurements on KEMAR.

Probe and Probe-Tube Microphone Measurements

As described in chapter 3, a microphone or flexible tubing with a microphone attached can be placed in an individual's earcanal between the tip of the earmold and the eardrum. With the probe microphone or probe-tube microphone, the SPL can be measured first without and then with the hearing aid. The first measurement reflects the earcanal resonance of that person's earcanal, and the second measurement reflects the total effect of (1) the sound reaching the hearing aid microphone, (2) the amplification provided by the aid, (3) the acoustic effects of coupling the aid to the earcanal (including loss of the normal resonance due to the earmold), and (4) the interaction between the acoustic immittance of the residual volume of air, the eardrum, and the middle-ear system, and the hearing aid output. The

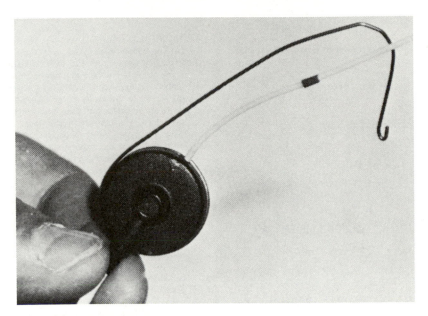

FIGURE 4.30. Preamplifier with reference microphone, probe microphone, and silicon tube for insertion into earcanal. From H. Birk-Nielsen 1985. "Hearing aid fitting based on insertion gain measurements." *Audecibel* 34(1): 16-19. Reproduced with permission of the author and publisher.

difference between the aided and unaided output is the *insertion gain* of a hearing aid. Insertion gain is a *physical measurement* in an individual's earcanal of the actual (real-ear) gain provided by a hearing aid.

As described in chapter 3, both the probe and probe-tube microphone systems have a control or reference microphone that samples the sound level on the individual's head (see figure 4.30), and a feedback circuit adjusts the sound produced by the loudspeaker so that it remains constant at the chosen test level (such as 60 dB SPL) for all frequencies *at the control microphone*. For probe-tube microphone systems, the SPL at the tubing tip is calibrated by placing the tip at the reference microphone and presenting a frequency sweep from the loudspeaker. The computer stores this information for subsequent testing. An example of the level of the initial frequency sweep from 125 to 8000 Hz measured at the reference and probe-tube microphone is shown in the bottom trace in figure 4.31A. The top trace shows the level equalized at 80 dB SPL input.

The probe microphone or probe-tube tip need to be placed 5 mm beyond the earmold tip. This placement avoids the pressure variations in the vicinity of the earmold tip. However, at 5 mm there are still significant variations in the sound pressure distribution above 3000 Hz at specific points in the space between the probe-tube tip and the eardrum. Consequently, the measurements for frequencies above 3000 Hz should be viewed

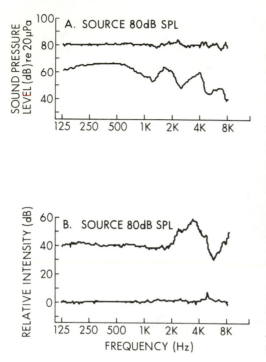

FIGURE 4.31.
(A) The bottom trace is the level of the initial frequency sweep from 125 to 8000 Hz measured at the reference and probe microphone (attached to the silicone tubing) held at approximately where the client will sit. The unequal levels are due to the room acoustics and tubing resonance. The top trace is the level of the second frequency sweep measured at the reference and probe microphone (attached to the tubing) held in the same position as for the first sweep; note that the computer has changed the output of the loudspeaker so that the level at the microphones is at approximately the same SPL at all frequencies. **(B)** The top trace is the level measured at the probe-tube tip (with the probe microphone) in the person's earcanal. It represents the open earcanal resonance when sound at the reference microphone (placed beside the head as shown in Figure 3.22) is approximately the same at all frequencies. The bottom trace is the open earcanal resonance set at 0 dB to represent the unaided condition. From E. R. Libby 1985. "State-of-the-art hearing aid selection procedures." *Hearing Instruments* 36(1): 30, 34, 36, 62. Reproduced with permission of the author and publisher.

with caution. In addition, the SPL measured at 5 mm beyond the earmold tip is approximately 2 to 10 dB lower than the SPL at the eardrum between 3500 and 9000 Hz (Sachs and Burkhard 1972).

For accurate comparison of unaided and aided measurements, the probe-tube tip (or probe microphone) needs to be at the same position in the earcanal. One way to accomplish this is by placing the probe tube beside the earmold and moving a marker so that it is flush with the outside surface of the earmold and the tip extends 5 mm beyond the earmold tip (see figure 4.32). Then the probe tube is placed in the individual's ear so that the marker is at the tragus. This marker is kept at the same position for both the unaided and aided measurements.

Before making any measurements, the individual's earcanal needs to have any cerumen, particularly soft cerumen, removed. If this is not removed, it will absorb some of the sound energy and give aberrant results.

It is important for the individual to keep his or her head in the same position for all the aided and unaided measurements. As shown in figures 4.12 and 4.13, changes in head position can make as much as 1 to 15 dB difference in the level in the earcanal.

The first measurement is usually unaided, with the probe or probe-tube microphone measuring the effect of the earcanal resonance. An example of this measurement is shown by the top curve in figure 4.31B. The input level was 80 dB SPL; in order to place it on the screen, the computer caused it to be centered at 40 dB on the graph in the low frequencies. By using the appropriate command, the computer can store this unaided measurement and convert it to a 0 dB reference curve, as shown in the bottom curve in figure 4.31B. Although this is useful for quickly viewing the difference between unaided and aided measurements (that is, the insertion gain), the actual SPL in the earcanal for these two measurements is not given. Sometimes it is important to see the relation between the actual unaided and aided SPLs in the earcanal, especially when earmold venting is used (Harford 1980). It is also helpful with people who have abnormal earcanal resonance due to middle-ear dysfunction or prior surgery. Their complaints about the amplified sound quality being intolerable can be supported by these data.

Several aided measurements can be made. The first one is with the volume wheel set so that speech is at the most intelligible, as well as comfortable level, and with the tone, SSPL90, and AGC settings chosen to give the desired output (an example of this is shown in figure 9.5). If the first aided measurement gives the prescribed insertion gain, then a frequency sweep can be made at 80 or 90 dB input level to determine whether or not the sound is uncomfortable. A decision is then made whether adjustments in the hearing aid output are indicated. The major advantage of this procedure is that the effect of successive adjustments can be measured in the individu-

FIGURE 4.32.   Silicone tube with red sleeve marking the desired insertion depth into the earcanal. The tip of the tube should be 5 mm deeper in the earcanal than the tip of the mold. From H. Birk-Nielsen 1985. "Hearing aid fitting based on insertion gain measurements." *Audecibel* 34(1): 16-19. Reproduced with permission of the author and publisher.

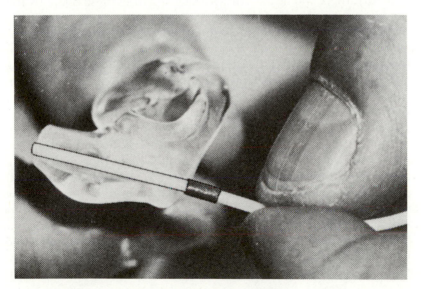

al's earcanal within a few minutes, and these physical measurements can be compared with the individual's subjective judgments about sound quality, sound clarity, and comfort. A printout of these measurements can then be compared with measurements made when the individual comes in for a recheck or complains that the hearing aid is not working well.

COMPARISON OF SUPRA-AURAL-EARPHONE, SOUND-FIELD, AND INSERT-EARPHONE MEASURES OF AN INDIVIDUAL'S AUDITORY AREA WITH HEARING AID OUTPUT

If an individual's auditory area (thresholds, MCLs, and UCLs for the audiometric frequencies) is obtained with a supra-aural earphone or in the sound field, then correction factors based on average data can be used to compare the results. The unifying concept is that the auditory sensitivity of any individual remains constant no matter how the sound is delivered. Consequently, the SPL associated with the average normal threshold at the eardrum (MAP) is a reference against which the SPL at the threshold in the sound field and 6-cc and 2-cc couplers can be compared (as done in tables 4.2 and 4.7). Another way to achieve this goal is to make a physical measurement of the SPL of a constant sound source at the reference point and at the eardrum (as done by Shaw 1966a and Sachs and Burkhard 1972). These correction factors have been used in tables 8.10, 8.11, and 8.12 in chapter 8 as a basis for estimating the 2-cc coupler gain and SSPL90 of a hearing aid that will provide the prescribed real-ear gain and SSPL90. It is important to remember that these correction factors are based on average data, and, consequently, there will be inaccuracies in estimating these relations for an individual.

When an insert earphone is used, an individual's auditory area can be compared directly with the output of a hearing aid because (1) the SPL from both is measured in an HA-1, 2-cc coupler, and (2) the sound source for both has high acoustic immittance. However, there are at least two variables that may not be taken into account. One is the effect of the earmold fit and venting, and the second is the possible difference between the acoustic immittance of the insert and that of the hearing aid earphones. Nevertheless, this comparison of insert earphone estimates of the auditory area with the hearing aid output produces more accurate results than does the use of correction factors for sound field and supra-aural earphone data.

An even more accurate method for comparing the auditory area with hearing aid output has been incorporated into the design and test protocol for a digital hearing aid developed jointly by Engebretson, Morley, and Popelka (1987). An insert earphone and probe microphone are imbedded in the earmold for this device. With the computer, sounds are presented through the insert earphone for obtaining auditory area data and the SPL of these is measured with the probe microphone. Based on these results, the frequency response, gain, and SSPL90 of the hearing aid are set according to fitting criteria and adjusted according to the SPL measurements made in the individual's earcanal. Since the insert earphone and earmold are the same as those used with the hearing aid, all the inaccuracies in estimating the resultant SPL in an individual's earcanal are eliminated. Although this aid and fitting system are not commercially available, it is highly likely that it will be in the future.

SUMMARY

There are standard procedures for measuring SPL from supra-aural earphones, insert earphones, and hearing aids, and a widely accepted protocol for measuring SPL from a loudspeaker in the sound field. However, the sounds from these sources are transmitted to an individual's eardrum in different ways. Consequently, for a given SPL measured in the 6-cc or 2-cc coupler or in the undisturbed sound field, the SPL at the eardrum will be different. A comparison can be made, based on average data, between sound delivered in each of these ways by calculating the difference in SPL at the reference point with the SPL at the eardrum as a function of frequency. Since this comparison is based on average data, there are inherent inaccuracies when it is applied to an individual. One way to avoid most of these inaccuracies is to use an insert earphone to obtain an individual's auditory area and to compare these data with the hearing aid output. This direct comparison is appropriate since the SPL for both sets of measurements are made in a 2-cc, HA-1 coupler.

   The real-ear gain and SSPL90 of a hearing aid worn by an individual cannot be predicted accurately from measurements in a test box with a 2-cc coupler or with KEMAR and a Zwislocki coupler in the sound field. A probe microphone or probe-tube microphone system can be used to measure the actual insertion gain and SSPL90 of a hearing aid in an individual's earcanal. With one of these systems the effects of various hearing aid settings and earmold configurations can be measured in a small amount of time.

Chapter Five
DETERMINING AN INDIVIDUAL'S AUDITORY AREA

The auditory area of an individual is the range of intensities between the threshold and the uncomfortable listening level (UCL) over the frequency range that can be heard. As mentioned in chapter 2, for hearing-impaired individuals the range between threshold and UCL probably reflects the composite effect of one or more sites of dysfunction in the auditory pathway, and these effects vary as a function of frequency. For example, the range may be normal in the low-frequency region (around 500 Hz) and reduced in the high-frequency region (around 4000 Hz), or it may be uniform across the frequency range from 250 to 6000 Hz. Somewhere above threshold and below UCL is a range of comfortable loudness levels bounded by a lower and an upper limit. The most comfortable loudness level (MCL) lies within this range.

The loudness of a sound can be directly related to its intensity by using the appropriate scaling procedures. The comfort of a sound is related to intensity in a complex way. That is, a person's judgment of comfort is based on the intensity as well as the sound quality (for example, pleasant versus harsh), the temporal sequence of the sound, the meaning of the sound for the individual, and other attributes. In determining an individual's auditory area, the focus is on loudness and not on sound quality in obtaining judgments of comfortable loudness levels and UCLs.

The values obtained for threshold, comfortable loudness levels, and UCL are based on the acoustical characteristics of the signal as well as on the individual's response criteria and the testing procedure. Since these values are used in a hearing aid evaluation, they need to be *reliable;* that is, the values for one measure (for example, threshold) obtained on two different occasions from the same person need to be nearly the same. These values also need to be *valid;* for example, when the maximum output of a hearing aid is set just below UCL, the amplified sound in real life should be limited before it becomes uncomfortably loud.

The reason for obtaining thresholds, MCLs, and UCLs, is to adjust the frequency response, gain, and maximum acoustic output (SSPL90) of hearing aids appropriately for each individual. With this goal in mind combinations of stimuli, instructions, and testing methods are used that are clinically effective.

Procedures for obtaining thresholds, MCLs, and UCLs with stimuli, audiometers, and sound-field equipment that are widely available today are described in the sections that follow. These procedures can be used with most children and adults; for those who cannot make MCL and UCL judgments, a method for estimating them from threshold and other audiometric information is described later in this chapter.

PROCEDURES

Stimuli

For three reasons, pulsed, pure tones (frequency modulated when presented in the sound field) are suggested for obtaining thresholds, MCLs, and UCLs. First, pure tones have a lower peak-to-rms difference than third-octave bands of noise or speech, and consequently they can be presented at a higher SPL (rms) than the noise or speech before causing nonlinear distortion in earphones or loudspeakers. This is important for UCL measurements with many individuals. Second, on the average MCLs and UCLs chosen by normal-hearing individuals are at approximately the same SPL for pulsed pure tones, pulsed noise bands, and third-octave bands of speech, as shown in table 5.1. Third, pulsed pure tones (200 msec. on and 200 msec. off) are generated by many audiometers now available. This suggestion to use pure tones to obtain UCLs may need to be revised if recent data by Byrne (1986a) are supported by other investigations.

Speech is used to obtain thresholds, MCLs, and UCLs for broad-band sound. Clinicians often use spondaic words (such as the CID W-1 word list) for thesholds and running speech for MCLs and UCLs. The overall SPL at which thresholds, MCLs, and UCLs are obtained is somewhat dependent on the spectral configuration of the speech. Some talkers speak with more high-frequency energy, and others speak with more low-frequency energy. To eliminate the variability associated with live-voice testing and different

TABLE 5.1. Mean MCLs and UCLs (dB SPL) Chosen by Normal-Hearing Listeners for Pulsed Pure Tones, Pulsed Third-Octave Bands of Noise, and Third-Octave Bands of Speech Presented Through Supra-Aural Earphones. Note That the Average Values for the Three Stimuli Are Close for Either MCL or UCL Within the Same Investigation. However, the Values for UCL Differ by Approximately 20 dB for the Two Investigations. The Higher UCL Values Were Obtained with a "Definitely Uncomfortable" Criterion, and the Lower UCL Values Were Obtained with a "Slightly Uncomfortable" Criterion. A Levitt (1978) Simple Up-down Adaptive Procedure Was Used in the Hawkins Investigation, and the Method of Adjustment Was Used in the Dawson Investigation.

				FREQUENCY (Hz)				
AUTHORS	LISTENERS	JUDGMENT	STIMULUS	250	500	1000	2000	4000
Hawkins	19	UCL	Pure tone	118	111	107	108	106
1980b			1/3-octave noise	117	111	112	108	108
			1/3-octave speech	115	112	110	109	108
Dawson	3	MCL	Pure tone	74	64	59	63	68
1981			1/3-octave noise	75	70	68	59	62
			1/3-octave speech	79	72	66	72	73
		UCL	Pure tone	93	84	84	85	82
			1/3-octave noise	99	89	87	82	82
			1/3-octave speech	96	88	85	88	83

talkers, tape recordings are recommended. If unaided judgments of MCL and UCL are going to be compared, one recorded speech sample should be used (for example, Fulton Lewis, Jr.'s, "Top of the Morning" passage; available from Technisonic Studios listed in Appendix 3A). The intensity of the chosen sample should be relatively constant over time to yield reliable MCLs and UCLs. Since the spectral configuration of speech is also affected by the way in which it is transformed on the way to a listener's eardrum, one should expect the MCL and UCL to be somewhat different depending on whether the speech is presented through an earphone, in the sound field, or through a hearing aid. These effects have been described in chapter 4.

Criteria for Judging Threshold, Comfortable Loudness Levels, and Uncomfortable Listening Levels

Threshold.   Two types of threshold—*detection* and *recognition*—are used in hearing aid evaluations. Detection thresholds are obtained for pure tones or narrow bands of noise and occasionally for speech when a listener cannot identify words (for example, infants or those with severe to profound hearing losses). For a detection threshold, an individual is instructed to respond whenever the sound is barely audible (or just different from silence). For a recognition threshold, an individual is instructed to report what s/he heard. For example, for a speech-reception threshold (SRT), the person identifies spondaic words. The threshold, for both detection and recognition thresholds, is the level at which an individual responds correctly 50 percent of the time (on two out of three or four trials). For speech, recognition threshold is approximately 6 to 10 dB higher than the detection threshold for normal-hearing listeners (Wilson and Margolis 1983).

Comfortable loudness level.   An individual's judgment of comfortable loudness levels is based on internal criteria derived from the instructions. Most clinicians ask for the level or range of levels that would be comfortable to listen to over a long period. The lower limit of the comfortable loudness range is the point at which sounds become soft, and the upper limit is the point at which sounds become loud. If one level is determined, this is often at the midpoint of the range and is called the most comfortable listening level (MCL). It is possible for MCL to fall close to the upper limit of the comfortable loudness range, depending on the instructions, the individual's response criteria, and the test procedure.

Uncomfortable listening level.   The UCL, also called the loudness discomfort level (LDL) or the threshold of discomfort (TD), has been defined according to three different criteria:

1. *Slightly Uncomfortable:* You would not be willing to listen to this for a long time but it would be okay for short sounds.

2. *Definitely Uncomfortable:* This level is louder than you would be willing to tolerate even for short sounds, but it is not painful.
3. *Painfully Loud:* This level makes your ear hurt. (Cox 1981b)

The average SPL at which speech is judged uncomfortably loud is lowest for the slightly uncomfortable criterion and highest for the painfully loud criterion, as shown in table 5.2; this relation also applies to other sounds. Since uncomfortably loud sound may cause damage to the inner ear, it is important to present high-level sounds as briefly as possible. For this same reason the painfully-loud criterion *should not be used* for obtaining UCL. Although further research is needed on whether the slightly uncomfortable or the definitely uncomfortable criterion gives the best estimate of UCL for setting the maximum acoustic output (SSPL90) of a hearing aid, many clinicians use the definitely uncomfortable criterion.

Methods for Presenting Stimuli and Obtaining Responses

To determine an individual's auditory area, the intensity level of frequency-specific sounds and speech are varied. Most testing is done with an *adaptive* procedure, in which each new presentation level depends on a listener's prior positive or negative responses. The first few stimuli are used for practice and to quickly reach the intensity range of interest (for example, that of threshold, MCL, or UCL). The levels of subsequent stimuli are changed in 5-, 2.5-, or 2-dB steps. These levels can be controlled by either the listener or the clinician as described in the following sections.

Clinician-controlled presentation.   There are several ways in which the adaptive procedure is applied in clinical situations: (1) an ascending approach; (2) a descending approach; (3) a bracketing approach; (4) a simple up-down procedure; and (5) rating the loudness of a sound on a continuum between too soft and too loud.

The Hughson-Westlake procedure (Carhart and Jerger 1959) is the most widely used *ascending approach*. When this procedure is used for determining detection thresholds, the first sound is presented at a clearly audible level, and listeners respond by raising their hands, saying that they hear it, or pressing a button. After this the intensity is decreased in 10-dB steps until the listeners no longer respond. The threshold determination begins at this point, and the intensity is increased (ascending approach) until the listeners respond. Following this the level is decreased in 10-dB steps and increased in 5-dB steps until a threshold is obtained. This is the lowest level at which three responses are obtained.

If an audiometer has 2.5-dB steps, the procedure can be modified to use 2.5- and 5-dB steps instead of 5- and 10-dB steps. In most clinics there is no nonauditory indication of when a sound is being presented, and most clinicians randomize the length of time between sounds to discourage listen-

TABLE 5.2. UCLs in dB SPL for Normal-Hearing Subjects Are Reported for Several Studies. The Investigations Are Arranged According to One of Five Categories (Initial Discomfort, Initial Discomfort/Discomfort, Discomfort, Tickle, or Pain) That Was Judged Most Appropriate, as Well as the Key Words or Phrases That Prompted This Categorization. The Psychophysical Method Is Also Briefly Described for Each Study. From R.C. Beattie, B.J. Edgerton, and D.W. Gagner 1979. "Effects of Speech Materials on the Loudness Discomfort Level." *Journal of Speech and Hearing Disorders* 44:435–58. Copyright 1979, American Speech-Language-Hearing Association, Rockville, Md. Reproduced with Permission of the Authors and Publisher.

INSTRUCTIONAL CATEGORY	INVESTIGATOR	KEY WORDS/PHRASES	UCL IN dB SPL	PSYCHOPHYSICAL METHOD
Initial Discomfort	McCandless and Miller (1972)	speech *first* becomes uncomfortable or annoying/level you would not care to listen to for any length of time	95	Method of limits in which the stimuli were gradually raised as a continuous function or in 2.5 or 5 dB steps.
	Denenberg and Altshuler (1976)	first point speech becomes uncomfortably loud	90.5	Method of limits in which connected discourse was increased in 5 dB steps. Three trials were averaged.
	Beattie, Edgerton, and Gagner (1979)	speech *first* becomes uncomfortable or annoying/level you would not care to listen to for any length of time	98.1	The stimuli were increased in 2 dB steps every 7 seconds. Three trials were averaged.
Initial Discomfort/ Discomfort	Olson and Hipskind (1973)	*first* expresses a feeling of discomfort	105.8	Method of constant stimuli in which the five-word sentence was randomly presented once at each of 16 predetermined intensities with 2 dB separating adjacent levels. Intervals of 3.5 seconds separated signal presentations.

(continued)

TABLE 5.2. (Continued)

INSTRUCTIONAL CATEGORY	INVESTIGATOR	KEY WORDS/PHRASES	UCL IN dB SPL	PSYCHOPHYSICAL METHOD
	Dirks and Kamm (1976)	level that is too loud, uncomfortably loud, or annoyingly loud/ to which you would not choose to listen for any period of time	97.0	Up-down adaptive procedure in which the stimuli were varied in 2 dB steps until eight reversals were obtained. Subject made two-alternative, forced-choice (Yes-No) to each spondee.
Discomfort	Silverman (1947)	uncomfortable/no longer care to listen/feel like removing the earphone	117.0	Method of limits in which the speech was initially presented at 100 dB SPL and, without interruption, increased 2 dB every 1.5 seconds. The increment size was changed to 1 dB for stimuli exceeding 130 dB SPL.
	Schmitz (1969)	uncomfortable/no longer care to listen	117.6+	Method of limits in which four-second samples of speech were presented in sound field in increasing 6 dB steps, with two-second off-times between presentations.
	McLeod and Greenberg (1977)	too loud or uncomfortably loud or not	102.7	Method of constant stimuli in which the speech was presented in 2 dB steps over a 16 dB range with 10 judgments per level.
Tickle	Silverman (1947)	feel a tickling sensation	129.3	See Silverman above.
Pain	Silverman (1947)	feel a sharp pain	137.9	See Silverman above.
	Denenberg and Altshuler (1976)	first point speech becomes physically painful	119.5+	See Denenberg and Altshuler above.

ers from responding spuriously. In my experience many listeners respond more reliably and efficiently when they know whether a sound is being presented. A small light connected to the stimulus-light circuit of the audiometer or a foot pedal can be used to deliver this information.

The ascending approach is often used for determining UCLs. With this approach clinicians first present sounds at a comfortable level and then increase the level until the person signals that it is uncomfortably loud. Following this the intensity is decreased 10, 15, or 20 dB and then increased in 5-dB steps until it is uncomfortable again. The UCL is the highest level the individual chooses on two out of three trials. If the UCL is obtained on several tests closely spaced in time, the UCL for many listeners increases until the third or fourth test. This increase in UCL is approximately 4 dB on the average, but it may be as much as 10 to 15 dB (see figure 5.1), particularly for those who have never worn a hearing aid. After the first few tests, however, it stabilizes and there is no further increase. For listeners who choose unusually low UCL levels, the UCL determination should be repeated until the level remains the same on two different tests.

The *descending approach* is often used for determining the speech-reception threshold (SRT). Wilson, Morgan, and Dirks (1973) have de-

FIGURE 5.1. **(A)** Change in mean UCLs (LDLs) between the first and successive trials for pure tones and wide-band noise presented through supra-aural earphones. From D. Morgan and D. Dirks 1974. "Loudness discomfort level under earphone and in the free field: The effects of calibration methods." *Journal of the Acoustical Society of America* 56: 172-78. Reproduced with permission of the authors and publisher. **(B)** Change in mean UCLs across trials for pulsed, third-octave bands of noise and third-octave bands of speech babble presented with an insert receiver attached to a personally fitted earmold. The dotted curve, labeled A, is for data obtained using a Békésy audiometer, and the solid curve, labeled B, is for data obtained with an ascending method like that of the Hughson-Westlake procedure (see text for description). From R. M. Cox 1981b. "Using LDLs to establish hearing aid limiting levels." *Hearing Instruments* 32(5): 16, 18, 20. Reproduced with permission of the author and the publisher.

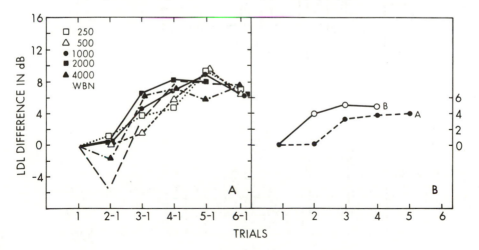

scribed one procedure in which they first familiarize the person with the words by presenting them at a comfortable loudness level. They obtain the level for starting the test by presenting one word at 30 to 40 dB above the expected threshold and descending in 10-dB steps until the person does not repeat a word correctly. The starting level is 10 dB above this. Then the intensity is decreased in 2-dB steps, with two words presented at each level. The measure is ended when the person misses five of the last six words presented. The level can also be decreased in 5-dB steps with five words presented at each level. The SRT is calculated as follows:

$$SRT_{50\%} = \text{Starting Level }_{dB\ HL} + 1/2 \text{ (decrement size }_{dB})$$
$$- \frac{(\text{decrement size }_{dB})(\text{number of correct responses})}{\text{number of words presented at each level,}}$$

where the decrement size is in 2-, 2.5-, or 5-dB steps.

An example of an SRT worksheet is shown in figure 5.2.

A descending approach can also be used to determine the upper limit of comfortable loudness (ULCL) by presenting a sound (for example, 4 or 5 pulses of a tone) that is loud but below UCL and then decreasing the level until the listener signals that it is first comfortably loud. This descending

FIGURE 5.2.   An example of a worksheet for obtaining spondaic word thresholds with a descending approach. The left panel is designed for 2-dB decrements, whereas the right panel is used for 5-dB decrements. An example of the calculation of SRT for the 2-dB increments is also shown. R. H. Wilson, D. E. Morgan, and D. R. Dirks 1973. "A proposed SRT procedure and its statistical precedent." *Journal of Speech and Hearing Disorders* 38: 184-91. Copyright 1973, American Speech-Language-Hearing Association, Rockville, Md. Reproduced with permission of the author and publisher.

INTENSITY			INTENSITY			INTENSITY					
0			40	✓	✓	0					
8			8	✓	✓	5					
6			6	✓	X	0					
4			4	✓	✓	5					
2			2	X	✓	0					
0			30	✓	X	5					
8			8	X	X						
6			6	X	X	0					
4			4			85	✓	✓	✓	✓	✓
2			2			0	✓	X	✓	X	✓
0			0			75	X	X	X	X	X
8			8			0					
6			6			5					

$SRT_{50\%} = 40 + 1/2\ (2) - 2(9)/2$

$= 41 - 9$

$= 32$ dB HL

sequence is repeated until the ULCL is determined. The ULCL is the highest level to which the listener responds that it is comfortable on two out of three trials (see Appendix A in Cox 1985).

A *bracketing approach* is usually used for obtaining one level (for example, MCL) within the comfortable listening range. With this approach the clinician increases the level of sounds until they are definitely loud and then decreases the level until the sounds are definitely soft. According to the listener's responses, the clinician increases and decreases the level over a smaller and smaller range until a single level is chosen. The bracketing approach, in which the clinician changes the sound level, is closely related to the *method of adjustment*, in which the listener changes the sound level.

Levitt's *simple up-down procedure* (1978) can be used to estimate the 50 percent response level for threshold, MCL, ULCL, and UCL. With this procedure the first few sounds are presented at a comfortable level, followed by sounds that are decreased or increased in relatively large steps (usually 10 dB) to the intensity region of interest. Then the sounds are increased and decreased in smaller steps (2 or 5 dB) within this intensity region. An example of the results from this procedure is shown in figure 5.3. Every time the listener responds (a plus sign on the figure), the intensity is decreased, and every time the listener does not respond (a minus sign on the figure), the intensity is increased. Each sound presentation is a trial, and each run is the successive trials in which the intensity is only decreased *or* only increased. To calculate the 50 percent response level, the first run is ignored and the levels of the midpoints for the next five to seven runs are averaged.

Rating the loudness of sounds on a continuum between too soft and too loud can be used to determine an individual's comfortable loudness range and UCL (Pascoe 1986). The listeners rate loudness according to a list of possible responses such as those shown in figure 5.4. They say the number or words that describe the loudness sensation. At Central Institute for the Deaf (CID), a response box is used (designed by Pascoe) that has ten buttons labeled according to the continuum shown in figure 5.4. When a listener presses a button, it lights up on both the listener's and the clinician's box. With this system a clinician can obtain data much more rapidly than if the listener responds verbally.

Pictures can be used to depict the loudness of sound for individuals, such as young children, who do not understand written or oral instructions but who can understand the concepts conveyed by pictures. An example of two sets of pictures is shown in figure 5.5.

To obtain reliable data, sounds are presented in an ascending-descending-ascending series of levels until the listener's rating of loudness at the upper and lower boundaries of the comfortable loudness range and at UCL are consistent. To check the stability of these judgments, Pascoe recommends alternating two tones in the same ear and seeing whether they retain the previous judgment of loudness. If they do not, he retests the tone that

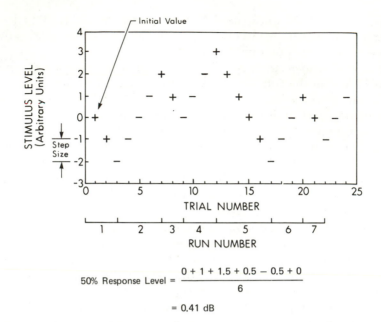

$$50\% \text{ Response Level} = \frac{0 + 1 + 1.5 + 0.5 - 0.5 + 0}{6}$$

$$= 0.41 \text{ dB}$$

FIGURE 5.3. Typical data record for the simple up-down procedure. The stimulus level (dB) is decreased after every positive response and increased after every negative response. A sequence of changes in one direction only is defined as a run. An example of the calculation of the 50 percent response level is also shown. From H. Levitt 1978. "Adaptive testing in audiology." In *Sensorineural Hearing Impairment and Hearing Aids*. Ed. C. Ludvigsen and J. Barfod. *Scandinavian Audiology*, supp. 6: 241-86. Reproduced with permission of the author and publisher.

differs. Binaural checks can be made if dynamic-range data have been obtained for both ears. To make these checks, Pascoe adjusts the intensity to MCL in each ear and asks the listener whether the tone that alternates from one ear to the other sounds equally comfortable. Although most people respond at consistent levels for the upper and lower boundaries of the

10	—	TOO LOUD
9	—	VERY LOUD
8	—	LOUD
7	—	COMFORTABLE BUT A LITTLE LOUD
6	—	COMFORTABLE
5	—	COMFORTABLE BUT A LITTLE SOFT
4	—	SOFT
3	—	VERY SOFT
2	—	TOO SOFT
1	—	NOTHING

FIGURE 5.4.
Words used to rate the loudness of sounds.

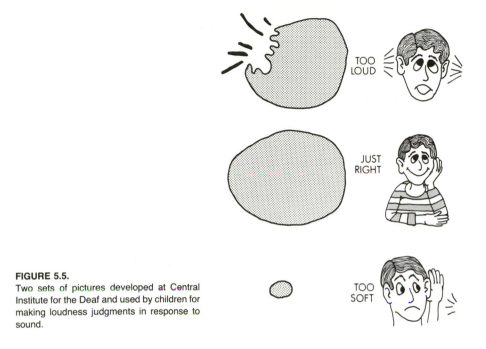

FIGURE 5.5.
Two sets of pictures developed at Central Institute for the Deaf and used by children for making loudness judgments in response to sound.

comfortable loudness range, some do not. However, these few usually respond at consistent levels for UCL.

Listener-controlled presentation.   Some clinicians use a Békésy audiometer to obtain thresholds, MCLs, or UCLs. With a Békésy audiometer the listener causes the intensity to decrease and increase by pressing and releasing the response button. If the sweep-frequency feature of the audiometer is used, measures of threshold, MCL, or UCL at frequencies between those usually tested are available. The sweep-frequency trace sometimes reveals large changes in threshold (and MCL or UCL) that are not evident when sounds are presented only at octave or half-octave intervals. This may be important information for setting the maximum acoustic output (SSPL90) of a hearing aid.

Occasionally an audiometer is adapted to include a listener-controlled attenuator such as that shown in Figure 5.6. When this attenuator is used to obtain threshold, MCL, or UCL, the clinician sets the level of the sound from the audiometer to the intensity region of interest and then asks the listener to adjust the attenuator so that the sound gets louder and softer until one level is chosen. Usually this procedure is repeated two or three times with different starting levels; the threshold, MCL, or UCL is the mean of the two or three levels obtained. This procedure, in which the listener changes the intensity level, is called the *method of adjustment*.

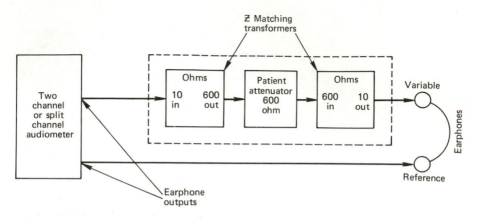

FIGURE 5.6.   Block diagram of one way to adapt a two-channel audiometer for the method of adjustment. The system within the dotted lines is inserted between the audiometer output (variable ear channel) and the earphone (variable earphone). Impedance-matching transformers are used because the output impedance in most audiometers is a nominal 10 ohms, but most attenuators have an impedance of 600 ohms. Note that the two transformers and the attenuator will insert approximately a 3-dB loss, which must be taken into account when the data are analyzed. If the transformer is not used and the 600-ohm attenuator is directly coupled with the audiometer and earphones, there will be a large voltage loss and distortion. From J. Katz 1978. *Handbook of Clinical Audiology*, 2nd ed. Figure 15.1 in "Loudness balance procedures" by W. F. Carver. Copyright 1978, Williams and Wilkins Co., Baltimore. Reproduced with permission of the author and publisher.

The method of adjustment is often used when an individual adjusts the volume wheel of a hearing aid so that speech presented in the field at 65 to 70 dB SPL is at MCL or a most-intelligible loudness level (MIL). This adjustment is made before aided thresholds are obtained or speech-discrimination tests are presented.

Instructions

The instructions for any test should convey to a listener information about the criterion for responding, the way to respond, the sounds, and the way in which they will be presented. Instructions should be stated clearly and succinctly, preferably in writing. Written instructions that are read either to or by the listener convey the needed information more consistently and with less bias than if the clinician repeats them from memory. This is particularly important for judgments of MCL or UCL that are strongly dependent on the listener's interpretation of the instructions.

Examples of instructions developed by clinicians for obtaining threshold, the upper limit of comfortable loudness (ULCL) and UCL with specific procedures are given below. The first example is for threshold obtained with an ascending method of presentation.

The purpose of this test is to see how well you can hear some faint tones. Each tone will be quite short. Some will be easy to hear. Others will be very faint. Whenever you hear one of these tones, no matter how faint it is, raise your finger. As soon as the tone goes off, lower your finger. (From R. Carhart and J. Jerger 1959. "Preferred method for clinical determination of pure tone thresholds." *Journal of Speech and Hearing Disorders* 24:330–45. Copyright 1959, American Speech-Language-Hearing Association, Rockville, Md. Reproduced with permission of J. Jerger and the publisher.)

A second example is of the ULCL obtained with a descending method of presentation.

The purpose of this test is to find the level of sounds which would be comfortable for you to listen to while you are watching television or listening to the radio. You will hear several sounds which will differ in loudness. Every time you hear a sound that is comfortably loud, please signal immediately by raising your hand. (From R.M. Cox 1985. "Hearing aids and aural rehabilitation: A structured approach to hearing aid selection." *Ear and Hearing* 6(5):226–39. Copyright by Williams and Wilkins, 1985. Reprinted with permission of the author and the publisher.)

A third example is of UCL obtained with an ascending method of presentation.

(Mr., Mrs., Miss) _____, now you will hear pulsing tones like those you heard before, but they will gradually become louder and louder. If they become so loud that they are uncomfortable to you just say "stop" and I'll turn them off. Don't say stop if the tones merely seem distracting but only when they first become uncomfortably loud. Consider the tones uncomfortable if you could not listen to them for 15 minutes or more. (From K.W. Berger, E.N. Hagberg, and R.L. Rane 1984. *Prescription of Hearing Aids: Rationale, Procedures and Results*, 4th ed. Kent, Ohio: Herald. Reprinted with permission of the authors and publisher.)

After giving instructions, it is important to ascertain whether the listener understands and clarify the instructions, if necessary.

Clinician Proficiency

A proficient clinician is one who gives instructions that are clear and gauged to each listener's level of understanding, who presents sounds at an optimum speed so that the listener is neither bored nor rushed, and who can detect whether a listener's responses are appropriate, indicate need of further training, or reflect lack of attention. A clinician who is proficient in giving one test may not be proficient in giving an unfamiliar test. Those who try new tests should not become discouraged when a listener does not give easily repeatable responses or when it takes longer than expected. It takes time and practice to become proficient.

Reliability of Threshold, MCL, and UCL Measures

An estimate of threshold, MCL, or UCL is meaningful only if it is *reliable*. For example, an estimate of threshold is reliable if the listener is just able to detect the tone at the same level, or close to it, on two or more occasions. If the threshold estimate, obtained by a well-trained clinician, differs markedly from one time to the next, then it is unreliable, and it is not clear what the listener's "true" threshold is.

A number of factors affect the reliability of measures of a listener's auditory area. These include the stimuli, equipment calibration, the method of presenting stimuli and obtaining responses, the clinician's proficiency, the instructions, the listener's internal criteria for responding, the status of the listener's hearing, and the listener's motivation and alertness. To evaluate the reliability of a listener's threshold (or other measures of auditory area), it is important to keep as many of these factors as possible constant for the different tests. For example, if pure tones were used the first time, then they should be used the second time, and they should be presented with the same audiometer, since the ANSI specifications allow as much as ±3 dB difference between the actual intensity and the nominal intensity (for tones between 500 and 3000 Hz). If an ascending procedure and specific instructions were used the first time, then the same procedure and instructions should be used the second time.

There are two measures used by those who have investigated the test-retest reliability of a listener's thresholds, MCLs, and UCLs. These are the *standard deviation* (SD) and the *range of score differences for a given percentage of subjects* in the group tested. If the reliability is expressed in SD units, it is assumed that the score differences are normally distributed and that statistically 67 percent of the listeners' difference scores would fall within ±1 SD and that 95 percent of the listeners' scores would fall within ±2 SD. For example, if the standard deviation is 4 dB, then for 95 percent of the listeners tested on two or more occasions, the test-retest difference of an individual's scores will not be greater than ±8 dB. When the results are expressed as the range of score differences for a given percentage of subjects, the actual value of the range is stated. For example, the test-retest difference was within ±5 dB for 91 percent of the listeners.

The data from a number of investigations indicate that listeners make more reliable responses at threshold (SD: 2 to 4 dB; see table 5.3) than at MCL (SD: 3 to 15 dB; see table 5.4) or UCL (SD: 4 to 6 dB; see table 5.5). This difference in reliability is probably related to the difference in the tasks. For threshold, a listener responds when the sound is barely detectible; that is, the sound is either detected or not detected. Furthermore, the range of intensities over which this is true is usually very small. For MCL and UCL, the instructions serve as a guide for the listener to judge the loudness of a sound;

TABLE 5.3. Repeatability of Thresholds*

AUTHORS	STIMULI	LISTENERS	SESSIONS	MEASURE OF VARIABILITY (dB)	PSYCHOPHYSICAL METHOD
Witting and Hughson 1940	PT 128–8192 Hz	18, Cond. HL 16–47 yrs	10 or more, over 2–28 months	SD = 3.8	Limits (ascending) 2.5-dB steps
Stephens et al. 1977	PT, pulsed 250 Hz 1000 Hz	10, Normal	4, 1–4 days apart	SD = 3.3 SD = 2.5	Békésy audiometer
Berger and Soltisz 1981	BBSpeech Babble	20, Normal	2, same day	TRDW ±4 in 80% of listeners; ±8 in 95% of listeners	Békésy audiometer
Byrne and Dillon 1981	Warble Tones 250–6kHz Earphone sound-field	7, Normal 3, SN HL	2, different days	SD = 4.1 SD = 4.6	Békésy audiometer
Dawson 1981	PT, pulsed NBN, pulsed NB Speech 250–4kHz. BBSpeech	3, Normals	5, over 2–3 weeks	SD = 3.7 SD = 3.4 SD = 3.9 SD = 3.3	Adjustment, 1-dB steps
Skinner et al. 1986	NBN 250–6kHz	21, SN HL	4, 1 day apart	SD = 2.7	Limits (ascending) 2.5-dB steps
Kwiecinski 1983	NBN, pulsed 250–6kHz BBN, pulsed	6, Normals	2, 1 day apart	SD = 2.4 SD = 1.9	Adjustment 1-dB steps
Matsumoto 1983	NBN, pulsed 250–6kHz BBN, pulsed	6, SN HL	2, 1–7 days apart	SD = 3.2 SD = 2.0	Adjustment 1-dB steps
Skinner and Miller 1983	NBN, pulsed 322–5242 Hz	7, SN HL	2, 1 day apart	SD = 2.7	Limits (ascending) 2-dB steps

*Listener's criterion for threshold was the just detectable presence of sound.
Abbreviations: PT = pure tones; NBN = third-octave bands of noise; NB speech=third-octave bands of speech; BBN = broad-band noise; BBSpeech = broad-band speech; Cond. HL = conductive hearing loss; SN HL = sensorineural hearing loss; TRDW: test-retest difference within; SD = standard deviation.

however, each listener forms an internal criterion for this judgment. This criterion may shift as a function of the preceding and succeeding sounds, and it may shift on different days of testing. If the individual is instructed to

TABLE 5.4. Repeatability of MCLs

AUTHORS	STIMULI	LISTENERS	SESSIONS	MEASURE OF VARIABILITY (dB)	PSYCHOPHYSICAL METHOD
Pollack 1952	PTs 125−1kHz 2−8kHz	33, Normals	2, different days	SD = 7.8−8.7 SD = 9.8−14.6	Adjustment MCL over moderate period of time
Ventry et al. 1971	PT NBN BBSpeech	64, Normals	2, different days	TRDW ±10 in 85% of listeners	Békésy audiometer
Stephens et al. 1977	PT, pulsed 250 Hz 1000 Hz	10, Normals	4, 1−4 days apart, same time of day	SD = 6.6 SD = 11.7	Békésy audiometer Level would like over long period of time
Ventry and Johnson 1978	Spondaic words	100, SN HL	2, different days	TRDW ±5 in 91% of listeners TRDW ±5 in 84% of listeners	Limits Descending Ascending
Berger et al. 1980	PT, pulsed 500−4kHz	7, Normals	2, 1 day apart	Mean diff = 4.3 − 12.9 Mean diff = 3.6 − 7.9	Limits 5-dB steps Comfort level Ascending Descending

choose one level (MCL that would be comfortable over a long period of time), a number of levels within a given intensity range may meet the listener's criterion. Therefore, on successive tests, the MCL chosen on two different occasions (SD: 3 to 15 dB; see table 5.4) differs more than does threshold. If more specific instructions are given for choosing a single level of MCL (such as the ULCL or the comfort level that is best for getting information), and these are coupled with a descending approach or method of adjustment, then the test-retest reliability (SD: 4 to 5 dB) is substantially better than for the less specific instructions. When MCL is obtained by rating the loudness and calculating the mean of the comfortable loudness range, the test-retest reliability (SD: 3 to 7 dB when the results are expressed in dB Sensation Level) is comparable to that when MCL is obtained with specific instructions for choosing a single level. Since it is important to obtain the most reliable values for MCL, specific instructions and the rating procedure are recommended to obtain the mean between the upper and lower limits of the comfortable loudness range.

TABLE 5.4. (Continued)

AUTHORS	STIMULI	LISTENERS	SESSIONS	MEASURE OF VARIABILITY (dB)	PSYCHOPHYSICAL METHOD
Christian and Byrne 1980	BBSpeech Babble	24, Normals	3, different days	TRDW ±10−14 in 92% of listeners (Mean = 5.3)	Békésy audiometer Level prefer over extended period of time
Cox and Bisset 1982	NBN NBSpeech Babble	16, SN HL		SD = 4.0 SD = 3.9	Bekesy (modif) Descending Upper limit of comfortable loudness
Pascoe et al. 1980	PT, pulsed 250−6kHz	18, SN HL	2, months apart	SD = 3.2−7.2 for SL SD = 4.4−12.5 for SPL	Rating loudness Mean of comfort range
Berger and Soltisz 1981	BBSpeech Babble	20, Normals	2, same day	TRDW ±12 in 75% of listeners TRDW ±20 in 90% of listeners	Békésy audiometer
Skinner and Miller 1983	NBN, pulsed 322−5242 Hz	7, SN HL	2, different days	SD = 4.1	Adjustment 1-dB steps Comfort level and get information

Abbreviations: PT = pure tones; NBN = third-octave bands of noise; NBSpeech = narrow-band speech; BBSpeech = broad-band speech; SN HL = sensorineural hearing loss; SD = standard deviation; TRDW = test-retest difference within; SL = data expressed in dB sensation level; SPL = data expressed in dB SPL.

Listeners vary widely in the reliability of their responses both at threshold and at MCL or UCL. Many are able to pay close attention to the sounds and respond consistently according to their internal criterion. Others allow their attention to drift and their criterion to change during the testing. A few have fluctuating hearing losses (such as those with Ménière's disease), and therefore, their auditory-area measures change concomitantly. After obtaining thresholds, each clinician needs to decide whether to obtain MCLs and UCLs. If a listener responds reliably at threshold and can understand either oral or written instructions for MCL and UCL, then it is important to obtain these suprathreshold values. Otherwise, the unaided MCLs and UCLs need to be estimated from the thresholds. This estimation is described later in this chapter.

TABLE 5.5.   Repeatability of UCLs

AUTHORS	STIMULI	LISTENERS	SESSIONS	MEASURE OF VARIABILITY (dB)	PSYCHOPHYSICAL METHOD
Stephens, et al. 1977	PT 1kHz	10, Normals	4, 1−4 days apart	SD = 5.2	Békésy audiometer Discomfort
Beattie et al. 1979	Speech	120, Normals	3, same day	TRWD ±6 in 85% of listeners	Limits (ascending) 2-dB steps Would not like to listen to it for any length of time
Dawson 1981	PT, pulsed NBN, pulsed NBSpeech 250−4kHz BBSpeech	3, Normals	5, different days	SD = 5.2 SD = 5.5 SD = 4.5 SD = 5.0	Adjustment 1-dB steps Would not like to listen to it for a long time
Kwiecinski 1983	NBN, pulsed BBN, pulsed	6, Normals	2, different days	SD = 4.7 SD = 2.0	Adjustment 1-dB steps Would not like to listen to it for a long time
Matsumoto 1983	NBN, pulsed 250−6kHz BBN, pulsed	6, SN HL	2, different days	SD = 5.4 SD = 2.8	Adjustment 1-dB steps Would not like to listen to it for a long time
Skinner and Miller 1983	NBN, pulsed	7, SN HL	2, different days	SD = 4.3	Adjustment 1-dB steps Would not like to listen to it for a long time

Abbreviations: PT = pure tones; NBN = third-octave bands of noise; NBSpeech = narrow-band speech; BBSpeech = broad-band speech; SN HL = sensorineural hearing loss; SD = standard deviation; TRDW = test-retest difference within; SL = data expressed in dB sensation level; SPL = data expressed in dB SPL.

Validity of These Measures

Measures of threshold, MCL, and UCL are valid if they enable us to meet the goals for fitting hearing aids. These goals are (1) to amplify conversational speech in specific frequency regions so that it is maximally intelligible and of acceptable sound quality and (2) to limit the maximum acoustic output so that the amplified sound does not surpass a listener's UCL.

One aspect of the validity of these measures is how well individuals function in their everyday lives with hearing aids adjusted according to measures obtained in sound-treated rooms. These adjustments include overall gain, frequency response, and SSPL90 of the aid. When listeners set the overall gain of a hearing aid so that speech presented at 70-dB SPL in the sound room is at MCL, this gain is very close to that which they use in everyday life (see table 5.6). Therefore, it is appropriate to use the 70-dB level in clinical evaluations, although this speech level is higher than that associated with average conversational speech (55- to 65-dB SPL).

The frequency response of a hearing aid can be chosen according to several different criteria that will be described in the next chapter. These criteria are used to estimate at what level in specific frequency regions a hearing-impaired individual can best process the acoustic cues of speech. At present the major issue is whether to use threshold or some MCL measure to determine the needed real-ear gain at each of the audiometric frequencies (that is, the frequency-gain characteristics of an aid) for an individual. Those who favor the threshold approach over the MCL approach argue that MCL measures are less reliable and more easily influenced by clinical procedures than are threshold measures. Those who favor using some measure of MCL believe that these measures cannot be predicted accurately from threshold data. Furthermore, they claim that these measures approximate the preferred listening levels associated with amplified broad-band speech more closely. Although further research is needed to resolve these issues, each criterion has been used for setting hearing aids in many clinics.

Because of loudness summation, comfortable loudness-level measures obtained with frequency-specific sounds may yield overestimates of the needed real-ear gain. Loudness summation, a concept described in chapter 2, occurs when the bandwidth of a complex sound exceeds some critical value. As the bandwidth is increased beyond a critical value and the level is kept constant, the loudness will increase. One can determine whether an individual is experiencing loudness summation by obtaining MCLs for frequency-specific sounds and comparing these levels with the third-octave-

TABLE 5.6. Mean Acoustic Gain (dB) Chosen by Hearing Aid Users for Speech Presented At 60 dB SPL in the Test Suite and for Daily Use in Their Everyday Lives on Four Different Days. If the Speech Is Presented at 70-dB SPL in the Test Suite, the Listeners Would Set the Overall Gain of Their Hearing Aids Approximately the Same as That They Choose for Daily Use. Adapted from B.E. Walden, G.I. Schuhman, and R.K. Sedge 1977. "The Reliability and Validity of the Comfort Level Method of Setting Hearing Aid Gain." *Journal of Speech and Hearing Disorders* 42:455–61. Copyright 1977, American Speech-Language-Hearing Association, Rockville, Md. Reprinted with Permission of the Authors and Publisher.

		DAILY USE			
	TEST SUITE	DAY 1	DAY 2	DAY 3	DAY 4
Mean Hearing Aid Gain	24.9	15.6	15.8	16.7	16.6

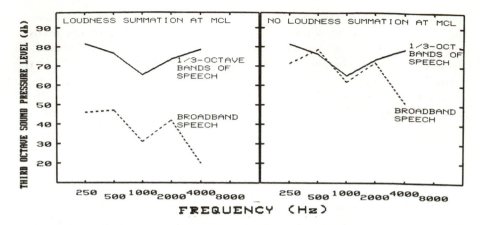

FIGURE 5.7.   Left panel: an example of loudness summation in a normal-hearing listener who adjusted third-octave bands of speech and broad-band speech (words of the California Consonant Test designed by Owens and Schubert 1977 and digitally re-recorded with no silent intervals by Skinner) to MCL while listening with earphones. After Dawson 1981. Note that the level judged as MCL for the broad-band speech is more than 30 dB lower than that for the third-octave bands of speech. Right panel: a hypothetical example of a listener with no loudness summation. For adjustments to MCL the third-octave bands of speech are at approximately the same level as third-octave bands within the broad-band speech.

band levels of a broad-band sound at MCL. This concept is shown in Figure 5.7.

In the left panel are plotted the MCLs for third-octave bands of speech for a listener with normal loudness summation. Note that when measurements were made of the broad-band speech (curve B), the level in third-octave bands is lower than that when separate third-octave bands of the speech were presented (curve A). If this listener had had no loudness summation, you would expect the results shown in the right panel. Since many hearing-impaired listeners experience some loudness summation, they will need less overall gain than would be predicted from the MCLs for third-octave-band sounds. Although there are no clinical procedures for determining the amount of loudness summation an individual experiences, the volume wheel of the hearing aid can be adjusted to compensate for this inaccuracy.

If an individual experiences loudness summation at UCL, the clinician must compensate by setting the SSPL90 of the aid lower than the UCLs for narrow-band stimuli. The amount of lowering is usually determined by presenting loud speech (about 85 dB SPL) in the sound field and adjusting the SSPL90 until the signal is no longer uncomfortable.

Several factors in addition to loudness summation must be considered in setting the SSPL90 so that amplified sound does not exceed UCL. These factors include a possible difference in calibration reference point (for example, 6-cc versus 2-cc coupler), the acoustic immittance of the hearing aid receiver, the acoustic immittance mismatch between this receiver and the individual's eardrum, and the difference between sounds used clinically to obtain UCLs and those which occur in everyday life. Since clinical procedures do not take all these factors into account, the SSPL90 may need to be reduced up to 10 dB if the noises of everyday life are too loud.

In summary, an insightful clinician can make appropriate adjustments in hearing aid settings even though the threshold, MCL, and UCL measurements on which they are based do not exactly reflect the overall gain, the frequency response, or the SSPL90 needed in everyday life.

Modes for Presenting Stimuli

The sounds used for obtaining thresholds, MCLs, and UCLs can be presented with supra-aural earphones, in the sound field, or through insert earphones. Each mode has its advantages and disadvantages.

The supra-aural earphone is available with all audiometers and is capable of delivering stimuli at high SPLs with little distortion. However, this mode of presenting sound does not directly relate to how a hearing-impaired person hears sound unaided in the sound field nor to how sound is delivered to the person's eardrum with a personally fitted earmold and hearing aid. Some clinicians also obtain UCLs in the field, but this mode is limited to individuals with low UCLs (90 dB HL and below).

In the past insert earphones have been used by a limited number of clinicians and researchers; however, the ER-3A insert earphones described in chapters 3 and 4 are commercially available and can be plugged into the supra-aural earphone jack of an audiometer. When this insert earphone is used to obtain the thresholds, MCLs, and UCLs, these data (expressed in dB SPL) are directly comparable to the output of a hearing aid measured with an HA-1 coupler. This direct comparison of auditory-area data with the output of the hearing aid eliminates many of the inaccuracies associated with estimating this relation indirectly as described in chapter 4.

COMPARING SUPRA-AURAL-EARPHONE, SOUND-FIELD, AND INSERT-EARPHONE RESULTS

The SPL values associated with an individual's thresholds, MCLs, and UCLs obtained with a supra-aural earphone are not at the same as those obtained in the sound field or with an insert earphone because the reference point for calibration and the sound delivered to the eardrum are different, as discussed in chapter 4. One way to express an individual's data with any of these modes of listening is to obtain all the behavioral measures (threshold, MCL, and UCL) with one mode and then use threshold measures obtained with the other two modes to derive the MCL and UCL values. Threshold measures are recommended since they are more reliable than MCL and UCL measures.

This derivation is based on the assumption that an individual's audi-

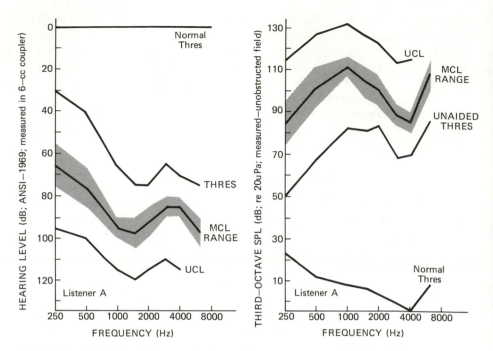

FIGURE 5.8. An example of the conversion from auditory-area measurements obtained with a supra-aural earphone (dB HL) to those in the sound field (dB SPL). See the text for an explanation of this calculation.

tory area remains constant regardless of the transducer through which the stimuli are presented. To derive sound-field data from supra-aural-earphone data, subtract the listener's earphone threshold from his or her MCL and UCL at each frequency to obtain MCLs and UCLs in dB SL. These values are then added to the sound-field thresholds to obtain the MCLs and UCLs in dB SPL in the sound field. An example of this derivation is summarized in the following formulas

$$\underset{\text{(earphone)}}{\text{MCL}_{\text{dB HL}}} - \underset{\text{(earphone)}}{\text{Threshold}_{\text{dB HL}}} = \text{MCL}_{\text{dB SL}}$$

$$\underset{\text{(field)}}{\text{Threshold}_{\text{dB SPL}}} + \text{MCL}_{\text{dB SL}} = \underset{\text{(field)}}{\text{MCL}_{\text{dB SPL}}}$$

and in figure 5.8. This derivation allows one to compare the individual's thresholds and MCLs in the sound field with the average level of conversational speech; this is the normal unaided condition. The derivation of sound-field values from insert-earphone values can be made in the same manner.

If insert-earphone data are not available, one can make an indirect approximation of the relation between the listener's UCL and the SSPL90 of an aid using the coupler gain and functional gain (that is, the difference between unaided and aided sound-field thresholds in specific frequency regions) or insertion gain. For example, an individual's unaided UCL at 4000 Hz expressed in dB SPL calibrated with a microphone in the unobstructed field is determined. The difference between the level at this microphone and that at an average individual's head at the front-facing microphone of a behind-the-ear hearing aid is approximately 0 dB; at this frequency there is no head-diffraction effect. Therefore, if the UCL in the field is 115 dB SPL, then the level at the hearing aid microphone is 115 dB SPL. The next step is to take into account alterations in the signal such as the acoustic leak of amplified sound from around the listener's earmold, and differences between the acoustic immittance of the coupler and that of the listener's ear. The functional gain (FG) (or insertion gain) is a composite of all these factors. Consequently, the functional gain (18 dB) is subtracted from the UCL value at the microphone of the hearing aid (115 dB SPL); this new value (97 dB SPL) may be thought of as the "aided" level at the microphone of the hearing aid. This is shown on the X axis of figure 5.9. The next step is to add the coupler gain (CG) obtained with a 60-dB input at 4000 Hz

FIGURE 5.9.   The input-output function at 4 kHz for an individual's hearing aid is shown in relation to threshold, MCL, and UCL. Also shown is the MPO (SSPL90) of the aid both at the input to the hearing aid microphone and at the output in the HA-2 coupler. From M. W. Skinner, D. P. Pascoe, J. D. Miller, and G. R. Popelka 1982. "Measurements to determine the optimal placement of speech energy within the listener's auditory area: A basis for selecting amplification characteristics." In *The Vanderbilt Hearing-Aid Report*. Ed. G. A. Studebaker and F. H. Bess. Upper Darby, Pa.: Monographs in Contemporary Audiology. Reproduced with permission of the authors and the publisher.

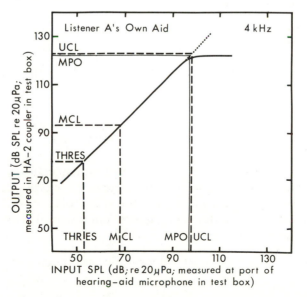

TABLE 5.7. Head and Body Baffle Effects Measured for Behind-the-Ear, In-the-Ear, In-the-Canal, and Body Hearing Aids. The Head or Body Baffle Effect Is Calculated by Subtracting the Level in dB SPL Measured in the Unobstructued Sound Field from That Measured at the Hearing Aid Microphone. Values Are Given for Sound Presented at 0° Azimuth and in the Diffuse Field.

	FREQUENCY (Hz)								
	250	500	750	1000	1500	2000	3000	4000	6000
Front-facing microphone, behind-the-ear aid[1]	0	1	0	−1	−2	2	0	0	—
Front-facing microphone, behind-the-ear aid[2]	0.5	1	1.5	2	2.5	3	2.5	2	1.5
Concha-filling, in-the-ear aid[3]	0.5	−1.5	—	1.5	2	4	4.5	3.5	−0.5
In-the-canal aid[4]	0.5	1	2	2.5	3	4.5	9	11	9
Body aid, front-facing microphone[5]	3	4	—	0	—	−4	0	0	0
Body aid, center chest position[6]	1	2	1	1	1	1	0	0	0

[1]Studebaker, Cox, and Formby 1980; 0° incidence (these values agree within 2.5 dB of Skinner et al. 1986).
[2]Kuhn 1979; diffuse field.
[3]Skinner et al. 1986; 0°incidence.
[4]Kuhn 1979; Killion and Monser 1980; diffuse field.
[5]Lybarger 1983 in Kuhn and Guernsey 1983; 0° incidence.
[6]Kuhn and Guernsey 1983; diffuse field.

to obtain the UCL value expressed in dB SPL measured with the microphone in the HA-2 coupler. The following equation summarizes this derivation.

$$\text{UCL}_{\text{field}} + \text{Head Baffle} - \text{FG} + \text{CG}_{\text{linear}} = \text{UCL}_{\text{HA-2 coupler}}$$
$$115 \text{ dB SPL} + (0 \text{ dB}) - 18 \text{ dB} + 25 \text{ dB} = 122 \text{ dB SPL}$$

This derivation is then repeated for the other frequencies using the average head-baffle data shown in table 5.7; this table also includes average head-baffle effects for other microphone positions. It is obvious that the time it would take to calculate this derivation makes it impractical to use for clinical procedures unless computers are available.[1]

[1]A calculation such as this is included in the computer program written by Popelka (1982).

ESTIMATING MCL AND UCL FROM THRESHOLD DATA

For individuals who cannot make MCL and UCL judgments but who need a hearing aid, MCLs and UCLs can be estimated from threshold and other audiometric data. Conditioned, behavioral thresholds that are reliable yield more accurate estimates of MCL and UCL than do thresholds based on observations of changes in behavior that occur when sounds are presented. Air-conduction thresholds obtained with brainstem-electric-response audiometry (BERA) can be used if one is alerted to the possible inaccuracy in predicting hearing sensitivity from these thresholds.

To estimate an individual's MCL and UCL from threshold, the growth of loudness needs to be estimated from information on the site(s) of dysfunction in the auditory system. As described in chapter 2, if an individual has a conductive hearing loss, the sound reaching the inner ear will be diminished by the amount of the loss; the growth of loudness above threshold will be similar to that in a normal ear. For an individual with a sensorineural hearing loss caused by hair-cell dysfunction, the growth of loudness above threshold will be greater than normal, and this is associated with a smaller than normal range between threshold and UCL. Most people with sensorineural hearing losses have a dysfunction at this site in the auditory pathway.

For people with less common dysfunction of the stria vascularis, spiral ligament, or neural pathways, the growth of loudness is probably slower than that associated with hair-cell dysfunction. Since clinically it is often very difficult to determine whether an individual with a sensorineural hearing loss has dysfunction at one or more of these sites, it is impossible to predict the growth of loudness exactly from threshold data. This is clearly shown in the large range of UCLs (for 500 Hz, 2000 Hz, and spondaic words) and MCLs (for 500, 1000, 2000, and 4000 Hz) associated with a single hearing threshold level (see figures 5.10 and 6.3). In tables 5.8 and 5.9 values for mean MCLs and UCLs from two studies are given as a function of hearing threshold (dB HL) for listeners with sensorineural hearing losses using supra-aural earphones.

To estimate MCLs and UCLs, it is important to know whether the individual's hearing loss is conductive, sensorineural, or mixed. This can be determined if reliable air- and bone-conduction thresholds are obtained. If no bone-conduction thresholds are available, then information from the case history, medical examination, and immittance values are important for determining whether there is a conductive hearing loss.

If an individual has a sensorineural hearing loss, MCL and UCL can be estimated from threshold using tables 5.10 and 5.11. These two tables are based on data from tables 5.8 and 5.9 as well as information cited at the bottom of the tables. For those with a conductive hearing loss, the MCL and UCL associated with a given hearing threshold level will be elevated above that for a sensorineural hearing loss by approximately one-quarter the difference between the air-conduction and bone-conduction thresholds (but

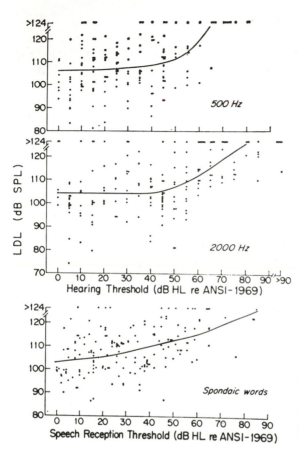

FIGURE 5.10.
Scatter plots of individual data and computer-generated best-fit curves for UCL (LDL) as a function of hearing threshold (ANSI S3.6-1969) for 500 Hz, 2000 Hz and spondaic words for listeners with sensorineural hearing losses. From C. Kamm, D. Dirks, and R. Mickey 1978. "Effect of sensorineural hearing loss on loudness discomfort level." *Journal of Speech and Hearing Research* 21: 668-81. Copyright 1978, American Speech-Language-Hearing Association, Rockville, Md. Reproduced with permission of the authors and publisher.

not more than 15 dB) at each frequency.[2] Acoustic reflex thresholds are not recommended for estimating UCLs. Although the acoustic reflex and UCL are both directly related to the intensity coding of sound, data collected from many hearing-impaired subjects indicate that the acoustic reflex cannot be used to predict the UCL reliably. This is shown by the scatter of data shown in figure 5.11 and the low correlation between these two measures.

[2]The rationale for this correction factor is as follows. Lybarger (1944) and Byrne (1983) have found that people with conductive hearing losses, when they set the volume wheel on their hearing aids so that conversational speech is comfortably loud, chose gain that was approximately the sum of (1) 0.5 multiplied by the threshold (dB HL) (this is the half-gain rule described in chapter 6), and (2) the air-bone gap (dB) multiplied by 0.25. Based on the experience of Lybarger and Byrne, it appears that people with conductive hearing losses have MCLs that are higher than MCLs chosen by people with sensorineural hearing losses by one-quarter of the air-bone gap (dB), since they choose this much additional gain. To approximate the elevation of MCLs and UCLs caused by conductive hearing loss, it is recommended that one-quarter of the air-bone gap (dB) be added to the values in tables 5.10 and 5.11. As more MCL and UCL data is gathered, these estimates may need to be modified.

145

TABLE 5.8. Estimates of MCL (dB HL) from Hearing Threshold (dB HL) for Pure Tones Presented Through Supra-Aural Earphones. The MCLs in the L Columns Are Based on Data from 106 Adults Between 51 and 94 years. For These Listeners the Average MCL Was 55 Percent of the Range Between Threshold and UCL. The Data Shown Here Were Calculated from the Average UCLs Shown in Table 5.9. From Leeds 1983. The MCLs in the K Columns Are Based on Data from 38 Adults. The Data Shown Here Represent the Midpoint Between the Best-Fit Functions for Ascending MCL and Descending MCL Measures. From Kamm, Dirks, and Mickey 1978.

HEARING THRESHOLD (dB HL)	FREQUENCY (Hz)					
	500 L	500 K	1000 L	2000 L	2000 K	4000 L
20	60	74	62	64	69	66
25	64	75	65	66	70	68
30	66	77	67	69	72	70
35	69	79	71	71	73	72
40	74	80	74	74	77	75
45	77	81	78	77	81	78
50	81	82	82	81	83	81
55	85	83	86	84	85	85
60	90	84	90	89	88	89
65	93	86	94	93	92	93
70	98	89	97	96		96
75	102	91	100	99		100
80			104	104		104
85			108	108		108
90			112			

TABLE 5.9. Estimates of UCL (dB HL) from Hearing Threshold (dB HL) for Pure Tones Presented Through Supra-Aural Earphones. The UCLs in the L Columns Are Based on Average Data for 106 Adults. From Leeds 1983. The UCLs in the K Columns Are Based on the Best-Fit Functions Shown in Figure 5.10. From Kamm, Dirks, and Mickey 1978.

HEARING THRESHOLD (dB HL)	FREQUENCY (Hz)					
	500 L	500 K	1000 L	2000 L	2000 K	4000 L
20	93	94	97	100	96	103
25	95	94	98	100	96	103
30	96	95	98	100	96	103
35	97	95	100	101	96	103
40	101	96	102	102	96	104
45	104	97	105	104	97	105
50	107	99	108	106	99	106
55	110		111	108	102	109
60	114		115	112	104	112
65	116		118	116	107	115
70	120		119	118	110	118
75	124		120	119	114	120
80			123	123	116	123
85			127	127		126
90			130			

TABLE 5.10. MCLs (dB HL) Predicted from Pure-Tone Thresholds (Obtained with TDH-Series Supra-Aural Earphone) for Individuals with Sensorineural Hearing Losses.[3] For Those with Conductive Hearing Losses, Divide the Amount of the Air-Bone Gap (dB) by 4 at Each Frequency and Add the Value to the Number for that Hearing Level and Frequency in the Table.[4]

HEARING THRESHOLD LEVEL (dB HL)	FREQUENCY (Hz)				
	250	500	1000	2000	4000
0	45	55	55	60	65
5	46	56	56	60	65
10	47	57	57	60	65
15	48	58	58	60	65
20	50	60	60	60	65
25	52	62	63	63	67
30	54	64	66	66	70
35	57	67	70	70	73
40	60	70	74	74	76
45	64	73	78	78	79
50	68	76	82	82	82
55	71	79	85	85	85
60	74	82	88	88	88
65	78	85	91	91	91
70	82	88	94	94	94
75	85	91	97	97	97
80	89	94	100	100	100
85	93	97	104	103	103
90	97	101	106	105	105
95		105	108	107	107
100		109	111	110	110
105		112	114	113	113
110		115	117	115	115

[3]The values in this table were derived from data from normal-hearing individuals (Mantevani, Pascoe, and Skinner 1978), from individuals with sensorineural hearing losses (Dirks and Kamm 1976; Kamm, Dirks, and Mickey 1978; Leeds 1983), and for the threshold levels between 90 and 110 dB, by placing the MCL so the speech spectrum would be approximately halfway between threshold and the estimated UCL level.
[4]See footnote 2 on page 144.

TABLE 5.11. **UCLs (dB HL) Predicted from Pure-Tone Thresholds (Obtained with TDH-Series Supra-Aural Earphones) for Individuals with Sensorineural Hearing Losses.[5] For Those with Conductive Hearing Losses, Divide the Amount of the Air-Bone Gap (dB) by 4 at Each Frequency and Add this Value to the Number for That Hearing Level and Frequency in the Table.[6]**

HEARING THRESHOLD LEVEL (dB HL)	FREQUENCY (Hz)				
	250	500	1000	2000	4000
0	78	90	93	91	90
5	78	90	93	91	90
10	78	90	93	91	90
15	78	90	93	91	90
20	78	90	93	91	90
25	78	90	93	91	90
30	79	91	94	91	90
35	79	91	94	91	90
40	80	92	95	91	90
45	82	92	95	93	93
50	84	93	97	95	95
55	86	95	99	97	97
60	88	97	101	99	99
65	90	99	103	101	101
70	92	101	105	103	103
75	95	103	107	105	105
80	98	105	109	107	107
85	102	108	111	109	109
90	105	111	113	111	111
95		114	115	113	113
100		117	118	115	115
105		119	121	117	117
110		120	124	119	119

[5]The values in this table were derived by setting the UCL at 100 dB SPL in the 6-cc coupler for 0-dB hearing-threshold level and approximately 130 dB SPL for 110 dB hearing-threshold level. These values agree fairly closely with data from Kamm, Dirks, and Mickey 1978; Martin et al. 1976; and Shapiro 1979.

[6]See footnote 2 on page 144.

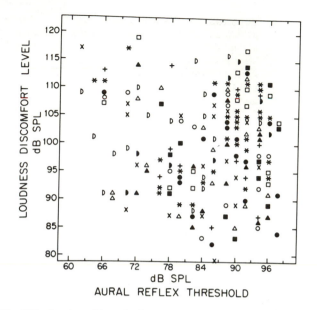

FIGURE 5.11.   UCLs (Loudness Discomfort Level) and aural-reflex thresholds for eleven normal-hearing individuals, for each of two trials and each of ten stimuli. The stimuli included consonant-vowel-consonant nonsense syllables, speech noise, and white noise. Each symbol represents a different stimulus. The * represents a level at which more than one data point was plotted. From D. Morgan, D. Dirks, D. Bower, and C. Kamm 1979. "Loudness discomfort level and the acoustic reflex threshold for speech stimuli." *Journal of Speech and Hearing Research* 22: 849-61. Copyright 1979, American Speech-Language-Hearing Association, Rockville, Md. Reproduced with permission of the authors and publisher.

SUMMARY

Thresholds, MCLs, and UCLs are obtained to estimate where the frequency response, gain, and maximum acoustic output (SSPL90) of hearing aids should be set for each individual. The values obtained depend on the acoustical characteristics of the signal as well as on the individual's response criteria and the testing procedure. Listeners make more reliable responses at threshold than at MCL or UCL. However, with the appropriate choices of criteria and test procedures, the reliability of MCL and UCL measures comes close to that for threshold. To maximize the validity of these measures, clinicians must be keenly aware of the relation between the values of threshold, MCL, and UCL obtained with their choice of instructions and test procedures and the criteria they use for adjusting the hearing aid for an individual. Modifications in the adjustment criteria may need to be made to provide amplification that is most useful to the individual in everyday life.

Chapter Six

CRITERIA FOR PRESELECTING REAL-EAR GAIN

A number of different commercial hearing aids can be adjusted to provide a hearing-impaired individual with acceptable sound quality, optimized speech intelligibility, and maximum sound output that is not uncomfortably loud. For a hearing aid evaluation to be clinically feasible, the clinician preselects and adjusts one or several aids for each individual. There are *comparative* and *prescriptive* approaches to this preselection and adjustment procedure. With the modified Carhart approach (described in Walden et al. 1983), a widely used comparative procedure, the criteria for preselecting and adjusting the aids are not specified but rather are based on the experience and judgment of the clinician. When criteria are not specified, it is difficult to develop the needed experience and impossible to verify whether a hearing aid has met criteria. With the prescriptive approaches, there are specified criteria for preselecting and adjusting aids that can be followed by any clinician. For these reasons, a prescriptive approach is recommended. This can be followed with a comparative approach for evaluating the aids that have been chosen.

In all prescriptive procedures the amount of real-ear gain prescribed in specific frequency regions is determined from either threshold or MCL/ULCL (most comfortable loudness/upper limit of comfortable loudness) data. *Real-ear gain* is defined as the actual gain provided by a hearing aid for an individual. Clinically, real-ear gain is estimated by obtaining functional-gain or insertion-gain measurements. *Functional gain* is the difference between the unaided and aided thresholds (for frequency-specific sounds) obtained with the same sound-field conditions. *Insertion gain* is the difference between the SPLs measured near the eardrum with and without a hearing aid; the same frequency-specific sounds are presented in the field for both measurements. A description of how functional and insertion gain are measured clinically and conditions that lead to inexact estimates of real-ear gain are described in chapter 9.

In this chapter all the criteria are based on real-ear gain. The relation between real-ear gain and coupler gain, which is so important for preselecting and adjusting hearing aids, will be described in chapter 8.

This chapter describes factors considered in prescribing real-ear gain, several procedures for prescribing it, bases for choosing one of these procedures, and suggestions for modifying the prescribed gain in special cases.

FACTORS CONSIDERED IN PRESCRIBING REAL-EAR GAIN

The major factors considered in prescribing the real-ear gain for an individual are the speech spectrum, the comfortable-loudness contour for speech for normal-hearing individuals, the preferred listening levels, the effect of low-frequency room noise, the relation between earphone and unaided field thresholds, and the prescribed real-ear gain that is intended to amplify the speech spectrum to an individual's preferred listening levels. These are described in the sections that follow.

Speech Spectrum

One factor that affects the amount of prescribed real-ear gain is the overall level and configuration of speech energy chosen to represent everyday speech. For hearing-impaired listeners, it is generally accepted that the overall level should be between 65 and 70 dB SPL. The speech spectra chosen for four prescriptive procedures (that incorporate it into their calculation of real-ear gain) are shown in figure 6.1. The speech spectra chosen by Pascoe (1978) and Cox (1983) are essentially identical, whereas those chosen by Byrne and Tonisson (1976) [note that this is the spectrum published by Byrne in 1977 and incorporated in a revised procedure; Byrne (1978)] and Byrne and Dillon (1986) of the National Acoustic Laboratories in Australia are of a different configuration. In the Byrne and Tonisson speech spectrum the level from 2000 to 6000 Hz is constant, whereas for the Pascoe and Cox spectra the level falls off 10 dB in the higher frequencies. In addition, the speech energy at 250 and 500 Hz in the Byrne and Tonisson speech sample is 15 dB higher than at 1000 Hz, whereas for the other two it is only 5 to 10 dB higher. If the overall level differencies are ignored, less real-ear gain will be needed at low (250 to 500 Hz) and high (3000 to 6000 Hz) frequencies relative to that in the midfrequency region (1000 to 2000 Hz) for the Byrne and Tonisson speech spectrum than for the Cox and Pascoe spectra. The Byrne and Dillon speech spectrum is intermediate between the others.

FIGURE 6.1.
Long-term rms levels of speech used to represent everyday speech in three procedures for prescribing real-ear gain for hearing aids. The speech spectrum for the Byrne and Tonisson procedure is based on measurements of Australian English spoken at 68 dB SPL made by Byrne (1977); the spectrum of Byrne and Dillon is based on more recent measurements. The speech spectrum for the Cox procedure is based on measurements of American English spoken at an overall level of 70 dB SPL. The speech spectrum for the Pascoe procedure is the sensation level at which normal-hearing persons hear third-octave bands of speech spoken by ten women and ten men (mixed electronically) when the overall level of the broad-band speech is presented at 65 dB SPL.

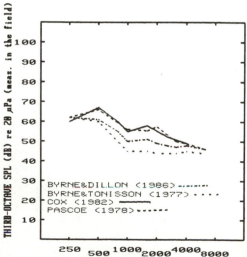

Later in this chapter there are examples of the amplified speech spectrum plotted in relation to an individual's auditory area. The amplified spectrum was calculated by adding the prescribed real-ear gain to the Pascoe speech spectrum. This spectrum was chosen for two reasons. First, it represents the sensation level at which normal-hearing listeners hear speech babble presented at an overall level of 65 dB SPL, and consequently it provides a perceptual as well as a physical basis for representing conversational speech. Second, the spectral shape is essentially identical not only to that of Cox (1983) but also to that of several others (for example, ANSI S3.5-1969; Pearsons, Bennett, and Fidell 1976). However, further research is needed to determine whether this is an appropriate choice.

Normal Comfortable-Loudness-Level Contour

Two of the prescriptive procedures incorporate estimates of the comfortable loudness levels for speech for normal-hearing individuals into the prediction of preferred listening levels for hearing-impaired individuals. In

FIGURE 6.2.   The Pascoe speech spectrum (dB HL) plotted in relation to the normal comfort range and the normal UCL range. The speech spectrum is the same as shown in figure 6.1 but converted to dB HL. The comfort and UCL ranges are based on data from ten normal-hearing young adults who labeled the loudness of pulsed, third-octave bands of noise presented in the sound field. The mean MCL is the mean of the normal comfort range.

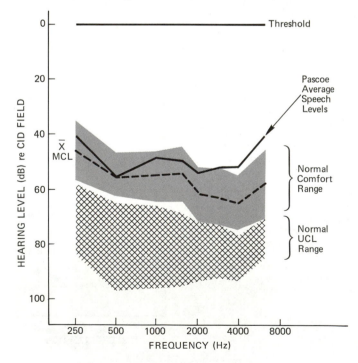

the Byrne and Tonisson procedure the 60-phon equal-loudness contour for pure tones was found to approximate the preferred listening levels for speech for normal-hearing listeners; consequently, a correction factor for this contour is included in the calculation of real-ear gain. In the Pascoe procedure an attempt is made to preserve the normal relation between the speech spectrum and the range of MCLs for normal-hearing individuals between 500 and 4000 Hz (see figure 6.2). As described above, the Pascoe spectrum represents the sensation level at which normal-hearing individuals perceive third-octave bands of speech babble. At 500 Hz this spectrum is at the midpoint of the normal comfort range (mean MCL) and within this range through 2500 Hz. It is slightly below this range at 4000 and 6000 Hz.

If the difference between threshold (0 dB HL) and the mean MCL is considered as 100 percent, then the level at 500 Hz is 100 percent of this difference, the levels at 1000, 1500, and 2000 Hz are approximately 90 percent of this difference, and the levels at 3000 and 4000 Hz are approximately 80 percent of this difference. These percentages are used in calculating the level at which the aided speech spectrum should fall within the auditory area of a hearing-impaired individual, to approximate the same relation that normal-hearing individuals have between the speech spectrum and mean MCL.

Preferred Listening Levels

In all prescriptive procedures it is assumed that there is a preferred listening level within the comfortable loudness range and that sound at this level provides the individual with a maximum amount of information. At the same time this level requires less effort to listen to than lower or higher levels. The preferred listening level will depend on each hearing-impaired individual's growth of loudness, and this level will often differ for specific frequencies between 250 and 6000 Hz. For broad-band sounds, such as speech, the preferred listening level will also depend on the individual's loudness summation, the frequency content of the speech, the frequency response of the hearing aid, and the relation of the amplified signal to the individual's auditory area.

In some prescriptive procedures measurements of one or more points in the comfortable loudness range are made for frequency-specific sounds from each individual. In the Pascoe procedure it is assumed that the preferred listening levels are in relation to the midpoint of the comfortable loudness range as described above, and in the Cox procedure it is assumed that they are at the midpoint of the range between threshold and the upper limit of comfortable loudness. These measurements are based on the growth of loudness experienced by the individual.

In other prescriptive procedures no direct measurements of comfortable loudness are obtained. The preferred listening levels are estimated

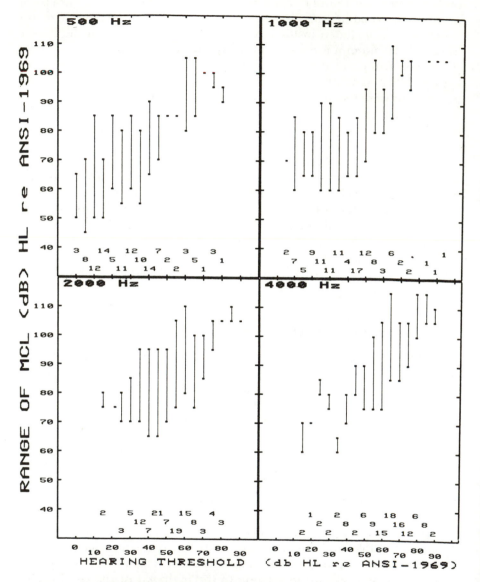

FIGURE 6.3.   Range of MCLs (mean of the comfort range) as a function of hearing-threshold level (dB HL re ANSI S3.6-1969) at 500, 1000, 2000 and 4000 Hz for 106 adults tested with the ascending-descending-ascending presentation and loudness-labeling procedure described in chapter 5. The number of data points for each hearing-threshold level are shown at the bottom of each panel. After Leeds 1983.

from pure-tone thresholds using formulas based on the average of preferred listening levels obtained from large groups of hearing-impaired
individuals, consisting mainly of those with sensorineural hearing loss.
These averages are often the mean of a 20- to 30-dB range (assuming that
preferred listening levels vary from one person to the next as much as MCLs
do; see figure 6.3). Consequently, an individual's *actual* preferred listening
level may differ by as much as ±15 dB from the average level. For example,
if the average preferred listening level is 80 dB HL for people with a
pure-tone threshold of 45 dB HL at 2000 Hz, one person may have an actual
preferred listening level as low as 65 dB HL and another have one as high as
95 dB HL.

Although further research is needed on more exact ways to determine
preferred listening levels, it is assumed that estimates based on a direct
determination of an individual's comfortable loudness range and a consideration of the normal comfortable-loudness-level contour will yield a closer
approximation of what they actually are than estimates based on threshold
data.

Low-Frequency Room Noise

Amplified low-frequency noise can be particularly annoying to hearing-
impaired listeners if it is of sufficient intensity to mask the speech energy at
higher frequencies. Since the level of noise in our everyday lives is usually
higher in the region of 125 to 400 Hz than at higher frequencies, all
prescriptive procedures recommend less gain at 250 Hz than would cause
the speech spectrum to reach the preferred listening levels. Some procedures recommend less gain at 500 Hz, particularly for mild to moderate
losses.

Earphone versus Unaided Sound-Field Thresholds

In clinical situations it saves time to obtain an individual's supra-aural
or insert earphone thresholds and assume that they are the same as the
unaided sound-field thresholds, *if* both are expressed in dB HL. On the
average this is true, but as described in chapter 4, individual variations result
in significant differences in the SPL at the eardrum, especially between 250
and 500 Hz and above 2000 Hz. Consequently, it is more accurate to
prescribe real-ear gain based on sound-field thresholds. If this is done, the
levels for the unaided thresholds, the speech spectrum, the prescribed real-
ear gain, and the prescribed aided thresholds are all referred to a single
calibration point—the microphone at the center of where the listener's
head would be in the sound field. Since the sound-level measurements are
referred to this one point, the auditory-area data and the aided speech levels
are directly comparable. In the procedures described below, these data have
been plotted in reference to the sound-field calibration.

Prescribed Real-Ear Gain: Speech Spectrum Amplified to Preferred Listening Levels

Ideally, the prescribed real-ear gain of a hearing aid should cause the long-term rms level of conversational speech to fall at an individual's preferred listening level in each frequency region between 250 and 6000 Hz. This concept is illustrated in figure 6.4, where the unaided field thresholds and preferred listening levels of a person with a moderate sensorineural hearing loss are plotted in relation to the speech spectrum. The real-ear gain is that needed to amplify the speech spectrum to the preferred listening levels. For this individual, 18 dB more gain is needed at 2000 Hz than at 500 Hz. This difference in gain is necessary to preserve the appropriate balance in the speech energy in the low- and high-frequency regions. This prescription of the particular configuration of real-ear gain is the most important aspect of the preselection process. The absolute value of the prescribed real-ear gain is considered approximate, since each person will adjust the overall sound output to a comfortable level and, therefore, compensate for unpredictable effects of loudness summation and other factors.

The Pascoe speech spectrum (shown in figures 6.1 and 6.2) and the thresholds, comfort range, and UCLs (obtained with Pascoe's ascending-descending-ascending presentation of pulsed pure tones and a labeling response, both of which were described in chapter 5) of a hearing-impaired individual will be used to demonstrate (1) how the real-ear gain prescribed by several procedures affects the configuration of the amplified speech spectrum and (2) how this amplified speech spectrum falls in relation to the comfort range. In calculating the amplified speech spectrum, it is assumed

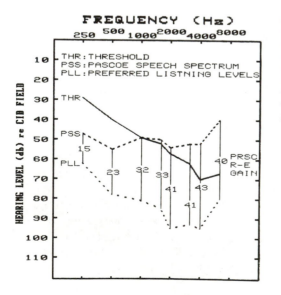

FIGURE 6.4.
The preferred listening levels and sound-field thresholds for a person with a sloping sensori-neural hearing loss are plotted in relation to the Pascoe unaided speech spectrum. The prescribed real-ear gain at each audiometric frequency is the difference between the preferred listening levels and the unaided speech spectrum.

that the hearing aid provides linear real-ear gain for the input levels of the Pascoe speech spectrum.

PROCEDURES FOR PRESCRIBING REAL-EAR GAIN

Since the 1930s many procedures have been devised for selecting the frequency responses and gain of hearing aids for hearing-impaired individuals. Of major clinical interest are those procedures in which *thresholds* (Lybarger 1944, 1955, 1963; Fletcher 1952; Byrne and Tonisson 1976, 1978; Berger et al. 1984; McCandless and Lyregaard 1983; Libby 1985 and 1986; Byrne and Dillon 1986), *MCLs* (Watson and Knudsen 1940; Victoreen 1960; Markle and Zaner 1966; de Vos 1968; Shapiro 1976; Pascoe 1978; Skinner, Pascoe, Miller, and Popelka 1982; Cox 1983, 1985; Leijon, Eriksson-Mangold, and Bech-Karlsen 1984), or *bisection of the range between threshold and UCL* (Balbi 1935; Wallenfels 1967) are used to prescribe the real-ear gain. Six of these procedures are described in the following sections.

Procedures Based on Threshold Data

Most threshold procedures are modifications of the *half-gain rule* developed by Lybarger (1944). This rule evolved from observations of the use-gain settings chosen by hearing aid wearers for whom the frequency response and gain had been adjusted to their comfort and satisfaction using trial-and-error methods. According to this rule an individual's audiometric thresholds (dB HL) obtained under earphones are multiplied by 0.5 between 1000 and 4000 Hz (and 0.3 at 500 Hz) to give the prescribed real-ear gain. This prescription is intended for those with sensorineural hearing losses. For those with a conductive hearing loss, Lybarger recommends additional gain (one-quarter the difference between the air-conduction and bone-conduction thresholds at each frequency).

POGO. In the "Prescription of Gain/Output (POGO) of Hearing Aids" procedure devised by McCandless and Lyregaard (1983), the half-gain rule is modified so that the gain at 500 and 250 Hz is reduced by 5 and 10 dB respectively; this provides less amplification of low-frequency room noise. These authors suggest that this procedure is appropriate for those with sensorineural hearing losses that are predominantly sensory and with thresholds no greater than 80 dB HL. At the present time POGO does not prescribe the additional gain needed by those with conductive hearing losses or for those with more severe hearing losses. The calculation of prescribed real-ear gain for someone with a moderate sensorineural hearing loss (listener 1) is shown at the bottom of figure 6.5. The authors recommend that these calculations be made with hearing thresholds expressed in dB HL and obtained with supra-aural earphones. At the bottom of figure 6.6 the calcu-

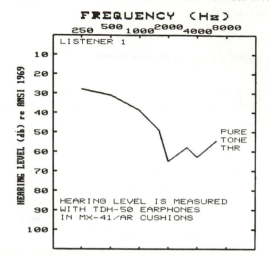

CALCULATIONS OF PRESCRIBED REAL-EAR GAIN FOR POGO PROCEDURE

	FREQUENCY (Hz)						
	250	500	1000	2000	3000	4000	6000
THRESHOLD HL (dB)	29	31	39	65	58	63	54
MULTIPLY BY 0.5	0.5	0.5	0.5	0.5	0.5	0.5	0.5
"½ gain"	14.5	15.5	19.5	32.5	29.0	31.5	27.0
CORRECTION FOR NOISE	−10	−5	0	0	0	0	0
PRESCRIBED REAL-EAR GAIN (dB)	4.5	10.5	19.5	32.5	29.0	31.5	27.0

FIGURE 6.5. Calculations of prescribed real-ear gain for the POGO procedure for listener 1, who has a sensorineural hearing loss whose pure-tone thresholds for the left ear are shown on the audiogram (dB HL re ANSI S3.6-1969).

lation of the prescribed aided field thresholds (dB HL) is shown, and at the top is a graph showing the earphone thresholds (dB HL), the unaided field thresholds (dB HL), and the prescribed aided field thresholds (dB HL). (If the unaided field thresholds had been used instead of the earphone thresholds in the calculation of the real-ear gain and prescribed aided thresholds, the aided thresholds would have differed by ±5 dB between 500 and 4000 Hz and by ±10 dB at 250 and 4000 Hz from those shown in figure 6.6.)

If a hearing aid is adjusted to give this prescribed real-ear gain, then the Pascoe speech spectrum should be amplified by the amounts shown in the left panel of figure 6.7. In the right panel of this figure the aided speech spectrum is shown in relation to the auditory area of listener 1.

CALCULATIONS OF PRESCRIBED AIDED FIELD THRESHOLDS FOR POGO

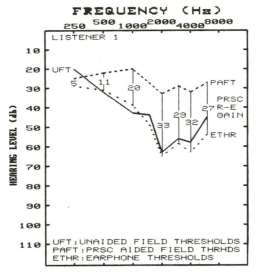

FIGURE 6.6. Calculations of the prescribed aided field thresholds for listener 1 for the real-ear gain prescribed by the POGO procedure. On the audiogram the earphone thresholds and the unaided field thresholds are both shown to indicate the differences that do occur for these two ways of delivering the sound.

FREQUENCY (Hz)	250	500	1000	2000	3000	4000	6000
THRESHOLD dB HL (EARPHONE)	29	31	39	65	58	63	54
PRESCRIBED REAL-EAR GAIN (dB) (Subtract)	4.5	10.5	19.5	32.5	29	31.5	27
PRESCRIBED AIDED FIELD THRESHOLDS (dB HL)	24.5	20.5	19.5	32.5	29	31.5	27

Berger et al. procedure. Berger, Hagberg, and Rane (1984) recommend using the half-gain rule (multiplying by 0.5) at 500, 4000, and 6000 Hz and more gain than this (0.59 to 0.67) between 1000 and 3000 Hz. This is called the *prescribed operating gain*; however, the calculation of prescribed aided thresholds suggests that operating gain is real-ear gain. Although the speech spectrum is not specified, these criteria for prescribing real-ear gain are intended to cause the amplified speech energy to be equally loud between 500 and 2000 Hz. Less gain is recommeneded at 4000 and 6000 Hz to avoid driving the damaged cochlea with high SPLs that might cause further distortion and reduced speech intelligibility.

For individuals with thresholds lower than 50 dB HL they recommend

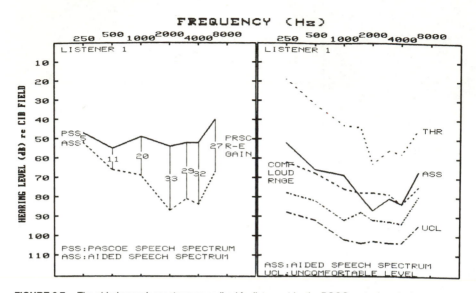

FIGURE 6.7.   The aided speech spectrum prescribed for listener 1 by the POGO procedure. In the left panel, the real-ear gain is denoted by the numbers on the vertical lines. This real-ear gain has been added to the unaided speech spectrum (Pascoe 1978) to obtain the prescribed aided speech spectrum. In the right panel, the aided speech spectrum has been plotted in relation to the threshold (THR), comfortable loudness range, and UCL contours for this listener.

less gain at 500 Hz (0.3 instead of 0.5, as shown in figure 6.8). In noisy or reverberant environments they have found these individuals prefer even less gain at 500 Hz (6 dB) and 1000 Hz (3 dB). Calculation of gain at 250 Hz is omitted in the formula because earphone thresholds are often an inaccurate indication of the field threshold and room noise is often high at this frequency. Although the authors note that the calculations of real-ear gain are more accurate if they are based on unaided field thresholds (dB HL), the earphone thresholds (dB HL) are often used because they have already been obtained as part of a routine hearing test.

Calculations of real-ear gain prescribed by the Berger et al. procedure and based on the unaided field thresholds for listener 1 are shown at the bottom of figure 6.8. The real-ear gain and the unaided and aided field thresholds are shown on the graph in the same figure. To simplify the procedure for clinical use with individuals with sensorienural hearing losses, the prescribed real-ear gain has been calculated as a function of frequency and hearing-threshold level and can be found in table 6.1. If a hearing aid is adjusted to give the real-ear gain for listener 1 as shown in figure 6.8, then the Pascoe speech spectrum should be amplified by the amounts shown in the left panel of figure 6.9. The aided speech spectrum is shown in relation to this listener's auditory area in the right panel of figure 6.9.

CALCULATION OF PRESCRIBED REAL-EAR GAIN AND AIDED FIELD THRESHOLDS FOR

THE BERGER ET AL. PROCEDURE

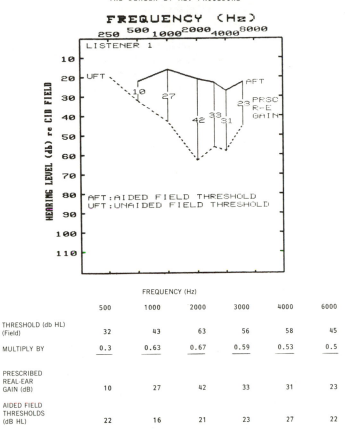

	FREQUENCY (Hz)					
	500	1000	2000	3000	4000	6000
THRESHOLD (db HL) (Field)	32	43	63	56	58	45
MULTIPLY BY	0.3	0.63	0.67	0.59	0.53	0.5
PRESCRIBED REAL-EAR GAIN (dB)	10	27	42	33	31	23
AIDED FIELD THRESHOLDS (dB HL)	22	16	21	23	27	22

FIGURE 6.8.   Calculations of the real-ear gain and aided field thresholds prescribed by the Berger *et al.* (1984) procedure for listener 1. The audiogram shows the unaided and aided field thresholds; the prescribed real-ear gain is denoted by the numbers on the vertical lines.

For two individuals with the same hearing thresholds, the one with a conductive hearing loss will need more gain than the one with a sensori-neural hearing loss. Berger et al. recommend that additional gain (0.2 multiplied by the difference between the air- and bone-conduction thresholds but not more than 8 dB) be added. An example of this calculation is shown in the bottom part of figure 6.10 for an individual who had the same air-conduction thresholds in the sound field and under earphones as listener 1 but who had the bone-conduction thresholds shown in the audiogram in the top part of figure 6.10.

TABLE 6.1. Prescribed Real-Ear Gain Calculated According to the Formulas Recommended By Berger et al. (1984) for Individuals with Sensorineural Hearing Losses. The Calculation Will Be Slightly More Accurate if Based on Hearing Thresholds (dB HL) Obtained in the Sound Field Than on Those Obtained with Earphones. For Hearing Thresholds Shown Below the Lines at 3000 Hz and Higher Frequencies, the Gain May Not Assist in the Reception of Speech Sounds at Those Frequencies Even if the Speech Is Loud. For Those with Conductive Hearing Losses Gain Should Be Calculated (HTL$_{AC}$ − HTL$_{BC}$/5) and Added to the Values in the Table. After Berger et al. 1984.

HEARING THRESHOLD (dB HL)	FREQUENCY (Hz)					
	500	1000	2000	3000	4000	6000
20	0	13	13	12	11	10
25	5	16	17	15	13	13
30	9	19	20	18	16	15
35	13	22	23	21	18	18
40	17	25	27	24	21	20
45	21	28	30	26	24	23
50	25	31	33	29	26	25
55	27	34	37	32	29	28
60	30	38	40	35	32	30
65	32	41	43	38	34	33
70	35	44	47	41	37	35
75	37	47	50	44	39	
80	40	50	53	47	42	
85	42	53	57	50	45	
90	45	56	60	53		
95	47	59	63	56		
100	50	62	67	59		
105	52	66	70			
110	55	69	73			

Byrne and Tonisson procedure (1976; revised by Byrne 1978). The predictions of real-ear gain in the Byrne and Tonisson procedure are derived from the preferred listening levels of speech chosen by children with sensorineural hearing losses who were wearing their own hearing aids. Byrne and Fifield (1974) found that the real-ear gain needed to amplify speech to the preferred listening levels was the hearing threshold level multiplied by 0.46 (a little less than 0.5, the factor of the half-gain rule) plus an appropriate constant at each frequency. In the B&T procedure revised by Byrne (1978), this constant is the sum of three correction factors: (1) the difference in loudness experienced by normal-hearing individuals at different frequencies as reflected in the 60-phon equal loudness contour; (2) the difference between the long-term rms level of speech in specific frequency

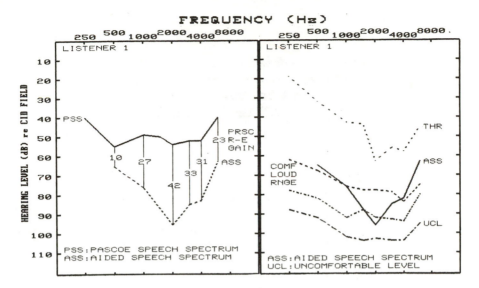

FIGURE 6.9. The aided speech spectrum prescribed for listener 1 by the Berger *et al.* procedure. In the left panel, the prescribed real-ear gain, denoted by the numbers on the vertical lines, has been added to the Pascoe speech spectrum to obtain the aided speech spectrum. In the right panel, this aided speech spectrum has been plotted in relation to the threshold, comfortable loudness range, and UCL contours for this listener.

regions (see the B&T speech spectrum in figure 6.1); and (3) additional gain (4 dB) needed to bring the overall level of speech to the preferred listening levels for normal-hearing individuals. These corrections are shown in table 6.2.

Calculations of real-ear gain prescribed by the B&T procedure for listener 1 are shown at the bottom of figure 6.11. The real-ear gain and the unaided and aided field thresholds are shown on the graph in the same figure. To simplify the procedure for clinical use with individuals with sensorineural hearing losses, the prescribed real-ear gain has been calculated as a function of frequency and hearing-threshold level as shown in table 6.3.

In figure 6.12 the real-ear gain calculated for listener 1 has been added to the Byrne and Tonisson and Pascoe speech spectra in the left and right panels, respectively, to obtain the aided speech spectra. The difference between these two speech spectra, both of which have been chosen to represent average conversational speech, is reflected in the aided speech spectra. When these aided spectra are plotted in relation to the auditory area of listener 1 (as shown in figure 6.13), the balance between the low- and high-frequency speech energy for the Byrne and Tonisson speech spectrum appears to follow the contour of the comfortable-loudness range reasonably

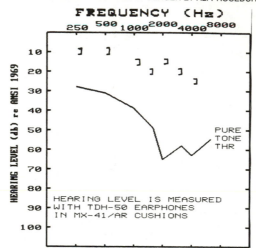

CALCULATIONS OF PRESCRIBED REAL-EAR GAIN FOR LISTENER WITH
CONDUCTIVE HEARING LOSS BY BERGER ET AL. PROCEDURE

FREQUENCY (Hz)

	500	1000	2000	3000	4000	6000
THRESHOLD (dB HL) (Earphones)	31	39	65	58	63	54
BONE-CONDUCTION THRESHOLDS (dB HL)	10	15	20	15	20	25
DIFFERENCE (dB) (AC-BC)	21	24	45	43	43	29
MULTIPLY BY 0.2	0.2	0.2	0.2	0.2	0.2	0.2
ADDITIONAL PRE-SCRIBED REAL-EAR GAIN (dB)	4.2	4.8	(9.0)	(8.6)	(8.6)	5.8
PRESCRIBED REAL-EAR GAIN FOR SN HEARING LOSS (dB)	10	27	42	33	31	23
TOTAL PRESCRIBED REAL-EAR GAIN (dB)	14	32	50	41	39	29

FIGURE 6.10. Calculations of real-ear gain prescribed by the Berger *et al.* procedure for listener 2, who has the same pure-tone thresholds as listener 1 but has a conductive instead of a sensorineural hearing loss. This listener's air-conduction and bone-conduction thresholds are shown on the audiogram (dB HL re ANSI S3.6-1969). According to this procedure no more than 8 dB additional gain is prescribed to compensate for the conductive hearing loss (see parentheses for the values at 2000, 3000 and 4000 Hz).

TABLE 6.2. **Correction Factors in Specific Frequency Regions for the 60-Phon Equal-Loudness Contour, the Long-Term rms Level of Speech Relative to the Real-Ear Gain at 1000 Hz, and Additional Gain Needed to Bring the Overall Level of Speech to the Preferred Listening Levels for Normal-Hearing Individuals. From Byrne and Tonisson 1976; Byrne 1978; Byrne 1983.**

	FREQUENCY (Hz)						
Correction Factors	250	500	1000	1500	2000	3000	4000
60-phon equal-loudness contour	−2	−4	0	0	−2	−7	−8
Average speech level	−17	−15	0	0	+1	+1	0
Additional gain	4	4	4	4	4	4	4
Total correction (dB)	−15	−15	4	4	3	−2	−2

well, whereas for the Pascoe speech spectrum there appears to be too much gain at 2000 Hz in relation to that at 500 Hz. It is important to realize that in evaluating the amount of real-ear gain prescribed by any procedure, the aided speech spectra depend on the specific speech spectrum used to represent conversational speech.

The Byrne and Tonisson procedure does not provide specific guidelines for calculating the additional gain needed for those with conductive hearing losses. From his experience Byrne (1983) suggests that Lybarger's one-quarter-gain formula is appropriate. That is, the amount of the conductive hearing loss (the air-conduction minus the bone-conduction threshold in decibels) is multiplied by 0.25, and this value is added to the real-ear gain obtained from table 6.3 for the air-conduction threshold at the appropriate frequency.

Byrne and Dillon procedure (1986).   Byrne and his colleagues at NAL have completed extensive studies to determine whether (1) the frequency-gain characteristics prescribed by the Byrne and Tonisson procedure did amplify low-, mid-, and high-frequency sound to comfortable loudness levels and (2) speech was more intelligible and sound quality more acceptable with the Byrne and Tonisson characteristics or with some other set of frequency-gain characteristics. The results of these studies indicated that for the majority of subjects the gain prescribed by the Byrne and Tonisson procedure was too little around 400 to 500 Hz compared to that at around 1250 Hz when the overall level of a broad-band sound was set at a comfortable loudness level. Furthermore, there was too much gain prescribed in the high frequencies relative to the mid and low frequencies for individuals with steeply sloping audiograms whose loss was predominantly in the high

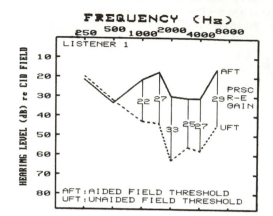

FIGURE 6.11. Calculations of real-ear gain and aided field thresholds for listener 1 prescribed by the Byrne and Tonisson procedure. The unaided and aided thresholds in the sound field are shown on the audiogram; the prescribed real-ear gain is denoted by the numbers on the vertical lines.

	FREQUENCY (Hz)							
	250	500	1000	1500	2000	3000	4000	6000
THRESHOLDS (dB HL) (Earphones)	29	31	39	49	65	58	63	54
MULTIPLY BY 0.46	0.46	0.46	0.46	0.46	0.46	0.46	0.46	0.46
	13	14	18	23	30	27	29	25
CORRECTION FACTORS	−15	−15	4	4	3	−2	−2	4
PRESCRIBED REAL-EAR GAIN (see Table 6-3)	−2	−1	22	27	33	25	27	29
UNAIDED FIELD THRESHOLDS (dB HL)	19	32	43	44	63	56	58	45
PRESCRIBED AIDED FIELD THRESHOLDS (dB HL)	21	33	21	17	30	31	31	16

frequencies (Byrne 1986a). Results of speech-recognition tests, speech-intelligibility ratings, and sound-quality ratings indicated that the frequency-gain characteristics prescribed according to the Byrne and Tonisson procedure were not optimal (Byrne 1986b).

Consequently, Byrne and Dillon have developed a new procedure to predict the real-ear gain needed to amplify the long-term rms levels of speech (Byrne and Dillon spectrum in figure 6.1) to MCL between 250 and 6000 Hz. The formulas they have derived are based on analyses of the relation between the slope of the audiogram and the slope of the optimal,

TABLE 6.3. Prescribed Real-Ear Gain as a Function of Hearing-Threshold Level for Frequencies 250 Through 6000 Hz from the National Acoustic Laboratories Aid Selection Table (Byrne and Tonisson 1976; Byrne 1978).

HEARING THRESHOLD (dB ISO)	250	500	1000	1500	2000	3000	4000	6000
0	−17	−15	4	4	3	−2	−2	4
5	−15	−12	7	7	6	1	1	7
10	−12	−10	9	9	8	3	3	9
15	−10	−8	11	11	10	5	5	11
20	−8	−6	13	13	12	7	7	13
25	−5	−3	15	15	14	9	9	15
30	−3	−1	18	18	17	12	12	18
35	−1	2	20	20	19	14	14	20
40	1	4	22	22	21	16	16	22
45	4	6	25	25	24	19	19	25
50	6	8	27	27	26	21	21	27
55	9	10	29	29	28	23	23	29
60	11	13	32	32	31	26	26	32
65	13	15	34	34	33	28	28	34
70	15	17	36	36	35	30	30	36
75	18	20	38	38	37	32	32	38
80	20	22	41	41	40	35	35	41
85	22	24	43	43	42	37	37	43
90	24	26	45	45	44	39	39	45
95	27	29	48	48	47	42	42	48
100	29	31	50	50	49	44	44	50
105	32	33	52	52	51	46	46	52

110 & over: benefit doubtful but table may be extended if desired.

real-ear frequency response of a hearing aid. The optimal response is defined as that which causes speech to be amplified to speech-band MCLs between 250 and 6000 Hz (Byrne 1984; Byrne 1986a), *or* that associated with the highest judged speech intelligibility (Byrne 1984; Byrne 1986a) or speech-recognition score (Levitt et al. 1978; Lippmann, Braida, and Durlach 1981; Skinner 1980). Linear regression analyses indicated that the response slope can be predicted reasonably well (within ±5 dB/octave; significant at the 0.05 level) from the audiogram slope (Byrne and Murray 1986). Therefore, regression equations from these analyses were used to derive the formulas for prescribing real-ear gain from supra-aural-earphone thresholds between 250 and 6000 Hz shown in table 6.4.

In these formulas the frequency-specific constants (e.g., −17 dB at 250 Hz in table 6.4) give the *relative*, real-ear gain at each frequency that the procedure predicts is optimal for someone with the same hearing threshold levels at all frequencies (dB HL). Note that the gain is maximal at 1000 and

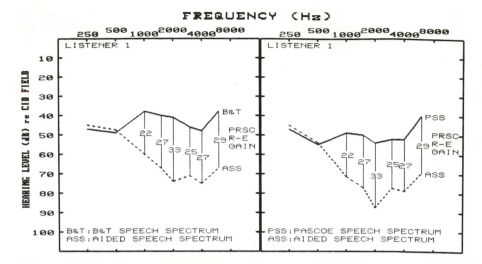

FIGURE 6.12. The aided speech spectrum prescribed for listener 1 by the Byrne and Tonisson procedure. In the left panel, the prescribed real-ear gain, denoted by the numbers on the vertical lines, has been added to the Byrne and Tonisson speech spectrum to obtain the aided speech spectrum. In the right panel, the prescribed real-ear gain has been added to the Pascoe speech spectrum to obtain the aided speech spectrum.

FIGURE 6.13. Two aided speech spectra, obtained by adding the real-ear gain prescribed by the Byrne and Tonisson procedure to the Byrne and Tonisson speech spectrum (left panel) and to the Pascoe speech spectrum (right panel), plotted in relation to the threshold, comfortable loudness range, and UCL contours of listener I.

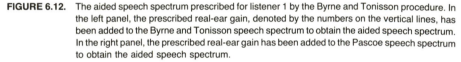

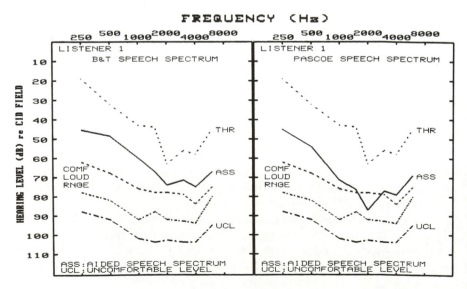

TABLE 6.4. **Formulas for Calculating Real-Ear Gain Prescribed at Specific Frequencies by the Byrne and Dillon Procedure When the Volume Wheel of the Hearing Aid Is Approximately 15 dB Below the Maximum Setting. Adapted from D. Byrne and H. Dillon 1986. "The National Acoustic Laboratories (NAL) New Procedure for Selecting the Gain and Frequency Response of a Hearing Aid." *Ear and Hearing* 7(4):257–65. Copyright 1986 by Williams and Wilkins. Reprinted with Permission of the Authors and Publisher.**

1. Calculate $X_{dB} = 0.05 \, (H_{500} + H_{1000} + H_{2000})$
    where H is the supra-aural earphone threshold (dB Hearing Level re the ISO standard) at the specified frequencies (Hz)

2. Calculate the prescribed real-ear gain (REG) at each frequency
REG_{250}	(dB) = $X + 0.31 \, H_{250}$	-17
REG_{500}	(dB) = $X + 0.31 \, H_{500}$	-8
REG_{750}	(dB) = $X + 0.31 \, H_{750}$	-3
REG_{1k}	(dB) = $X + 0.31 \, H_{1k}$	$+1$
$REG_{1.5k}$	(dB) = $X + 0.31 \, H_{1.5k}$	$+1$
REG_{2k}	(dB) = $X + 0.31 \, H_{2k}$	-1
REG_{3k}	(dB) = $X + 0.31 \, H_{3k}$	-2
REG_{4k}	(dB) = $X + 0.31 \, H_{4k}$	-2
REG_{6k}	(dB) = $X + 0.31 \, H_{6k}$	-2

1500 Hz, and that the gain in the low frequencies, especially at 500 Hz, is significantly more than in the Byrne and Tonisson procedure. The thresholds at specific frequencies are multiplied by a slope value of 0.31, the mean value from regression analyses of five studies for predicting the real-ear frequency response from the audiogram slopes (Byrne and Murray 1986). Since a wealth of clinical experience with the Byrne and Tonisson procedure indicated that hearing-aid wearers chose overall gain was very close to that prescribed (0.46 times the hearing threshold level), the formulas in the Byrne and Dillon procedure were adjusted so that the overall gain at 500, 1000, and 2000 Hz was the same as prescribed by the Byrne and Tonisson procedure.

Calculations of real-ear gain prescribed by the Byrne and Dillon procedure for listener 1 are shown at the bottom of figure 6.14. The real-ear gain and the unaided and aided field thresholds are shown on the graph in the same figure.

In figure 6.15 the real-ear gain calculated for listener 1 according to the Byrne and Dillon procedure has been added to the Byrne and Dillon and Pascoe speech spectra in the left and right panels, respectively, to obtain the aided speech spectra. When these aided speech spectra are plotted in relation to the auditory area of listener 1 (as shown in figure 6.16), the balance between the low- and high-frequency speech energy for the Byrne and Dillon speech spectrum appears to follow the contour of the comfortable loudness range reasonably well, whereas for the Pascoe speech spectrum there appears to be too much gain at 2000 Hz in relation to that at 500 Hz. In both cases the overall level falls below the comfortable loudness range.

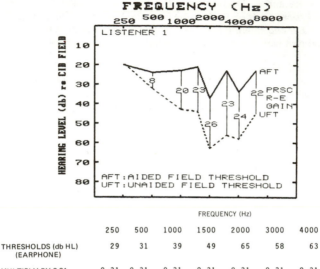

CALCULATIONS OF PRESCRIBED REAL-EAR GAIN BY THE BYRNE AND DILLON
PROCEDURE

	FREQUENCY (Hz)							
	250	500	1000	1500	2000	3000	4000	6000
THRESHOLDS (db HL) (EARPHONE)	29	31	39	49	65	58	63	54
MULTIPLY BY 0.31	0.31	0.31	0.31	0.31	0.31	0.31	0.31	0.31
	9.0	9.6	12.1	15.2	20.2	18.0	19.5	16.7
ADD OVERALL GAIN [0.05 (31 + 39 + 65)]	6.8	6.8	6.8	6.8	6.8	6.8	6.8	6.8
ADD FREQUENCY SPECIFIC CONSTANT (TABLE 6-4)	-17	-8	+1	+1	-1	-2	-2	-2
PRESCRIBED REAL-EAR GAIN (dB)	-1	8	20	23	26	23	24	22

FIGURE 6.14. Calculations of real-ear gain and aided field thresholds for listener 1 prescribed by the Byrne and Dillon procedure. The unaided and aided thresholds in the sound field are shown on the audiogram; the prescribed real-ear gain is denoted by the numbers on the vertical lines.

Byrne and Dillon have designed this procedure for those with mild to moderately severe sensorineural hearing losses. For those with conductive hearing losses, additional gain is needed at each frequency, equal to one-fourth of the difference between air-conduction and bone-conduction thresholds. If this procedure is used for those with severe or profound hearing losses, the real-ear gain will not be sufficient to make all speech sounds audible. In addition, it will not take into account amplifying only in frequency regions where there is useful hearing function.

Unaided speech-reception threshold. A widely used approximation of the half-gain rule to estimate the average gain needed in the mid-frequency range between 500 and 2000 Hz is based on the unaided speech-reception threshold (SRT; dB HL). The unaided SRT, usually obtained with earphones, is multiplied by 0.5 and the result is the average real-ear gain.

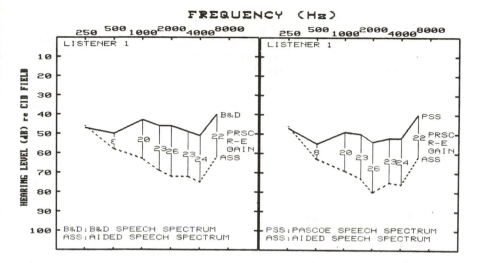

FIGURE 6.15. The aided speech spectrum prescribed for listener 1 by the Byrne and Dillon procedure. In the left panel, the prescribed real-ear gain, denoted by the numbers on the vertical lines, has been added to the Byrne and Dillon speech spectrum to obtain the aided speech spectrum. In the right panel, the prescribed real-ear gain has been added to the Pascoe speech spectrum to obtain the aided speech spectrum.

FIGURE 6.16. Two aided speech spectra, obtained by adding the real-ear gain prescribed by the Byrne and Dillon procedure to the Byrne and Dillon speech spectrum (left panel) and to the Pascoe speech spectrum (right panel), plotted in relation to the threshold, comfortable loudness range, and UCL contours of listener 1.

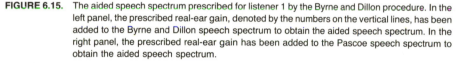

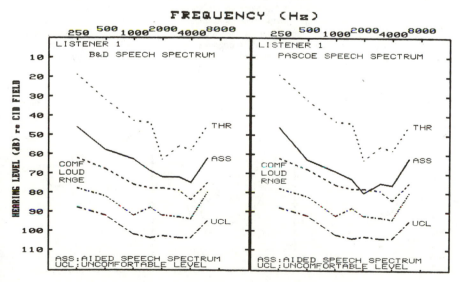

Procedures Based on MCL or ULCL Data

Pascoe procedure. In this procedure (Pascoe 1978; Skinner, Pascoe, Miller, and Popelka 1982) a hearing-impaired individual's preferred listening levels for speech are assumed to be a certain percentage of the difference between threshold and the midpoint of the comfortable loudness range between 500 and 4000 Hz. As described in the section above on the normal comfortable-loudness-level contour, this calculation of the preferred listening levels is intended to approximate the same relation between the speech spectrum and the MCL that normal-hearing individuals have. These preferred listening levels are the prescribed aided speech spectrum. At 250 and 6000 Hz the prescribed aided speech levels are 50 percent of the distance between an individual's threshold and her or his MCL, which is less than that for normal-hearing individuals (see figure 6.2). At 250 Hz this means that room noise is not amplified as much and therefore causes less upward spread of masking. At 6000 Hz, where the relevant acoustic cues for speech are often brief and the peak levels are higher than the average speech level, the speech energy is audible. It is hoped that the amplified sound in this frequency region does not cause excessive distortion in the ear and provides sound quality that is acceptable; if not, the gain can be reduced.

The estimate of where the aided speech spectrum should fall within the auditory area of listener 1 is shown in the left panel of figure 6.17. In the middle panel the real-ear gain, shown by the numbers on the vertical lines, represents the amount of gain needed to amplify the Pascoe speech spectrum to the aided speech spectrum. In the right panel the prescribed aided

FIGURE 6.17. The aided speech spectrum, real-ear gain, and aided thresholds prescribed by the Pascoe procedure for listener 1. **(A)** The aided speech spectrum is plotted in relation to the comfortable loudness range according to the criteria described in the text. **(B)** The aided speech spectrum is plotted on the same graph as the Pascoe speech spectrum; the numbers on the vertical lines denote the real-ear gain necessary to amplify speech to the aided speech spectrum. **(C)** The aided field thresholds were obtained by subtracting the real-ear gain, denoted by the numbers on the vertical lines, from the unaided sound-field thresholds.

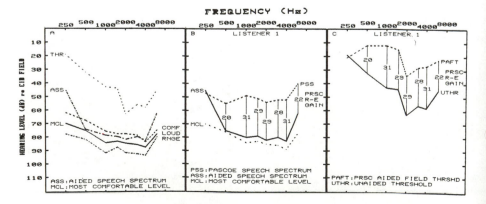

thresholds are derived by subtracting the real-ear gain at each frequency from the unaided field thresholds. Clinically, all this information can be plotted on the same audiogram form.

A computer program has been written by Popelka (1982, 1983-Hewlett-Packard version, available from CID) that facilitates the prescription of the aided speech spectrum, real-ear gain, and aided field thresholds. The actual steps in the calculation of these values are shown in figure 6.18. The calculations in panels A and B (including conversion of MCL to dB SL and multiplication by the Pascoe weights) allow one to place the aided speech spectrum within the listener's auditory area according to the criteria listed above.

Since this procedure is based on a direct determination of MCL, it is applicable to any hearing-impaired individual regardless of the degree of hearing loss or the sites of dysfunction along the auditory pathway. For example, no correction needs to be added for those with conductive hearing losses whose comfortable loudness range is elevated when compared to those with a cochlear hearing impairment (as shown in figure 2.7). If there is a neural component to the sensorineural hearing loss and the MCL is also elevated (see figure 2.7), this is measured directly and the needed real-ear gain prescribed.

Cox procedure. The preferred listening levels for speech in the Cox procedure (1983, 1985) are assumed to be at the midpoint of the range between the upper limit of comfortable loudness (ULCL) and threshold for individuals with a sensorineural hearing loss. This assumption is based on data from adults who adjusted the overall gain of hearing aids so that speech was most intelligible as well as comfortable for long periods of time (Cox and Bisset 1982). Their ULCLs were obtained with a descending procedure and the instructions given in chapter 5. Although Cox recommends using thresholds and ULCLs obtained with the individual's earmold and an insert receiver, sound-field data have been used for figure 6.19 so that the results can be compared with those of other procedures described in this chapter.

The thresholds and high MCLs of listener 1 are shown in panel A of figure 6.19. The high MCLs were obtained with the Pascoe ascending-descending-ascending, labeling procedure instead of with Cox's ULCL procedure. Consequently, they may not be the same as listener 1's ULCLs. However, they can serve to demonstrate the method by which Cox predicts

---

FIGURE 6.18. (overleaf, pp. 174–175). Calculations of the aided speech spectrum, real-ear gain, and aided thresholds prescribed by the Pascoe procedure for listener 1. **(A)** The calculation of MCL in dB SL is shown graphically and numerically. **(B)** The calculation of the aided speech spectrum, which is based on a multiplication of the MCL (dB SL) by a weighting factor and then converting this value from SL to HL, is shown graphically and numerically. **(C)** The calculation of the real-ear gain by subtracting the Pascoe speech spectrum from the aided speech spectrum is shown graphically and numerically. **(D)** The calculation of the aided field thresholds by subtracting the real-ear gain from the unaided field thresholds is shown graphically and numerically.

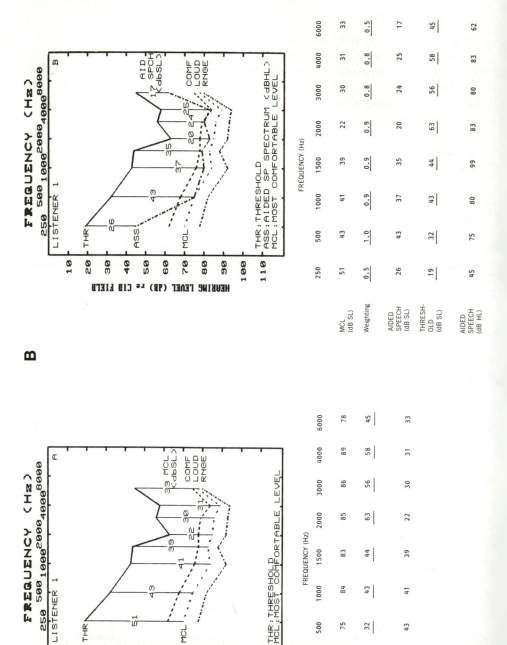

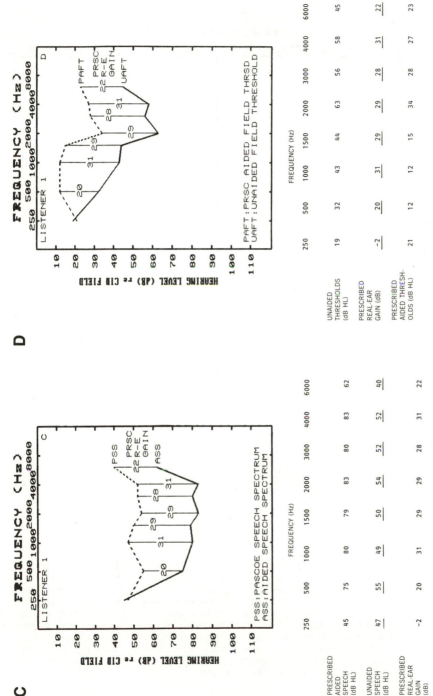

D

FREQUENCY (Hz)	250	500	1000	1500	2000	3000	4000	6000
UNAIDED THRESHOLDS (dB HL)	19	32	43	44	63	56	58	45
PRESCRIBED REAL-EAR GAIN (dB)	-2	20	31	29	29	28	31	22
PRESCRIBED AIDED THRESHOLDS (dB HL)	21	12	12	15	34	28	27	23

PAFT:PRSC AIDED FIELD THRSD
UAFT:UNAIDED FIELD THRESHOLD

C

FREQUENCY (Hz)	250	500	1000	1500	2000	3000	4000	6000
PRESCRIBED AIDED SPEECH (dB HL)	45	75	80	79	83	80	83	62
UNAIDED SPEECH (dB HL)	47	55	49	50	54	52	52	40
PRESCRIBED REAL-EAR GAIN (dB)	-2	20	31	29	29	28	31	22

PSS:PASCOE SPEECH SPECTRUM
ASS:AIDED SPEECH SPECTRUM

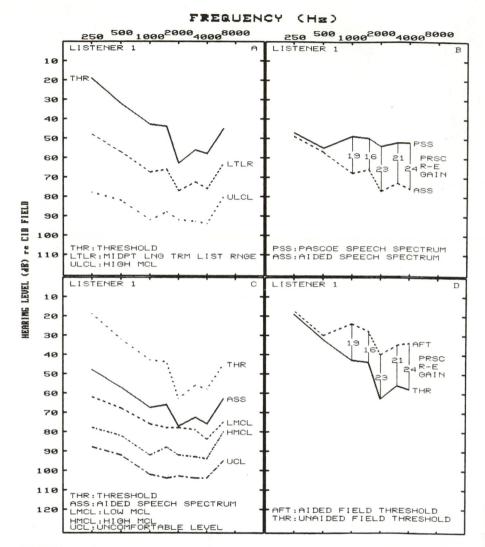

FIGURE 6.19. Calculation of the aided speech spectrum, real-ear gain, and aided field thresholds prescribed by the Cox procedure for listener 1. **(A)** The midpoint of the long-term listening range (LTLR), which is bounded by the threshold and high MCL contours (ULCL, or upper limit of comfortable loudness), is the prescribed aided speech spectrum (denoted by the dashed line). **(B)** The real-ear gain, denoted by the numbers on the vertical lines, is the difference between the unaided speech spectrum (these are the Pascoe values; the Cox values are within two dB of the Pascoe values, as shown in figure 6.1). **(C)** The aided speech spectrum is shown in relation to listener 1's threshold, comfortable loudness range, and UCL contours. **(D)** The aided field thresholds are obtained by subtracting the real-ear gain, denoted by the numbers on the vertical lines, from the unaided field thresholds.

real-ear gain. The dashed curve in panel A of figure 6.19 joins the midpoints of the range between threshold and ULCL (called the long-term listening range). These midpoints are the prescribed aided speech spectrum as shown in panel B. The real-ear gain needed to amplify the Pascoe speech spectrum to these midpoints is shown by the numbers within the vertical lines. The aided speech spectrum is shown in relation to the auditory area of listener 1 in panel C; note that it follows the contour of the range between low and high MCL (that is, the lowest and highest levels consistently labeled comfortable) except at 2000 Hz, where the threshold is particularly high, and this affected the midpoint level. The aided field thresholds are obtained by subtracting the real-ear gain from the unaided field thresholds. This is seen in panel D.

BASES FOR CHOOSING A PRESCRIPTIVE PROCEDURE

A prescriptive procedure should be chosen based on how well it meets the following two goals. The primary goal is to prescribe the *configuration* of real-ear gain in specific frequency regions that will be the best compromise between the most intelligible speech and acceptable sound quality in everyday life. As described in chapter 2, audibility, an effective bandwidth that is as wide as possible (between 250 and 6000 Hz), the appropriate balance between low- and high-frequency energy, and output limiting at UCL are the major factors contributing to maximally intelligible speech. The factor most closely related to the configuration of real-ear gain is the *balance* between the low- and high-frequency speech energy.

A second goal of prescriptive procedures is to specify the amount of *overall gain*. Since almost all hearing aids have a volume wheel with which the wearer can adjust the overall level over a 25- to 30-dB range, it is not critical that any procedure predict the overall gain exactly. However, if the procedure is based on substantially lower estimates of overall gain than are actually used, the configuration of real-ear gain may include more gain in the high frequencies (for people with greater hearing impairment in this region) than if higher estimates of overall gain were used. The converse of this is also true. Consequently, the amount of overall gain prescribed needs to be reasonably close to that used in everyday life. In addition, the aid that is recommended should have approximately 10- to 15-dB reserve gain above the setting at which moderate levels of broad-band sound are comfortable for the individual.

Research Results

Configuration of real-ear gain.   In recent years a number of investigators have explored the issue of what configuration of real-ear gain will make speech most intelligible for hearing-impaired individuals. For those with audiometric configurations that slope gently down toward the high frequencies, amplified speech is most intelligible when there is between 5 and 15 dB more gain at 2000 Hz than at 500 Hz (Pascoe 1975). For those with steeply sloping, high-frequency hearing losses who listen to speech at comfortable loudness levels, the real-ear gain at 2000 Hz should be at least 15 dB but no more that 35 dB higher than at 500 Hz; if it is greater than this, word-recognition scores decrease (Barfod 1972; Skinner 1980; Lippmann, Braida, and Durlach 1981). Other investigations with individuals with this same type of hearing loss have shown that these individuals prefer the sound quality of amplified speech when the real-ear gain at 2000 Hz is between 15 and 25 dB greater than that at 500 Hz (Punch and Beck 1980; Beck, Leatherwood, and Punch 1980; Punch and Beck 1986); the sound quality associated with larger differences is less acceptable.

If there is an inappropriate balance between the low- and high-frequency gain, the individual will set the overall gain at a comfortable loudness level and the speech energy will be at too low a level or inaudible in some parts of the spectrum. This is shown clearly in figure 2.11, where there is as much as a 30 percent decrease in word-recognition scores for those with steeply sloping hearing losses when the balance is inappropriate. In another example, adults with gently and steeply sloping hearing losses correctly identified significantly more words with their own hearing aids (fit according to the Pascoe procedure) than with a speech audiometer when the overall level of the speech was set to be most intelligible (Skinner et al. 1986).

For individuals with steeply sloping hearing losses who have normal or near-normal hearing either in the low frequencies (for example, 250 to 500 Hz) or high frequenices (for example 2000 Hz and above), speech will be most intelligible if there is sufficient gain in the frequency region of the steep slope. That is, the gain should emphasize the speech spectrum in the frequency region of the steep slope and extend at least a half octave toward the region of normal hearing. This hypothesis is based on research in which the gain at the steep slope was varied for people who have high-frequency (Barford 1972; Skinner 1980; Lippmann, Braida, and Durlach 1981) and low-frequency hearing losses (Collins 1985).

In a recent investigation the speech spectrum was amplified to each hearing-impaired individual's MCL contour and speech-recognition scores obtained for this condition for several different configurations of balance (between the low- and high-frequency gain) as well as overall level. Most performed best with the configuration of real-ear gain that caused the speech to be amplified to the MCL contour (Sullivan, Neuman, and Levitt 1983). In another investigation in which twelve elderly individuals were fitted with binaural experimental aids for which the bass-cut at 500 Hz could be adjusted over a 20-dB range both in the laboratory and in everyday use, these individuals preferred more gain at 500 Hz relative to that at 2000 Hz than was prescribed by the Byrne and Tonisson procedure (Leijon, Eriksson-Mangold, and Bech-Karlsen 1984). These findings are in agreement with those of Byrne (1984; 1986b) and Byrne and Murray (1986) mentioned earlier in this chapter, which led to the development of the Byrne and Dillon procedure. In a validation study of the Byrne and Dillon procedure with 44 people, most of them judged that speech was as intelligible or more so with the Byrne and Dillon-fitted hearing aid than with speech filtered according to other frequency-gain characteristics. The majority found the quality of speech in noise was as good with the Byrne and Dillon-fitted hearing aid as with the other filtered conditions or better. In addition, the gain chosen as comfortable agreed closely with the prescribed gain averaged over 500, 1000, and 2000 Hz (Byrne and Dillon 1986).

Overall gain.   There have been several studies of overall gain chosen by hearing-aid wearers as their preferred hearing levels. Among experienced hearing-aid wearers who have the same mean hearing threshold (i.e., 500, 1000, and 2000 Hz), the range chosen by individuals may differ 20 to 25 dB (Brooks 1973; Martin et al. 1976). This is reasonable in view of the range of MCLs for a given hearing threshold level (e.g., figures 5.10 and 6.3) and the differing amounts of loudness summation between individuals. Some studies have shown that people with mild to moderately severe sensorineural hearing losses on the average choose gain that is approximately half the mean hearing threshold level (for example, the validation study of Byrne and Dillon 1986; Skinner et al. 1986). In addition, the half-gain rule of Lybarger (1944) and the POGO procedure is based on this assumption. Other studies, such as that of Leijon, Ericksson-Mangold, and Beck-Karlsen (1984), indicate that some individuals choose real-ear gain that is less than half the mean hearing threshold level. The third-gain rule of Libby (1985a) is consistent with this assumption. Although a number of inexperienced hearing-aid wearers and those with mild to moderate sensorineural hearing impairment may choose volume wheel settings that are one-third of their mean hearing threshold, the research by Byrne and Dillon (1986) suggests that the half-gain rule reflects the use-gain of the majority of hearing-aid wearers better than the third-gain rule.

Examples of Prescribed Real-Ear Gain

In this section the real-ear gain prescribed for three individuals with different threshold configurations (steeply sloping, gently sloping, and flat), different comfortable loudness ranges, and different degrees of sensorineural hearing loss will be compared for the six procedures. Since these differences are shown clearly in figures in which the aided speech spectrum is plotted in relation to an individual's auditory area, the data will be presented in this form first and then in terms of the associated real-ear gain.

Listener 1.   The aided speech spectra prescribed by the POGO, Berger et al., Byrne and Tonisson, Byrne and Dillon, Pascoe, and Cox procedures are shown in relation to the threshold, comfortable loudness range, and

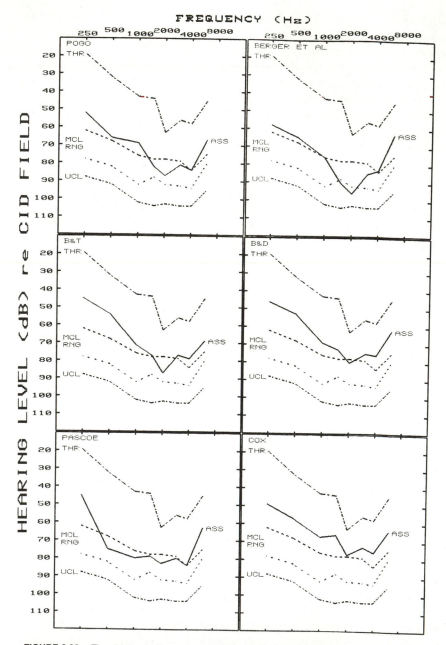

FIGURE 6.20.   The aided speech spectra prescribed by the POGO (1983), Berger *et al.* (1984), Byrne and Tonisson (B&T; 1976), Byrne and Dillon (B&D; 1986), Pascoe (1978), and Cox (1983) procedures shown in relation to the threshold, comfortable loudness range and UCL contours of listener 1. The Pascoe speech spectrum was added to the prescribed real-ear gain to obtain the aided speech spectra.

UCL contours of listener 1 in figure 6.20. This listener has a mild to moderate steeply sloping sensorineural hearing loss. The Berger et al. and Byrne and Tonisson procedures recommend 22 to 24 dB higher speech levels at 2000 Hz than at 500 Hz when compared with the Pascoe procedure. The POGO, Byrne and Dillon, and Cox procedures recommend 8 to 13 dB higher speech levels at 2000 Hz than at 500 Hz when compared with the Pascoe procedure. There are several reasons for these differences. First, for individuals with hearing thresholds that slope down toward higher intensities for the higher frequencies, such as listener 1, the prescriptions based on threshold data (POGO; Berger, et al.; Byrne and Tonisson; Byrne and Dillon; and to some extent Cox, since the preferred listening levels are the mean of the range between ULCL and threshold) prescribe more gain in the higher frequencies than the prescriptions based only on MCL data (Pascoe), the contour of which usually slopes more gently than that of the threshold contour. Second, as noted above, the Byrne and Tonisson speech spectrum has more energy at 500 Hz than at 2000 Hz compared to the Pascoe or Cox speech spectrum. This difference results in more gain prescribed at 2000 Hz by the Byrne and Tonisson procedure than by the Pascoe and Cox procedures. In the Berger et al. procedure proportionally more gain is prescribed at 2000 Hz than at any other frequency to adjust for the speech spectrum. A third reason for these differences is the Pascoe criterion of amplyfing the speech spectrum at 500 Hz to an individual's MCL. This results in more gain being prescribed at 500 Hz than with any other procedure. Consequently, there is less difference in gain between 500 and 2000 Hz for the Pascoe procedure than for others.

If the relation between the aided speech spectrum and the comfortable loudness range in figure 6.20 is examined, all the aided speech spectra enter the range of comfortable loudness in at least one frequency region except in the Cox procedure. In fact, in the Berger et al. prediction the speech spectrum at 2000 Hz surpasses the upper limit of comfort. For the Cox procedure the speech spectrum falls entirely below the comfortable loudness range.

The real-ear gain prescribed for listener 1 by each procedure is shown in figure 6.21. The difference in real-ear gain at 500 and 2000 Hz is shown by the number within the vertical line in each panel.

Listener 2. The aided speech spectra prescribed by the six procedures are shown in relation to the threshold, comfortable loudness range, and UCL contours of listener 2 in figure 6.22. This listener has a sensorineural hearing loss with an audiometric pattern that slopes more gently than that of listener 1. The Berger et al. and Byrne and Tonisson procedures prescribe 19 and 24 dB higher speech levels respectively at 2000 Hz than at 500 Hz, for the Byrne and Dillon procedure the speech level is 10 dB more at 2000 Hz than at 500 Hz, and for the POGO, Pascoe, and Cox procedures the

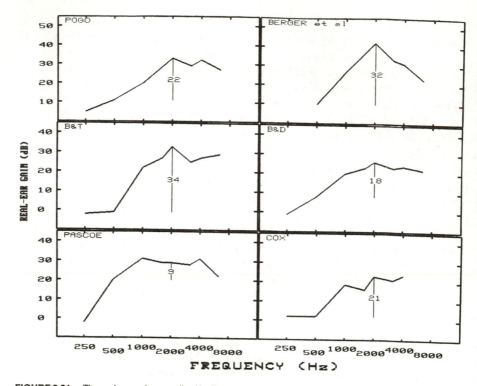

FIGURE 6.21.   The real-ear gain prescribed for listener 1 by the six procedures. The difference in gain between 500 and 2000 Hz is denoted by the numbers on the vertical lines.

speech levels are within ±5 dB at 2000 and 500 Hz. Because the slope of listener 2's threshold contour is less steep than listener 1's, the aided speech spectra for the POGO and Pascoe procedures are quite similar for listener 2 (see figure 6.20). The real-ear gain prescribed by each of the six procedures is shown in figure 6.23.

The comfortable loudness range and UCL contour for listener 2 are at lower HLs than for listener 1. For this reason, the aided speech spectra, except for the Cox spectrum, fall within or above the comfortable loudness range. The speech spectra for the threshold procedures (POGO, Berger et al. and Byrne and Tonisson) fall above the comfortable loudness range because these estimates of the preferred listening levels are based on average threshold data and not on measurements of MCL or UCL for the individual listener. For the Berger et al. prediction, listener 2 would probably turn down the overall gain because the aided speech spectrum is so close to the UCL contour at 2000 and 3000 Hz. For the Cox prediction this listener may find the overall level too low unless there is a significant amount of loudness

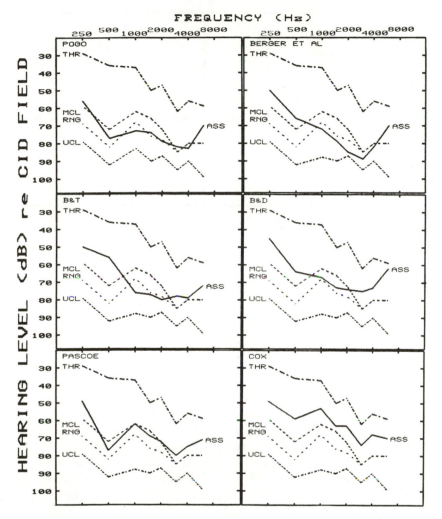

FIGURE 6.22.   The aided speech spectra prescribed by the six procedures are shown in relation to the threshold, comfortable loudness range, and UCL contours of listener 2.

summation. If there is significant loudness summation, the Pascoe proce-dure may prescribe too much overall gain.

Listener 3.   The aided speech spectra prescribed by the six procedures are shown in relation to the threshold, comfortable loudness range, and UCL contours of listener 3 in figure 6.24. This listener has a severe sensori-neural hearing loss with a flat audiometric configuration and approximately a 30-dB range between threshold and UCL. The Byrne and Dillon, Berger et al. and Byrne and Tonisson procedures prescribe 7, 13, and 19 dB higher

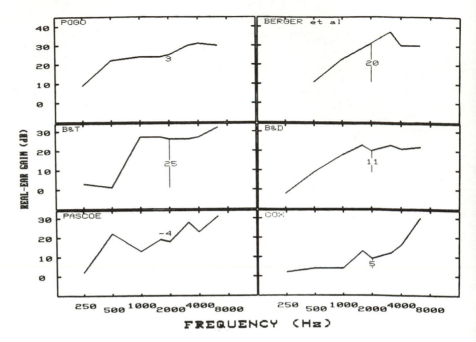

FIGURE 6.23.   The real-ear gain prescribed for listener 2 by the six procedures. The difference in gain between 500 and 2000 Hz is denoted by the numbers on the vertical lines.

speech levels, respectively, at 2000 Hz than at 500 Hz, whereas the speech levels are approximately the same (±5 dB) at 500 and 2000 Hz for the POGO, Cox, and Pascoe procedures. For this listener the balance between the low- and high-frequency energy becomes more critical than for those with larger dynamic ranges because if there is too much gain in the high frequencies (around 2000 Hz), the overall gain may have to be turned down to make the speech comfortable. This may cause the low-frequency speech energy to be close to threshold or inaudible. If this happens, it is likely that there will be a marked decrease in speech intelligibility. The real-ear gain prescribed by each of the six procedures is shown in figure 6.25.

For this severe hearing loss the POGO, Byrne and Tonisson, and Byrne and Dillon procedures predict aided speech spectra that are closer to threshold than to MCL in many frequency regions, and for the Byrne and Tonisson procedure the speech spectrum falls below threshold at 250 and 500 Hz (note that the real-ear gain was added to the Pascoe spectrum instead of the Byrne and Tonisson spectrum to obtain this aided spectrum). However, if the hearing aid has sufficient additional gain, this listener could adjust the overall level so that speech is heard at a comfortable level higher than that prescribed. This may also be necessary with the Cox prescription, unless there is a significant amount of loudness summation. If there is

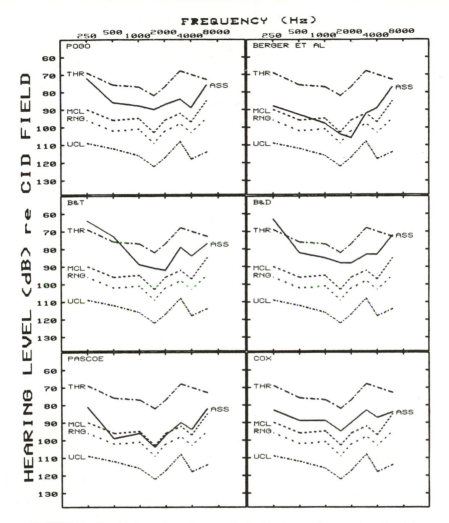

FIGURE 6.24. The aided speech spectra prescribed by the six procedures are shown in relation to the threshold, comfortable loudness range, and UCL contours for listener 3.

loudness summation, this listener may want to turn down the gain for the Pascoe or Berger et al. prescriptions.

Comparison of Prescriptive Procedures

Given the information that is available, the important clinical decision is what procedure to choose. There are several observations that can be made based on the research and examples described above and on a comparison of six threshold procedures made by Byrne (1987). These are

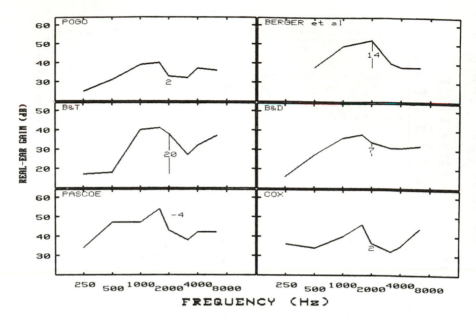

FIGURE 6.25.   The real-ear gain prescribed for listener 3 by the six procedures. The difference in gain between 500 and 2000 Hz is denoted by the numbers on the vertical lines.

1. The *Byrne and Tonisson* and *Berger et al.* procedures prescribe more gain at 2000 Hz relative to 500 Hz for all audiometric configurations than is optimal.

2. The *Pascoe* procedure prescribes more real-ear gain at 500 Hz than do all the other procedures; this gain probably needs to be reduced. In addition, the overall gain may need to be reduced to account for loudness summation.

3. The *POGO* procedure prescribes more gain at 2000 Hz relative to 500 Hz than is optimal for those with steeply sloping audiograms and greater loss in the high frequencies. It also prescribes less gain in the high frequencies than is optimal for those with low-frequency hearing loss and near-normal hearing in the high frequencies.

4. The *Byrne and Dillon* procedure prescribes less gain at 250 and 500 Hz than the Pascoe and Cox procedures for all audiometric configurations because of the differences in speech spectra on which these procedures are based.

5. The *Cox* procedure prescribes overall gain that may cause the aided speech spectrum to fall below the comfortable loudness levels at specific frequencies. With loudness summation this real-ear gain may make speech comfortably loud. If not, more overall gain may be needed.

6. The *Libby* (1985) procedure prescribes real-ear gain that is one-third of the hearing threshold level, with 3 and 5 dB less than this at 500 and 250 Hz. Less overall gain and less difference in gain as a function of change in audiogram slope is prescribed by this procedure than by any of the other threshold procedures.

7. The *Pascoe* and *Cox* procedures are based on direct judgments of comfortable loudness levels from individuals, and therefore they can be used with people with any etiology or amount of hearing impairment.

8. The threshold procedures can be used for those with sensorineural hearing impairment (and corrected for conductive impairment) with thresholds up to approximately 80 dB HL. The prescription of real-ear gain is based on average data instead of individual judgments of comfortable loudness levels.

9. The real-ear gain prescribed by any procedure may need to be modified. Several reasons for modifying the prescription are described in the next section. In addition, changes in the overall gain or the amount of low- or high-frequency gain may need to be made once the individual is evaluated with a hearing aid set for the prescribed characteristics.

The procedure that is chosen should prescribe a configuration of real-ear gain that is appropriate for the majority of individuals with hearing impairment. The proponents of MCL/ULCL procedures believe that the direct estimates of an individual's MCLs or ULCLs will give a better prediction of the configuration of real-ear gain than will using a threshold procedure that predicts preferred listening levels from average data. In some cases only thresholds are available, so preferred listening levels are estimated from average data. There are proponents of threshold procedures who point to the reliability and efficiency of basing a prescription on thresholds; however, there are data to support the reasonably good reliability of the Cox and Pascoe procedures for obtaining MCL and ULCL. In addition, the MCL/ULCL procedures are applicable to people with any etiology or amount of hearing impairment, whereas the threshold procedures are intended for those with up to moderately severe, sensorineural hearing impairment. All of these considerations need to be weighed by the individual clinician in choosing one or a combination of prescriptive procedures. After making this choice, it is important to know the limitations of a particular procedure, and, if necessary, to modify it for the hearing-impaired individual. In the future, further modifications or a change in procedure may be indicated based on clinical experience and/or research.

MODIFICATION OF PRESCRIBED REAL-EAR GAIN

It may be neither feasible nor advisable to try to find commercial hearing aids coupled with earmolds that will give the *exact* values of prescribed real-ear gain. The prescribed values may have to be modified to: (1) smooth the frequency response, (2) reduce the predicted gain at 3000 to 6000 Hz if it is much greater (for example, 15 to 30 dB) than at the lower frequencies, (3) reduce the difference in gain between 500 and 2000 Hz to less than or equal to 35 dB, (4) adjust the overall gain so that moderate sound levels are comfortably loud when the volume wheel is set at less than full, and (5) adjust the prescribed values for those with severe to profound hearing losses so that speech is audible but not markedly distorted by limiting.

An example of how the prescribed real-ear gain may need to be "smoothed" is shown in the bottom panel of figure 6.26 for listener 4, an

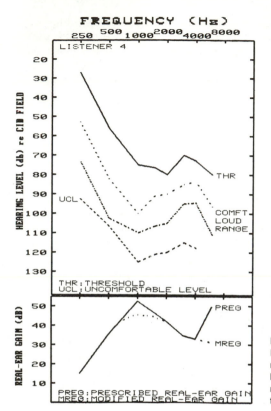

FIGURE 6.26.
Example of how the prescribed real-ear gain may need to be modified (bottom panel) for listener 4 whose threshold, comfortable loudness range and UCL contours are shown in the top panel.

individual whose threshold, comfortable loudness range, and UCL contours are shown in the top panel of the figure. The real-ear gain prescribed by the Pascoe procedure calls for 20 dB more gain at 1000 Hz than at 4000 Hz. If the gain at 1000 Hz is reduced 5 to 10 dB, the 30-dB range of speech will still be audible (so that speech intelligibility is not reduced), and the sound quality should be more acceptable. In addition, the prescription of 17 dB more gain at 6000 Hz than at 4000 Hz cannot be achieved with commercially available hearing aids, and it may cause more distortion than when less real-ear gain is used. Consequently, the gain at 6000 Hz should be reduced.

For individuals with steeply sloping hearing losses, the prescribed difference in real-ear gain between 500 and 2000 Hz may be greater than 35 dB. It is important to reduce this recommended difference in gain to less than 35 dB to avoid a decrease in speech intelligibility and unacceptable sound quality. An example of the prescribed speech spectrum and the recommended speech spectrum for an individual with a noise-induced hearing loss are shown in figure 6.27 (listener 5). Note that the recommended speech spectrum is such that there is additional energy at the steep slope of the threshold contour but the energy above 3000 Hz is inaudible.

Individuals with severe or profound sensorineural hearing losses often have a small range between threshold and UCL, as shown by the threshold and UCL contours for listener 6 in figure 6.28. With a dynamic range between 15 and 25 dB, it is impossible to amplify the 30-dB range of speech spoken at one vocal effort so that it is all audible unless a compression hearing aid is used. For this individual the maximum acoustic output must be limited at or slightly below the UCL contour and the prescribed aided speech spectrum should be approximately halfway between threshold and UCL. This compromise makes the speech audible but may result in some distortion when the aided speech level is less than 12 dB below UCL at a specific frequency. If speech energy is audible out to 4000 or 6000 Hz and there is enough residual hearing to process this information, the person will be able to understand speech more readily and monitor his or her own speech more accurately.

FIGURE 6.27. The prescribed and recommended aided speech spectra shown in relation to the threshold, comfortable loudness range, and UCL contours of listener 5. In the left panel, the aided speech spectrum was calculated by adding the Pascoe speech spectrum to the real-ear gain prescribed by the POGO procedure; the difference in real-ear gain between 500 and 2000 Hz is 39 dB. In the right panel, the recommended aided speech spectrum is very close to that associated with the highest word-identification score this listener obtained on the Pascoe High-Frequency Word List when tested with forty different combinations of frequency-gain characteristics and overall gain (Skinner 1980); the difference in real-ear gain between 500 and 2000 Hz is 20 dB.

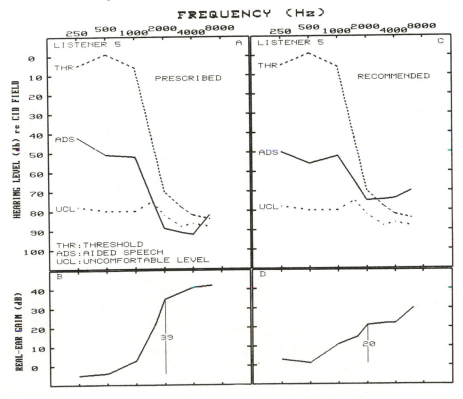

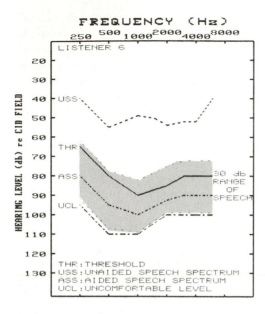

FIGURE 6.28.
The recommended aided speech spectrum for listener 6, who has a severe sensorineural hearing loss and a dynamic range of 15 to 25 dB. The aided speech spectrum is placed so that it is approximately halfway between the threshold and UCL at each frequency. The 30-dB range of speech includes the variation in level associated with the long-term rms level. This range, which is denoted by the shaded area, should extend approximately 18 dB below and 12 dB above the long-term rms level. In this case the upper bound of this 30-dB range would exceed this listener's UCL contour and consequently needs to be output limited. Although this may cause some distortion, it is an important compromise that must be made to make the speech audible and at a level at which the listener can best perceive the acoustic cues.

For some individuals there is no measurable hearing at the limits of the audiometer for some or all of the frequencies between 250 and 8000 Hz. Some clinicians select and adjust hearing aids to provide gain mainly at the frequencies at which responses were obtained with the audiometer. For example, some individuals with profound hearing losses and audiometric thresholds only at 125, 250, and 500 Hz have been fitted with powerful, low-frequency hearing aids. This fitting is based on the rationale that amplification should be concentrated in the frequency region at which there is some residual hearing and that trying to amplify the higher frequencies, so that they are audible, will overdrive the cochlea, cause distortion, and generate acoustic feedback. Other clinicians believe that a powerful, broad-band hearing aid should be tried. With this aid they want to determine whether (1) aided thresholds can be obtained for frequency-specific sounds in regions at which there was no response under earphones and (2) the amplified sound with the broad-band hearing aid is more useful in everyday life than with an aid that has a narrower bandwidth. Because both views are reasonable, both types of aids may be tried if sufficient time is available and the person is willing to try them.

SUMMARY

The prescriptive approach to preselecting and adjusting hearing aids is based on specified criteria that can be verified. For this reason, this approach is recommended instead of a comparative approach for preselecting aids.

The usefulness of the comparative approach for evaluating several aids chosen by the prescriptive approach will be described in chapter 9.

Six prescriptive procedures (POGO; Berger et al.; Byrne and Tonisson; Byrne and Dillon; Pascoe; and Cox) were described in this chapter. All these procedures prescribe aided speech spectra that fall within an individual's auditory area, but the overall level and the balance between low-frequency (around 500 Hz) and high-frequency (around 2000 Hz) speech energy differs.

A description of this balance in the configuration of real-ear gain prescribed by each of the procedures is summarized in the section, "Comparison of Prescriptive Procedures." There are also descriptions of some arguments for and against a threshold or a MCL/ULCL procedure. This information needs to be considered in choosing one or a combination of prescriptive procedures. After making a choice, it is important to know the limitations of a particular procedure. Modifications in the prescribed real-ear gain may be needed to adjust for ways in which a particular procedure does not prescribe an optimal response, smooth the frequency response, reduce gain at 3000 to 6000 Hz, or adjust for individual needs. In the future, further modifications or a change in procedure may be indicated based on clinical experience and/or research.

Chapter Seven
CRITERIA FOR PRESCRIBING MAXIMUM ACOUSTIC OUTPUT (SSPL90)

The maximum acoustic output of a hearing aid varies as a function of frequency. On many aids the overall output can be adjusted over approximately a 20-dB range. As described in chapter 4, the maximum acoustic output of a hearing aid is measured by presenting tones at 90 dB SPL and measuring the output in a 2-cc coupler. This output is called the *saturation sound-pressure level*, or SSPL90. The reference point for this measurement is the microphone in the coupler. It is important to note that this reference point is different from that for the calibration of supra-aural earphones, with which many UCL measurements are obtained. Consequently, correction factors must be used to compare UCLs obtained with supra-aural earphones directly with the SSPL90 of a hearing aid. Direct comparison can be made when insert earphones are used to obtain UCLs and the output of the earphone and hearing aid are both calibrated in an HA-1, 2-cc coupler.

For an individual to derive the most benefit from a hearing aid, the SSPL90 should be adjusted so that amplified sound does not become uncomfortably loud when the volume wheel is set to hear speech at a comfortable level. This chapter will describe factors considered in prescribing the SSPL90 for an individual and procedures for prescribing it.

FACTORS CONSIDERED IN PRESCRIBING SSPL90

Relation of Amplified Sound to Individual's Auditory Area

Amplified sound.   Hearing aids amplify sound between approximately 200 and 6000 Hz. Within this range the sounds in our world can occur over a large range of intensities (approximately 160 dB). Many of the sounds of importance to us occur between approximately 30 and 90 dB SPL. Environmental sounds provide many clues to what is happening in the world around us. Some of them, when amplified, can be irritating (for example, silverware clinking, wind rushing, the babble of many people talking) or uncomfortable (for example, a door slamming, an airplane flying overhead). The irritation may be reduced by choosing a hearing aid with low distortion and adjusting the frequency response so that the sound quality is acceptable. The discomfort and distortion can be minimized if the SSPL90 is set appropriately.

When speech is amplified with a hearing aid, the level reaching the microphone may be as low as 40 dB SPL (very soft conversational speech) or as high as 85 dB SPL (very loud conversational speech or the voice of the person who is wearing an ear-level aid). The average level of speech spoken to a normal-hearing person is about 60 dB SPL at the ear. Speech spoken to someone with a hearing loss is usually a little louder (70 dB SPL).

As described in chapter 2 (see figure 2.2), the level of speech in specific frequency regions varies over a 30-dB range when someone is speaking at a constant overall level (for example, at an average level of 70 dB SPL). For speech to be most intelligible, it must be audible and not uncomfortably loud. Consequently, as much as possible of the 30-dB range of speech energy should be amplified so that it is audible and not uncomfortably loud.

Individual's auditory area.   The auditory area covers the region between threshold and UCL, which is the dynamic range, and between 250 to 6000 Hz, which is the frequency range. An individual's dynamic range may be quite wide (60 to 80 dB) or quite narrow (5 to 10 dB); in addition, this range may vary as a function of frequency. If other people's speech is amplified so that its average spectrum is close to the MCL contour, the upper level of the 30-dB range will fall well below the UCL contour of listener A (figure 7.1A), who has a wide dynamic range. It will fall just below and above the UCL contour of listener B (figure 7.1B), who has a narrow dynamic range. If the SSPL90 is set at the UCL contour for these two people, the contour representing the highest levels of the speech range does not reach the SSPL90 for listener A but exceeds it for listener B between 1000 and 6000 Hz. If the speech spectrum of an individual's own voice is amplified at a

FIGURE 7.1.   Relation of amplified speech to the auditory area of two listeners with sensorineural hearing losses. **(A)** The threshold (THR) and UCL contours for listener A have been plotted in relation to the long-term average level of the aided speech spectrum (ASS). The vertical lines represent the 30-dB range of the speech energy at each of the measured frequencies. This speech represents that spoken by other people to listener A. **(B)** The same information is plotted for listener B.

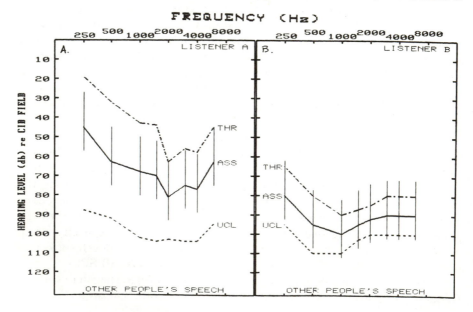

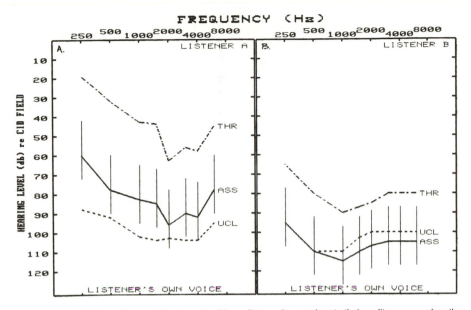

FIGURE 7.2. Relation of the amplified speech of these listeners' own voices to their auditory areas when the volume wheel of a hearing aid is set to amplify other people's speech to MCL. **(A)** The threshold and UCL contours of listener A plotted in relation to this aided speech spectrum. **(B)** The same information plotted for listener B.

gain setting chosen to make other people's speech comfortable, the overall level at the hearing aid microphone is approximately 15 dB higher. In figure 7.2 the aided speech spectrum for listener A's and listener B's own voices are plotted on the same graph as their threshold and UCL contours. For listener A, only the energy at 2000 Hz surpasses UCL, whereas for listener B, much of the energy would surpass UCL if the SSPL90 were set high enough.

Range of Possible SSPL90 Levels

For an individual with a wide dynamic range it may be feasible to set the SSPL90 of an aid at any level between a minimum at the upper level of the amplified speech contour and a maximum at the UCL contour (see listener A's data in figure 7.3A). With the aid set at the minimum SSPL90 setting, other people's speech is relatively undistorted and louder sounds are limited well below UCL; however, listener A's own speech would be distorted. To prevent this distortion, the SSPL90 would need to be set higher. If an individual has a dynamic range of 30 dB or less, like listener B, then the maximum and minimum SSPL90 settings would be the same (see figure 7.3B), to prevent sounds from being uncomfortably loud.

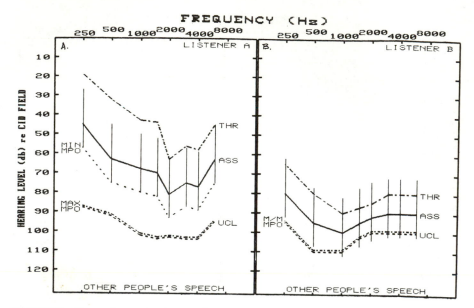

FIGURE 7.3. The maximum acoustic output (MPO, which is another name for SSPL90) of a hearing aid set at minimum and maximum levels and plotted in relation to the amplified speech spectrum and the listeners' UCL contours. **(A)** The minimum MPO is set at the highest level of the 30-dB range of speech, and the maximum MPO is set at the UCL contour for listener A. **(B)** The minimum and maximum MPO are both superimposed on the UCL contour; this is caused by the small dynamic range of listener B.

Loudness Summation

When the SSPL90 of a hearing aid is set based on UCLs measured for frequency-specific stimuli, no allowance is made for the loudness summation most hearing-impaired individuals experience when listening to broadband sound. Consequently, the SSPL90 may need to be reduced to prevent loud, broad-band amplified sound such as speech from being uncomfortably loud. Since there is no clinically efficient way to determine an individual's loudness summation, the SSPL90 is usually set to limit the amplified sound at or below the UCL contour. After putting on the hearing aid, the person adjusts the volume wheel so that speech spoken at a conversational level is comfortably loud. Then speech and other broad-band sounds are presented at 85 to 90 dB SPL; if they are uncomfortably loud the SSPL90 is reduced. If hearing aids are fitted at both ears, the SSPL90 of both aids may need to be reduced because of the binaural summation of loudness. For these reasons, hearing aids that are preselected should have SSPL90s that can be reduced to allow for monaural and binaural summation effects.

Relation Between UCL and SSPL90

Criterion for UCL.   As described in chapter 5, an individual sets a criterion for UCL based on the instructions given and an internal interpretation of these instructions. People sensitive to loud sound tend to choose low UCLs; others who are less sensitive choose substantially higher UCLs. Their choices are also affected by the spectral, temporal, and amplitude characteristics of the signal, the testing procedure, and prior experience with amplified sound. Although a hearing aid may be adjusted in the clinic to prevent sounds from being intolerably loud, the SSPL90 may need to be adjusted either up or down as the individual adapts to the amplified sounds of everyday life.

Calibration of signal for obtaining UCL.   Clinically, UCLs are obtained with supra-aural earphones, in the sound field, and with insert receivers. As described in chapter 4, the lack of a common reference point for sound calibration makes it inaccurate to compare the SPL value for UCLs from a supra-aural earphone (or sound field) directly with the SSPL90 of a hearing aid. However, one can directly compare the UCL (dB SPL) obtained with an insert earphone with the SSPL90 of an aid, if both are calibrated in an HA-1, 2-cc coupler. With this coupler the output of in-the-ear and in-the-canal aids, as well as other aids attached to the individual's earmold, can be measured.

In chapter 5, one method is described for using correction factors to convert UCLs (dB SPL) obtained under earphones to UCLs (dB SPL) referred to the 2-cc coupler so that they can be compared directly with the SSPL90 of a hearing aid. With this method the UCLs (dB sensation level) are added to the unaided thresholds in the field to obtain UCLs in dB SPL referred to the sound-field calibration. Then a stock hearing aid is chosen, the volume wheel set so the overall level of speech is at MCL, and aided thresholds are obtained. The functional gain (FG) is calculated by subtracting the aided from the unaided thresholds at the audiometric frequencies. Without changing any of the hearing aid settings, the coupler gain (CG) of the hearing aid is measured. Then the following equation is used to calculate the UCL (dB SPL) referred to the 2-cc coupler:

$$\text{UCL}_{field} + \text{Head Baffle} - \text{FG} + \text{CG}_{linear} = \text{UCL}_{\text{HA-1 coupler}}$$

Average values for the head baffle effect associated with the position of the microphone for behind-the-ear, in-the-ear, in-the-canal, and body hearing aids are given in table 5.7. After these calculations are made at each frequency, the SSPL90 of the test aid is adjusted so that it is at or below the UCLs. Although these calculations can be done quickly with a computer, it is more efficient to use an insert receiver because the UCLs (dB SPL) are directly comparable with the SSPL90 of the hearing aid. Therefore, they can be used to set the SSPL90 of the hearing aid before aided thresholds are obtained. In addition, possible inaccuracies in using functional and coupler gain as correction factors are avoided.[1]

Frequency-specific adjustment of SSPL90.   On most commercial hearing aids the potentiometer for adjusting the SSPL90 causes a change in the output that is essentially equal at all frequencies. The highest level to which the SSPL90 can be set without exceeding the individual's UCLs is dependent on the frequency or frequencies at which the SSPL90 is closest to the individual's UCL. If this frequency is at the 1-kHz resonant peak caused by the earhook and earmold tubing, then an acoustic damper can be placed in the earhook to lessen or eliminate it. Then the SSPL90 may be raised so that all frequencies are closer to the UCL contour without the amplified sound becoming uncomfortably loud.

PROCEDURES FOR PRESCRIBING SSPL90

The SSPL90 of a hearing aid can be prescribed based on direct measures of UCL for speech and frequency-specific sounds or on estimates of UCL derived from threshold data and the amount of any conductive component to the hearing loss.

Prescribed SSPL90 Based on Direct Measures of UCL

Most adults and children who are able to understand the instructions and procedures can judge when sounds are definitely uncomfortable. These judgments are the basis for a number of procedures for prescribing the SSPL90 of hearing aids. The criterion for judging UCL, the procedure, the transducer for obtaining UCL and its calibration, the stimuli, and correction factors for eight procedures are described in table 7.1.

The clinical procedure used most widely in the United States is that of Berger, Hagberg, and Rane (1984). In this procedure it is assumed that the calibration of the output of the supra-aural earphone in a 6-cc coupler is equivalent to the calibration of the hearing aid output in a 2-cc coupler; that is, the calibrated SPL represents the same level at the person's eardrum for both the supra-aural earphone and the hearing aid. For this reason, the UCL is converted from dB HL to dB SPL by using the ANSI (S3.6-1969) calibration values for supra-aural earphones. As shown in table 4.2, this conversion

---

[1]The measured functional gain may be lower than the actual functional gain if the ambient noise of the room or the noise floor of the hearing aid are above threshold. For hearing aids with automatic-gain-control circuits, it may be impossible to obtain an estimate of the linear gain; to get an accurate value would necessitate a complex computer interface and program to use the appropriate hearing aid input-output values.

TABLE 7.1. Procedures for Prescribing Maximum Acoustic Output (SSPL90) of Hearing Aids from UCLs or ULCL.

AUTHORS	UCL CRITERIA	PROCEDURE	TRANSDUCER	STIMULI	CORRECTION FACTORS
Berger, Hagberg, and Rane (1984)	When sounds first become uncomfortably loud	Start at level halfway between threshold and 110 dB HL. Level raised 5 dB every 5 seconds until UCL or audiometer limits reached.	Supra-aural earphones calibrated in 6-cc coupler (speech and tones measured in dB SPL and converted to dB HL)	Speech (person speaking or reading)	
				Pulsed pure tones	*Maximum SSPL90 setting in dB SPL re 2-cc coupler*
				500 Hz	UCL (dB HL) + 11 dB (or 115 dB SPL; the lower one)
				1000 Hz	UCL (dB HL) + 7 dB
				2000 Hz	UCL (dB HL) + 9 dB
				4000 Hz	UCL (dB HL) + 9 dB
					Minimum SSPL90 setting
				500 Hz	Real-ear gain + 75 dB
				1000 Hz	Real-ear gain + 75 dB
				2000 Hz	Real-ear gain + 72 dB
				4000 Hz	Real-ear gain + 70 dB
POGO (McCandless and Lyregaard 1983)	Uncomfortably loud to listen to for any length of time	Not stated	Supra-aural earphones calibrated in a 6-cc coupler (tones measured in dB SPL and converted to dB HL)	Pure tones: 500, 1000, 2000 Hz	UCL (dB HL) at 500 + 1000 + 2000 Hz/ 3 + 4 dB = Mean SSPL90 (dB SPL)
Leijon (1983)	Sounds are uncomfortably loud	Not stated	Supra-aural earphones calibrated in a 6-cc coupler (tones measured in dB SPL and converted to dB HL)	Pure tones	UCL with corrections from 6-cc coupler for earphone to 2-cc coupler for hearing aid output; SSPL90 less if this setting does not distort person's own voice

(continued)

TABLE 7.1. (Continued)

AUTHORS	UCL CRITERIA	PROCEDURE	TRANSDUCER	STIMULI	CORRECTION FACTORS
Pascoe (1978, 1980, 1986)	Sounds judged to be "too loud"	Loudness of sounds rated on a scale between too soft and too loud. See chapter 5 for more complete description of this procedure.	Supra-aural earphones calibrated in 6-cc coupler (tones measured in dB SPL and converted to dB HL)	Pulsed pure tones: 250, 500, 1000, 1500, 2000, 3000, 4000, and 6000 Hz	See Chap 5. for correction factors to express UCL in dB SPL re 2-cc coupler; SSPL90 should be 3 dB lower than UCL or 15 dB above aided speech level, whichever is lower
Byrne (1978)	Not stated	Not stated	Insert earphone and person's earmold calibrated with 1" of #13 tubing on 2-cc coupler (dB SPL)	Pulsed pure tones: 500, 1000, 2000 Hz and frequency of peak of hearing aid SSPL90 contour if different	UCL (dB SPL) − 5 dB if dynamic range > 35 dB; UCL if dynamic range <25 dB
Cox (1981b)	Lowest level which they would not tolerate even for sounds lasting a few seconds	Sound increased in 5 dB steps until UCL reached; decrease 10, 15, or 20 dB and increase in 5-dB steps until UCL reached; repeat until no further elevation in UCL. UCL is the highest level chosen in two out of three trials.	Insert earphone and person's earmold calibrated with 25 mm of #13 tubing on 2-cc coupler (dB SPL)	Pulsed pure tones: 500, 1000, 2000 Hz	UCL (dB SPL) + 3 dB + insert receiver correction or lower

Reference	Measure/Definition	Procedure	Calibration	Stimuli	Conversion
Cox (1983)	ULCL. (dbSPL)	Present 4 or 5 pulses of a tone at each level. Start at a level that is loud and descend in 5-dB steps to the first level that is comfortable. ULCL is highest level in two out of three trials.	Insert earphone and person's earmold calibrated with 25 mm of #13 tubing on an HA-2, 2-cc coupler (dBSPL)	Pulsed $\frac{1}{3}$-octave bands of noise or pure tones: 250, 500, 800, 1600, and 4000 Hz 1000 Hz 2500 Hz	ULCL. + dB12 = SSPL90 ULCL + 10 dB = SSPL90 ULCL + 17 dB = SSPL90
Hawkins (1980a)	Sound is definitely uncomfortable; it is louder than they would want to listen to even briefly.	Békésy audiometer— individual presses button when sound is uncomfortable and releases it when it is loud. Intensity increases and decreases automatically.	Insert earphone and person's earmold calibrated with 25 mm of #13 tubing on an HA-2, 2-cc coupler (dB SPL).	Pulsed pure tones: 250, 500, 1000, 2000, 4000 Hz	UCL (dB SPL) = SSPL90

is inaccurate because the difference (dB) between the average SPL in the 6-cc coupler and at the eardrum is not the same as the difference between the average SPL in the 2-cc coupler and at the eardrum. In addition, no allowance is made for differences between hearing aid output and supra-aural-earphone output at the individual's eardrum caused by leaks around the supra-aural earphone or by the earmold coupling of the hearing aid and the acoustic immittance at the eardrum. For these reasons, the prescribed SSPL90 may be higher or lower than the individual's UCLs. These authors include frequency-specific estimates of SSPL90. In addition, they have described the concept of a minimum and a maximum setting of SSPL90, with the minimum setting such that loud speech is not distorted.

POGO (Prescription of Gain/Output for Hearing Aids) is the second procedure described in table 7.1. With this procedure a mean SSPL90 is prescribed based on UCLs for pure tones in the frequency range (500 to 2000 Hz) at which the highest output of commercially available hearing aids is found. The correction from dB HL to dB SPL includes not only the ANSI calibration values (S3.6-1969) for earphones but other adjustments that the authors do not describe. Their value is 5 dB lower than the average maximum SSPL90 setting suggested by Berger, Hagberg, and Rane (1984), if it is assumed that the tones were pulsed and the same UCL criterion and procedure were used.

The procedures by Leijon (1983) and Pascoe (1980) include a correction for the difference in the SPL at the eardrum between UCL obtained with a supra-aural earphone and that with hearing aid and earmold. Both procedures recommend setting the SSPL90 below UCL, if the dynamic range is wide enough. For the Pascoe procedure, the minimum setting is chosen, to prevent distortion of other people's speech; that is, the SSPL90 is set so that it is at least 15 dB above the long-term speech spectrum at all frequencies. For the Leijon procedure, the minimum SSPL90 is set so that the individual's own speech is not distorted.

The last four procedures described in table 7.1 are based on direct measures of UCL with an insert earphone. Use of the insert earphone and the earmold that will be worn with the hearing aid gives a much closer approximation of the individual's UCLs to the SSPL90 of a hearing aid measured with a 2-cc coupler than the Berger, Hagberg, and Rane and POGO methods do. Although the acoustic immittance of the insert earphone used for testing may be different from that of a given hearing aid, the resulting differences in dB SPL usually amount to only 1 to 2 dB.

In the procedure described by Byrne (1978), the maximum SSPL90 at UCL is recommended for those with dynamic ranges of less than 25 dB and a minimum SSPL90 at 5 dB below UCL for those with dynamic ranges greater than 35 dB. He also recommends measuring UCL for the frequency at the peak SSPL90, if it is not one of the usual test frequencies.

The two procedures by Cox (1981b, 1983) have different UCL criteria and test protocols. In the earlier one (1981b), 3 dB is added to the UCL because the level chosen on the first day of testing is usually lower than that obtained on subsequent days. In the later one (1983), the ULCL is obtained and average correction values are used to estimate UCL.

In the procedure by Hawkins (1980a) the SSPL90 is set at UCL for the audiometric frequencies between 250 and 4000 Hz. If UCL is measured with speech, Hawkins (1983) suggests that this corresponds to the UCLs between 500 and 1000 Hz. The initial setting of the SSPL90 is changed if loud speech (85 to 90 dB SPL), spoken while the person wears the aid set at the highest volume-wheel setting without acoustic feedback, is uncomfortably loud. As an alternative to delivering sound with an insert earphone, Hawkins (1985) has described a procedure for using a high-output, linear-gain hearing aid, attached to the individual's own earmold, for obtaining UCLs.

Each of the procedures described above is useful in setting the initial SSPL90; some are more exact and/or efficient for prescribing this initial setting than others. By choosing aspects of several, the following procedure is recommended for individuals who can give reliable UCL estimates. Ask the person to label the loudness of the sounds on a scale from "okay" to "too loud." Present pulsed, pure tones in several ascending series (in 5-dB steps) at each audiometric frequency until the same level is judged too loud at least twice; this level is the UCL. Use an insert earphone (calibrated with the HA-1, 2-cc coupler used for measuring the SSPL90 of the hearing aid) and the person's own earmold (or a temporary mold and tubing similar to the one that will be made). Set the SSPL90 of the hearing aid at UCL (for the frequency at which they are closest) for individuals with dynamic ranges that are narrow (less than 25 dB) and 5 dB below UCL for those whose dynamic ranges are greater than 35 dB. Have the person put on the hearing aid and set the volume wheel so that continuous discourse at 70 dB SPL is comfortably loud; then speak loudly (85 to 90 dB SPL) and find out whether it is too loud. If so, lower the SSPL90 until the amplified speech is not too loud.

Prescribed SSPL90 Data Based on Estimates of UCL from Threshold Data

Infants, small children, and other difficult-to-test individuals (such as those who are profoundly retarded, psychotic, or senile) cannot understand the instructions or give the appropriate responses to directly obtain UCLs. If the SSPL90 is too high and amplified loud sound surpasses their UCLs, they may respond by wincing, crying, or taking off the earphone or hearing aid, or they may have vestibular symptoms of dizziness or nystagmus when the amplified sound is too loud. These responses indicate that the SSPL90 should be set below the level that caused them; however, it is not clear how much lower.

Since direct measures of UCL are not available, the prescribed SSPL90 is estimated from threshold data and knowing whether the hearing loss is sensorineural, conductive, or mixed. For those with sensorineural hearing losses, table 5.11 gives estimates of UCL for the audiometric frequencies derived by setting the UCL at 100 dB SPL in the 6-cc coupler for 0 dB hearing-threshold level and approximately 130 dB SPL for 110 dB hearing-threshold level. The values in this table agree fairly closely with data collected from hearing-impaired adults with sensorineural hearing losses. For individuals who have a conductive hearing loss, the amount of the air-bone gap (dB) may be divided by 4 (if this value exceeds 15 dB, then use 15 dB) and added to the UCL estimates for a given hearing-threshold level (air-conduction) in table 5.11.[2]

When UCLs (dB HL) are obtained with supra-aural earphones, the values in table 7.2 may be used to estimate the SSPL90 (dB SPL). The conversion from UCL (dB HL) to SSPL90 takes into account the minimum audible pressure (MAP) at the eardrum for normal-hearing people and the difference between the eardrum and 2-cc coupler measurements. These estimates of SSPL90 are for setting the maximum output of the hearing aid attached to the person's own earmold, which is then coupled to an HA-1, 2-cc coupler. In this way, the acoustic effects of the earmold are included in the measurement.

The estimates of SSPL90 in table 7.2 are for older children and adults. These estimates have to be reduced for infants and small children because the volume of air between the earmold tip and the eardrum is significantly smaller and consequently the SPL will be higher than for adults. It is recommended that 6 dB be *subtracted* from the SSPL90 for infants (0 to 2 years of age), and 3 dB subtracted for children 2 to 5. For binaural hearing aids, 5 dB can be subtracted from the SSPL90 of each aid to account for loudness-summation effects (Byrne 1981) for people of any age.

When an insert earphone is used to obtain UCLs, the UCLs (dB SPL) can be compared directly with the SSPL90 of the hearing aid *if* (1) the output of the hearing aid (attached to the person's own earmold) and the output of the insert earphone (attached to tubing or earmold used for testing) are both measured in an HA-1 coupler, or (2) the output of the hearing aid and insert earphone are both measured in an HA-2 coupler and the insert earphone is attached to the person's own earmold for obtaining UCLs.

The SSPL90 setting may need to be changed based on the response of the hearing-impaired individual as the aid is worn. Since the relation between UCL (and particularly UCL estimated from threshold) and SSPL90 is not fully understood, it is better to be conservative and estimate a low SSPL90 when first fitting an aid. Furthermore, the individual should carefully observe (or be observed by a parent or caregiver) in a variety of listening situations (soft sounds and loud sounds) to determine whether the SSPL90 is

---

[2]The rationale for this correction of the estimated SSPL90 for individuals with conductive hearing loss is given on page 144.

TABLE 7.2.   Estimated SSPL90 (dB SPL) for UCLs (dB HL). For UCLs Obtained with TDH-Series Supra-Aural Earpones, Use Person's Own Earmold and Measure the Hearing-Aid Output in a HA-1 Coupler and Adjust It to These Levels. (See A below).

UCL (dB HL)	FREQUENCY (Hz)						
	250	500	1000	2000	3000	4000	6000
70	85	78	74	77	76	71	69
75	90	83	79	82	81	76	74
80	95	88	84	87	86	81	79
85	100	93	89	92	91	86	84
90	105	98	94	97	96	91	89
95	110	103	99	102	101	96	94
100	115	108	104	107	106	101	99
105	120	113	109	112	111	106	104
110		118	114	117	116	111	109
115		123	119	122	121	116	
120			124	127	126	121	
125			129	132	131	126	

A.   These estimates of the SSPL90 (dB SPL) associated with UCLs (dB HL) are based on the following calculation of correction factors.

	FREQUENCY (Hz)						
	250	500	1000	2000	3000	4000	6000
MAP at the eardrum (dB SPL)[1]	19	12	9	15	16	13	13
Difference: 2-cc coupler/ eardrum[2]	−4	−4	−5	−8	−10	−12	−14
Correction	15	8	4	7	6	1	−1

[1]Killion 1978.
[2]Sachs and Burkhard 1972 (in Levitt, Pickett, and Houde 1980).

too high (and needs to be turned down) or is too low (and the person is not getting enough gain for sound to be meaningful) or the sound is very distorted.

SUMMARY

The maximum acoustic output (SSPL90) of a hearing aid must be set so that amplified loud sound is not uncomfortably loud when the volume wheel is set to hear speech at a comfortable listening level. Since an individual's UCLs vary as a function of frequency, it is important to measure UCL at frequencies between at least 500 and 3000 Hz instead of just for speech. If an individual's dynamic range is large (approximately 50 dB), then the SSPL90 can be set below UCL at all frequencies and still not cause undue distortion to other people's speech or the person's own voice. However, if the dynamic range is narrow (approximately 10 to 25 dB), the SSPL90 will need to be set at or just below UCL. Since most hearing-impaired individuals experience monaural and binaural loudness summation at UCL, it is important to adjust the initial setting of SSPL90 (based on the frequency-specific UCLs) so that loud, broad-band sound such as speech is not uncomfortably loud.

Procedures for prescribing SSPL90 that are based on direct measures of UCL take into account the effects of conductive, cochlear, and neural sites of dysfunction as well as individual differences in tolerance for loud sound. However, for individuals who cannot give reliable valid responses to UCL testing, UCLs are estimated from threshold data.

Supra-aural earphones are universally available with audiometers and, therefore, convenient to use to obtain UCLs. However, when these UCLs are used to prescribe SSPL90, they do not yield as accurate a setting of SSPL90 as using an insert earphone (calibrated in the 2-cc coupler) and the person's own earmold. Although correction factors can be used (Pascoe 1980; Leijon 1983), this takes more time than using the insert earphone. For this reason, the insert earphone is recommended.

Chapter Eight
PRESELECTION OF A HEARING AID AND EARMOLD

HEARING AIDS

Types
Air-Conduction Aids
Bone-Conduction Aids
Hearing Aid Options
Tone Controls
SSPL90 Control
Compression
Directional Microphone
Direct Audio Input
Telecoil/FM Communication Systems
Color

EARMOLDS

Earmold Materials
Parts of the Earmold
Modifying Acoustic Output with the Earmold
Damping Resonant Peaks
Amount of High-Frequency Gain
Amount of Low-Frequency Gain
Average Corrections in Hearing Aid Output for
Earmold Modifications
Ways To Prevent Acoustic Feedback

CROS FITTINGS

BINAURAL VERSUS MONAURAL FITTING

Advantages of Normal Binaural Condition
Advantages of Binaural Hearing Aid Fitting
Monaural Instead of Binaural Fitting
Creating a Binaural Listening Condition
When To Fit a Second Hearing Aid
Criteria for Gain and SSPL90 for Binaural Fitting

NONACOUSTIC NEEDS OF THE INDIVIDUAL
Interpersonal Communication
Sound Environment
Physical Limitations
Cosmetic Appearance
Financial Limitations

PRESELECTION OF A HEARING AID AND EARMOLD
Prescribe Real-Ear Gain
Obtain Thresholds
Obtain or Predict MCLs and UCLs
Select Criteria for Prescribing Real-Ear Gain
Prescribe Aided Sound-Field Thresholds
Select Type of Hearing Aid
Select Earmold
Predict 2-cc Coupler Gain
Predict SSPL90
Select Specific Hearing Aid and Adjust It in the Test Box
Selected Cases
SUMMARY

Many models of hearing aids are commercially available. The task is to preselect one (or several) and an earmold that will meet both the acoustic and the nonacoustic needs of the individual. This preselection requires weighing and balancing a number of different factors that will be described in this chapter.

HEARING AIDS

Types

There are air-conduction and bone-conduction hearing aids. Air-conduction aids are coupled to the individual's earcanal and pinna so that amplified sound is delivered acoustically to the eardrum. Bone-conduction aids deliver the amplified signal to a vibrator that is placed on the skull, usually on the mastoid process. The vibrator is held against the head with a headband or with an eyeglass frame, and the vibrations are transmitted to the inner ear through the bones of the head. The types of hearing aids and the degree of hearing loss for which each type is indicated are listed in table 8.1. A picture of each type is shown in figure 8.1.

Air-conduction aids. There are two major types of air-conduction hearing aids: body aids and ear-level aids. Most body aids are worn by people with profound hearing losses because the aids can produce higher SPL outputs than ear-level aids. Furthermore, the distance between the microphone (on the chest) and the receiver (at the ear) of body aids reduces the possibility of acoustic feedback at these high output levels. The body-baffle effect, which is caused by wearing the microphone on the chest, enhances sound by approximately 3 to 4 dB between 250 and 750 Hz and deemphasizes it 4 to 6 dB between 1000 and 2000 Hz compared to measurements in the unobstructed sound field (see figure 4.21). For individuals who need more gain in the high frequencies than in the low, this is not the appropriate frequency response. However, for those who have no hearing above 1000 Hz, this shift of the input sound level does not seriously affect the perceived signal. Body aids are also worn by people with mild to severe hearing losses when (1) they cannot reach up to the ear to manipulate the hearing aid controls, or (2) they spend most of the time lying in bed (and there is feedback because the pillow is so close to the microphone and receiver of an ear-level aid). In 1984 less than one percent of the hearing aids sold in the United States were body aids (Mahon 1985).

There are four types of ear-level, air-conduction hearing aids: canal, in-the-ear, behind-the-ear, and eyeglass aids (see figure 8.1). The major limiting factor in choosing from among these is the amount of real-ear gain needed. Behind-the-ear and eyeglass aids can provide 60 to 65 dB real-ear gain between 500 and 4000 Hz, which is sufficient for those with severe and

TABLE 8.1.   Types of Hearing Aids and the Type and Degree of Hearing Loss for Which They Are Indicated.

TYPE OF HEARING AID	TYPE AND DEGREE OF HEARING LOSS
I. Air conduction	All types and degrees of hearing loss.
A. Body	Profound hearing losses and those with mild, moderate, or severe hearing losses if the person (1) is in bed most of the time (e.g., young infants or those who are ill) or (2) needs large controls and batteries because of difficulty with fine motor control.
B. Ear level	Mild, moderate, or severe conductive, mixed, or sensorineural hearing losses.
1. Canal	Mild to moderate hearing losses. Cannot use for "Contralateral Routing of Signals" (CROS) fitting.
2. In-the-ear	Mild to moderately severe hearing losses. Cannot use for CROS fitting.
3. Behind-the-ear	Mild, moderate, or severe hearing losses. Can use for CROS fitting either with hard-wire or radio-frequency transmission.
4. Eyeglass	Mild, moderate, or severe hearing losses. Well-suited for hard-wire CROS fitting and for open-mold fitting.
II. Bone conduction	Mild to moderate conductive hearing loss caused by chronically draining middle ear or atresia of the earcanal.
A. Body	Body aid can provide sufficient power to drive bone-conduction vibrator.
B. Ear level	Powerful ear-level aids can provide sufficient gain.
1. Behind-the-ear	Headband gives reasonable coupling of vibrator to head.
2. Eyeglass	Eyeglass frame does not provide sufficient pressure of vibrator against the head.

profound hearing losses; these aids can also be adjusted to provide less gain for those with mild or moderate hearing losses. In addition, they are large enough to house a variety of adjustable features: low- and high-frequency tone controls, adjustments for compression and SSPL90, directional microphone, microphone/telephone switches and telecoil amplifiers, and an audio input. The flexibility these features allow is highly desirable for adjusting the aid for an individual at the initial evaluation and subsequently as adaptation to the amplification occurs or the hearing loss changes.

In recent years the number of eyeglass aids sold has decreased to 1.5

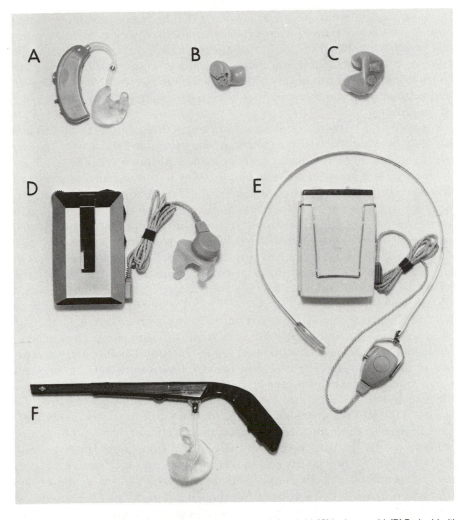

FIGURE 8.1.   Types of hearing aids. **(A)** Behind-the-ear aid; **(B)** Canal aid; **(C)** In-the-ear aid; **(D)** Body aid with external receiver; **(E)** Body aid with bone-conduction vibrator; **(F)** Eyeglass aid.

percent of the U.S. hearing aid sales (Mahon 1985). Two possible reasons for this decline are that it is more cost-effective to manufacture and fit behind-the-ear aids that can be worn by people whether or not they wear glasses, and that it often takes much time and cooperation between the hearing aid dispenser and the optician to fit the glasses so that they are comfortable.

Despite all the features available on the behind-the-ear aids, many people want canal or in-the-ear aids because they are smaller and more cosmetically acceptable. Acoustically, there are advantages and disadvantages in choosing an in-the-ear or a canal aid. The major advantage is that some of the normal pinna and concha resonances are preserved by positioning the microphone in the center of the pinna (in-the-ear aids) or at the entrance of the earcanal (canal aids). Therefore, sound at the hearing aid microphone is higher than for the behind-the-ear aid in the high frequencies (see table 5.7), and this gain does not have to be provided by the hearing aid amplifier.

Canal and in-the-ear aids have two major disadvantages. The first is that they provide less real-ear gain than the other air-conduction hearing aids because acoustic feedback occurs at a lower output level. The feedback is caused by the microphone port being closer to the sound-outlet port of the receiver. The second disadvantage is that few changes can be made by the dispenser (or wearer) in the acoustic output of the aid. The small size of the in-the-ear and canal aids limits the circuitry and space for external adjustments. On almost all canal aids there is room for only the volume wheel; the SSPL90 and frequency response are set by the manufacturer. On in-the-ear aids, the number of adjustments depends on the size of the individual's concha and earcanal. For some there may be room for only a volume wheel. For others there may be room for one or two controls. Since the manufacturers can only approximate the appropriate hearing aid characteristics from the individual's data, often one or more parameters need to be adjusted to make speech more intelligible, the sound quality more acceptable, or the output-limiting level appropriate. This may need to be repeated several times. If this can be done by turning a screw or adjusting a switch, it will take much less time and be more exact than sending it back to the factory. To try to resolve this problem, several manufacturers have developed a range of different circuits, parts, and faceplates that can be stocked and inserted by the dispenser in in-the-ear and canal aids. However, one needs to develop the expertise to make modifications efficiently.

In summary, the advantages and disadvantages of each type of air-conduction hearing aid are listed in tables 8.2 and 8.3. These should be considered in relation to the needs of the hearing-impaired individual in selecting one type of aid.

Bone-conduction aids.   It takes substantially more energy to deliver a bone-conducted vibration to the cochlea than an air-conducted sound to the eardrum. Consequently, it is necessary to use a powerful hearing aid to drive the vibrator. Only people with conductive hearing losses whose sensorineural hearing sensitivity is normal or minimally impaired will hear the bone-conducted sound at a comfortable loudness level.

There is a paucity of data on the real-ear gain provided by an air-conduction compared to a bone-conduction aid, and a body-level versus an ear-level, bone-conduction aid. The major concern is to provide a broadband (200 to 6000 Hz) signal that has sufficient gain in the high frequencies. Since

TABLE 8.2. Advantages of the Five Types of Air-Conduction Hearing Aids.

HEARING AID CHARACTERISTIC	TYPE OF HEARING AID				
	CANAL	IN-THE-EAR	BEHIND-THE-EAR	EYEGLASS	BODY
Microphone placement	Microphone in the ear-canal enhances sound between 1500 and 6000 Hz by 5 to 10 dB; this provides efficient delivery of high-frequency energy.	Microphone in the pinna enhances sound between 1500 and 4000 Hz by 5 dB; this provides efficient delivery of high-frequency energy.	Microphone is either at top of pinna or at bottom of aid behind the pinna; the top location gives better reception of sound.	Microphone is on temple piece in front of pinna.	Microphone is on body, usually at top of aid. It is usually covered by clothing, which can rub against the microphone and create noise. If it is at top, small children may drop food into it.
	Can take advantage of changes in sound at microphone as head is moved; this helps localize the sound source.	Can take advantage of changes in sound at microphone as head is moved; this helps localize the sound source.	Can take advantage of changes in sound at microphone as head is moved; this helps localize sound source.	Can take advantage changes in sound at microphone as head is moved; this helps localize sound source.	
Real-ear gain	Up to 25 dB.	Up to 45 dB.	Up to 65 dB.	Up to 65 dB.	Up to 70 dB.
Modification of acoustic output	None can be made by dispenser, without purchase of system with variety of circuits.	SSPL90, AGC, and tone controls can be ordered on some models; ear-canal must be large enough to accommodate them. Range of adjustment more restricted than on larger hearing aids.	Number of models have AGC, SSPL90, and low and high tone controls that can be finely adjusted over useful range. The frequency response and SSPL90 can be changed over 5–15 dB range with earmold modifications and acoustic dampers. All these adjustments can be made by dispenser.	On the few models available, can make SSPL90 and tone-control adjustments. Frequency response and SSPL90 can be changed over 5–15 dB range with earmold modifications and acoustic dampers. All these adjustments can be made by dispenser.	Most models have SSPL90, AGC, and tone controls. The frequency response and SSPL90 can be changed by choice of external receiver and to a small extent by configuration of bore in earmold.

(continued)

TABLE 8.2. (Continued)

HEARING AID CHARACTERISTIC	TYPE OF HEARING AID				
	CANAL	IN-THE-EAR	BEHIND-THE-EAR	EYEGLASS	BODY
Acoustic feedback	Microphone is within ¾" of receiver; aid must fit snugly in the earcanal, and there cannot be a vent if more than 5 dB real-ear gain without feedback is desired.	Microphone within 1" of receiver; although large vents can be used, this severely limits the real-ear gain because of feedback. It must fit snugly and have no vent to achieve 45 dB real-ear gain.	Microphone is further away from amplified sound than in in-the-ear aids, so can get greater real-ear gain before feedback occurs. To get the maximum gain (65 dB), the earmold must fit very snugly in earcanal and a vent cannot be used.	Microphone is further away from amplified sound than in behind-the-ear aids, so greater real-ear gain can be obtained before feedback occurs. To get maximum gain (65 dB), the earmold must fit very snugly in earcanal, and a vent cannot be used.	Microphone is 8" to 12" from the amplified sound, which reduces possibility of feedback (with a severe hearing loss or if patient is bedridden), compared with the other aids.
Venting	Cannot use larger than a capillary vent.	Can use both capillary vents and low-frequency vents.	Can use a vented or open earmold.	Can use a vented or open earmold.	Can use a small vent with mild or moderate gain.
Fitting with CROS aids	Cannot fit.	Available but not practical.	Can fit CROS aids with either hard-wire or radio-frequency transmission.	CROS aids fit with hard-wire through frame; use of open molds for CROS aid most satisfactory with eyeglass aids.	Cannot fit.
Ease of manipulation	If person can hold aid in fingertips, aid is easily inserted.	If person can hold aid in fingertips, aid is relatively easy to insert.	Inserting battery and adjusting controls easier than with canal and in-the-ear aids.	Easier to put on aid and adjust controls than behind-the-ear aids. Batteries usually larger and easier to insert than in in-the-ear aids.	Controls easily accessible and large enough for those with coordination problems. Battery large and easy to insert.

Directional microphone	Not available.	Available on some models if aid is large enough.	Available on many models.	Available on some models.	Not available.
Direct acoustic input	Not available.	Not available.	Available on some models.	Not available.	Available on some models.
Telecoil	Not available.	Available on some models.	Available on many models	Available on many models.	Available on some models.
Cosmetic appeal	Most cosmetically appealing of all aids; least conspicuous.	Many people believe this aid is less conspicuous than behind-the-ear aid; however, it is more conspicuous except on those with hair that covers the aid.	Cosmetically acceptable, particularly for those whose hair covers the aid.	Cosmetically more acceptable to some people than behind-the-ear aids.	Not cosmetically acceptable to most people.
Durability	Most fragile of all aids.	More fragile than behind-the-ear and body aids.	Reasonably durable.	Reasonably durable.	Reasonably durable.
Repair	Canal aids are in custom molds and cannot be used in other ear except stock models.	Person can wear loaner aid with own earmold when hearing aid sent for repair.	Person can wear loaner aid with own earmold when hearing aid sent for repair.	Person can wear loaner aid with own earmold when hearing aid sent for repair.	Person can wear loaner aid with own earmold when hearing aid sent for repair.
Use at other ear	In-the-ear aids are in custom molds and cannot be used in other ear.	Can wear hearing aid at other ear with custom earmold.	Can wear hearing aid at other ear with custom earmold.	Can wear hearing aid at other ear with custom earmold.	Can wear hearing aid at other ear with custom earmold.

TABLE 8.3. Disadvantages of the Five Types of Air-Conduction Hearing Aids.

HEARING AID CHARACTERISTIC	TYPES OF HEARING AID				
	CANAL	IN-THE-EAR	BEHIND-THE-EAR	EYEGLASS	BODY
Microphone placement		Microphone may pick up wind noise.	May pick up wind noise.	May pick up wind noise.	Microphone on body prevents using head movements for localizing sound source. Clothing rubbing against microphone can cause noise that will mask some sounds the person wants to hear. Microphone on chest enhances reception of low-frequency sound before it is amplified.
Real-ear gain	Maximum limited to 25 dB.	Maximum limited to 45 dB.			
Modification of acoustic output	Adjustments in SSPL90 or frequency response can be made by dispenser only by changing the circuits.	Small physical size limits number of adjustments to 1 or 2; e.g., SSPL90, frequency response or telecoil.	Tubing resonances may create unacceptable sound quality, and when damped with acoustic dampers may require greater battery consumption.	So few models manufactured that it may be difficult to get the SSPL90, frequency response, and gain needed to meet the acoustic needs of the patient.	

	Cannot use acoustic dampers to modify frequency response. Difficult to convey to manufacturer the SSPL90 and frequency response needed to obtain prescribed real-ear gain and maximum acoustic output.	Foam to damp resonant peaks may not be as effective as fused mesh acoustic dampers. Difficult to convey to manufacturer the SSPL90 and the frequency response needed to obtain prescribed real-ear gain and maximum acoustic output.		
Ease of manipulation	Small size makes them hard to manipulate, especially the battery and controls.	Small controls, battery, and battery case may be difficult to use.	Putting in earmold and placing aid behind ear without twisting tubing may be difficult.	
Size	Earcanal must be large enough for the canal aid.	Earcanal and pinna must be large enough for the in-the-ear aid.		
Wearing comfort	Usually cannot vent for pressure equalization and preventing hollow sound of one's own voice (occlusion effects).		Aid may not remain comfortably on top of and behind pinna for those who are physically active or those with small pinnas. Aid may not be comfortable worn with eyeglasses.	Hearing aids and lenses may be too heavy for comfort (especially those with bifocal or cataract lenses). Frames need special adjustments for optimum placement of lenses for vision and for comfortable distribution of weight on bridge of nose and top of ears.	Weight of receiver, length of cord against neck, and hearing aid case on chest may not be comfortable to some people.

(continued)

TABLE 8.3. (Continued)

TYPES OF HEARING AID

HEARING AID CHARACTERISTIC	CANAL	IN-THE-EAR	BEHIND-THE-EAR	EYEGLASS	BODY
Durability	Relatively fragile.				Cords break easily and need to be replaced.
				Wires placed in aid for CROS fitting may break. (Also need to send frame to manufacturer for the initial wiring.)	
Repair	Requires more repair than other aids. When send in for repair, cannot use same model aid as a loaner; need earmold and another aid.	When send aid in for modification or repair, cannot use same model aid as a loaner; need earmold and another aid.		Frame hinges become loose more readily than with eyeglasses alone. When send hearing aid(s) in for repair, need another pair of temples to use glasses.	
Use at other ear	Cannot use at other ear.	Cannot use at other ear.		Cannot use at other ear.	

those with long-standing middle-ear disease often have bone-conduction thresholds that are abnormal at 3000 and 4000 Hz, it is not clear whether the frequency response of the aid can be adjusted to give sufficient real-ear gain when a bone-conduction vibrator is used. Eyeglass bone-conduction aids are rarely used because it is difficult to get (1) sufficient pressure of the vibrator against the mastoid, and (2) a good positioning of the vibrator even though the temple pieces come in ten different lengths.

For the above reasons, bone-conduction hearing aids are indicated only for people with conductive hearing losses who cannot wear an air-conduction hearing aid. This includes people who have no external ear-canals (due to congenital or traumatic causes) and those who have chronic drainage from the middle ear. For these people, a bone-conduction aid makes the low- and mid-frequency speech sounds comfortably loud and consequently is definitely beneficial.

Within the last few years a new surgical technique has been developed in which the bone vibrator can be coupled to the skull by snapping it onto an implanted titanium post or embedding the vibrator in the mastoid process.[1] This coupling is more efficient, and less energy is needed to drive the vibrator than when it is coupled to the skull with a headband. This increased efficiency means that the vibrator can be driven by an ear-level aid. Since this aid requires surgical implantation, only people with chronic middle-ear disease or bilateral atresia of the earcanal are considered candidates at the present.

Hearing Aid Options

A number of options are available on hearing aids. These should be considered in selecting a hearing aid for an individual.

Tone controls. Many hearing aids have a tone control that affects the amount of gain in the frequencies below 1000 Hz; this is usually adjusted by changing the position of a screw. Recently, some aids have been manufactured that have tone controls for both low- and high-frequency gain; the range over which both low- and high-frequency gain can be changed in a representative hearing aid is shown in figure 8.2. On some aids the wearer can change the position of a switch to decrease low-frequency gain in noisy listening situations.

---

[1] A bone-conduction hearing aid, in which the vibrator is snapped onto a titanium post implanted in the mastoid process of the skull, has been developed by Hakansson and colleagues in Sweden. The design for this aid and results from a number of patients are described in Hakansson, Tjellstrom, and Rosenhall (1984) and Hakansson et al. (1985). Another bone-conduction aid, in which the magnetic vibrator is fully implanted in the region of the mastoid process and driven by an external inductive coil, has been developed by Hough and colleagues in Oklahoma and Oregon. The design for this aid and results from nine patients are described in Hough et al. (1986).

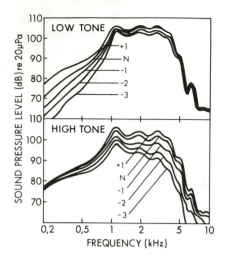

FIGURE 8.2.

Example of the range over which the low- and high-frequency output can be changed with the low- and high-frequency tone controls of a behind-the-ear hearing aid. Redrawn courtesy of Bernafon, Inc.

SSPL90 control.   Almost all body and behind-the-ear hearing aids have potentiometers to change the maximum acoustic output of the hearing aid over a 10- to 20-dB range (see figure 8.3). Unless the SSPL90 of a hearing aid is set so that high input sounds do not become too loud, the individual will reduce the gain and thereby make speech too soft, wear the aid only in quiet places, or not wear the aid. On the other hand, if the SSPL90 is set too low, the individuals's own speech may be severely distorted. Since the setting of the SSPL90 must be verified with the aid and the custom earmold, the ability to adjust the aid at the time of fitting is important. Readjustment of the SSPL90 may also be necessary after the person has worn the aid in everyday life. For these reasons, it is advantageous to choose an aid that has an adjustable SSPL90 control.

The output limiting in most hearing aids is accomplished with *peak clipping*. Peak clipping occurs when the output SPL surpasses the saturation point, and there are no significant increases in SPL output corresponding to increases in SPL input. The peaks of the output waveform are clipped, resulting in harmonic and intermodulation distortion that degrades the amplified sound. Although some peak clipping does not interfere with

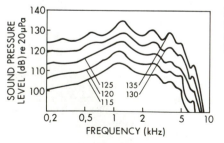

FIGURE 8.3.

Example of the range over which the SSPL90 can be changed with a control on a behind-the-ear hearing aid. Redrawn courtesy of Bernafon, Inc.

perceiving the sound, severe peak clipping, particularly with hearing aids that amplify sound through 6000 Hz, makes the sound distortion unacceptable. Hawkins (1986) has suggested that when the gain of the hearing aid plus the input SPL of one's own voice (approximately 80 dB) is equal to or greater than the SSPL90 of a hearing aid (set just below the individual's UCL), limiter compression should be considered to prevent peak clipping.

Compression. In limiter compression there is a level-detecting device that reduces the gain of the hearing aid when the output signal reaches a certain SPL (knee point), which is set to prevent the maximum output from exceeding the individual's UCLs. This gain reduction (called output compression) prevents the amplified sound from being peak-clipped, even when the input SPL is high. Since the output waveform is not peak-clipped, harmonic and intermodulation distortion caused by peak clipping is avoided. However, there is temporal distortion caused by the compression circuit. To minimize temporal distortion, prevent sudden loud sounds from being uncomfortable, and keep the gain of the aid from changing rapidly, Walker and Dillon (1982) suggest an attack time (that is, the time between the onset of a loud sound and the reduction of gain) of between 2 and 5 msec and a release time of between 60 and 150 msec. Walker and Dillon also suggest a compression ratio (that is, the ratio of the increment in input SPL to the increment in output SPL) of greater than 10 to 1.

Compression circuits (often called automatic gain control or AGC circuits) also can be used to reduce the range of output SPLs in relation to the range of input SPLs. The major reason for using compression in this way is to make both soft and loud speech cues audible and not uncomfortable so that one's own voice as well as another person speaking at a distance will both be heard. For this application, the knee point of the compression is set lower than for limiter compression and the compression ratio is lower, perhaps 2 to 1. On AGC hearing aids this knee can be set at a certain level, such as 70 dB SPL. If an input compression circuit is used, the level-detecting device monitors the SPL at the input to the hearing aid, and when this input surpasses the knee, the gain is reduced. An increase in the volume-wheel setting will cause an increase in the output SPL. If an output compression circuit is used, the level-detecting device will monitor the SPL at the output of the device. Depending on the choice of input versus output compression, the knee point, and the compression ratio, all or part of the typical range of inputs will be compressed.

Clinical guidelines for making these choices are not clear. If an individual has a dynamic range that is less than 40 dB or complains that momentary sounds are loud and irritating despite the fact that the SSPL90 has been set so that broad-band sound is not too loud, a compression hearing aid should be considered. When fitting an AGC aid, the clinician and hearing-impaired individual should listen to speech (and other sounds) through the aid, as the volume-wheel and compression knee settings are varied, before choosing an AGC setting and recommending the aid.

Directional microphone.   Most hearing-aid microphones are *omnidirectional*, that is, they are equally sensitive to sound coming from all directions. Directional microphones are more sensitive to sounds coming from in front of rather than from behind a person. They have two sound ports, one facing to the front and the other facing to the rear. There is typically a 58 μsec. delay in the sound reaching the microphone diaphragm from the rear port. This delay, which is caused by acoustic resistance and an air cavity on the back of the microphone diaphragm, is purposely set for the amount of time it takes sound to travel from the rear to the front port. Sound occurring behind the person will arrive from each port at the diaphragm of the microphone simultaneously, and consequently will be cancelled (Lybarger 1985b). Sound occurring in front will reach the microphone diaphragm approximately 116 μsec. before it reaches the diaphragm from the rear port. For this reason, there will be no cancellation. From measurements with directional aids on KEMAR, Lybarger (1986b) has found that the maximum directional response of the hearing aid is at 45° instead of 0°. Nevertheless, a carefully engineered directional microphone can make sounds from the front approximately 3 dB more intense than from the rear in rooms with relatively short reverberation times, for example 0.6 sec. (Beck 1983). In situations where the noise is from the rear and someone is speaking in front of a hearing-impaired individual, the improvement in understanding sentences can be as much as 20 to 30 percent over that which the individual would get with an omnidirectional microphone (Hawkins 1986). For these reasons, a directional microphone can provide substantial benefit for those who attend mostly to sounds that occur in front of them, particularly people speaking to them. An omnidirectional microphone is more appropriate for people, such as taxi drivers, who need to listen to speech spoken from behind them.

Direct audio input.   For people who have moderate or severe hearing losses and can understand speech better when someone talks directly into a separate microphone, a hearing aid with a direct audio input is helpful. The hearing aid has a jack to which a wire from a small hand-held microphone is attached. This arrangement improves the signal-to-noise ratio and eliminates the adverse effect of room reverberation on speech. If the person speaking and the person wearing the hearing aid are willing to use this somewhat restrictive system, the hearing-impaired person can understand speech more clearly and with less fatigue.

Telecoil/FM communication systems.   A telecoil provides induction pick-up from electromagnetic signals such as the strong magnetic field produced by some telephone receivers such as the U-type magnetic receiver used for many years by the Bell telephone system. The major advantage of the telecoil is that it is not sensitive to air-borne acoustic signals. Therefore, when a hearing aid is set for telecoil (and not microphone) input, the person hears the telephone signal without the degrading effect of room noise or the acoustic feedback caused by getting the microphone and amplified sound close to the telephone receiver.

The frequency response and gain of a hearing aid set for the telecoil cannot necessarily be predicted from that of the microphone. The gain is usually lower with the telecoil, and the frequency response may be the same or different. Of course, frequency response should be the same and the gain sufficient to provide the needed benefit. If the amplifier in the hearing aid is not sufficient or if the stray magnetic field of the telephone receiver is too small, then an acoustic-to-magnetic converter (a device strapped to the telephone receiver) can be used to boost the level of the signal so it can be heard at a comfortable level (see figure 8.4A). This converter can also be attached to the outside of a TV loudspeaker. Then a wire is placed between this converter and a *silhouette inductor*, which is placed alongside an ear-level hearing aid, or a *teleloop*, which is placed around the neck. Both these devices produce a magnetic field that activates the telecoil of the hearing aid (see figure 8.4B).

A telecoil is recommended for people who wear a hearing aid at the ear they use with the telephone and who either need their aids to hear over the telephone or do not want to take off their aids each time they use it.

A telecoil also may be needed for those who use it as part of an FM communication system—in a classroom, in meetings, or while listening to television. The major advantages of using an FM system are (1) it will pick up a person's voice close to the sound source so the level is high in relation to the background noise and there is no chance for the voice to reverberate in the room, and (2) it will deliver this signal directly to the hearing aid. With this system (see figure 8.4 B), a microphone is placed close to the sound source (for example, near the person's lips or on the TV loudspeaker), and a transmitter processes the signal and sends it by radio frequency to a receiver worn by the person with the hearing aid. This signal can be received in three ways: (1) a direct audio input (bypassing the telecoil) with a jack into the hearing aid from an FM receiver box; (2) a silhouette inductor that activates the telecoil of the hearing aid; or (3) a teleloop that also activates the telecoil. Since a person's voice (or the TV audio) is about 15 dB higher near the source than at the microphone of a hearing aid 6 ft. away, and the background noise remains approximately the same, this FM system provides a much better signal-to-noise ratio than a hearing aid microphone. Since the signal is 15 dB higher, the gain needed may be less by this amount. If the person wearing the hearing aid is even farther from the sound source, the advantage of the FM system with respect to signal-to-noise ratio is greater. Infrared systems provide the same benefit as EM systems by transmitting infrared instead of radio frequency signals.

A

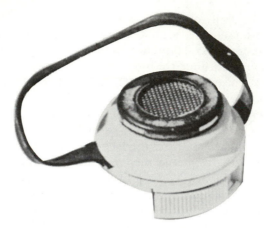

B

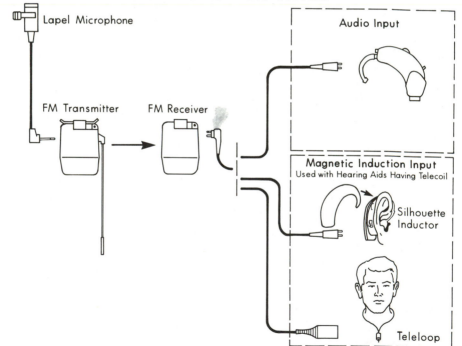

FIGURE 8.4. Devices to assist with reception of signals by the telecoil of a hearing aid. **(A)** Acoustic-to-magnetic converter for a telephone receiver (AT&T device). From S. F. Lybarger 1982. "Telephone coupling." In *The Vanderbilt Hearing-Aid Report*. Ed. G. A. Studebaker and F. H. Bess. Upper Darby, Pa.: Monographs in Contemporary Audiology. Reproduced with permission of the author and publisher. **(B)** FM communication system with microphone and FM transmitter for the person who is speaking and an FM receiver for the person wearing a hearing aid. The transmitted signal is received and may be sent as a direct audio input to the hearing aid, or an electromagnetic field can be set up by a silhouette inductor or teleloop that activates the telecoil in the hearing aid. Reproduced courtesy of Phonic Ear, Inc.

Some hearing aids have a three-position switch for microphone, microphone and telecoil, and telecoil. The mixed microphone and telephone input enables the person wearing the aid to hear his or her own voice and other people, who do not have the FM microphone close to their lips. This is helpful when the background noise is very low but not when it is high. In the latter case, the switch should be set for the telecoil alone.

If a person has a moderate, severe, or profound hearing loss and it is important to hear the TV or people talking at a better signal-to-noise ratio, an aid with direct audio input or that is part of an FM or infrared communication system may provide significant benefits.

Color.   Most models of behind-the-ear, in-the-ear, and canal hearing aids can be ordered in several colors to blend with one's skin or hair color. This is an important consideration for those who are concerned with cosmetic appearance. Eyeglass aids usually come in only black and/or brown, and a particular model of body aid usually comes in only one color.

EARMOLDS

Earmolds are used to couple air-conduction hearing aids to the pinna and ear canal so the amplified sound is directed into the earcanal. For body, behind-the-ear, and eyeglasses hearing aids, a custom-made earmold is made and attached to the hearing aid. With in-the-ear and canal aids, the outer casing of the hearing aid is the "earmold."

Earmold Materials

Earmolds can be made of several different materials. *Hard acrylic* is used most often because it is nonporous and can be buffed to form a very smooth surface. Both these properties make it more comfortable to wear, particularly in hot weather, than some of the other materials. It is also more durable and is generally nonallergenic. In addition, the hard acrylic earmolds can be modified more easily than earmolds made of soft materials. Soft materials, such as *flexible acrylic, polyvinyl chloride,* and *silicone,* are used (1) for young children (to prevent injury if the ear is hit) and (2) to achieve a tight acoustic seal with high-gain hearing aids. This seal is possible because the body heat causes the material to expand slightly. If someone has a severe allergic reaction to earmolds made of the hard acrylic or soft materials, *polyethylene* can be used. This semihard material is the least durable of all those mentioned.

Parts of the Earmold

The parts of an earmold are labeled in figure 8.5. Two ways of coupling an earmold to a hearing aid are with a *snap ring* or with *tubing.* The standard earmold shown here has a medium-length canal and a sound bore

PARTS OF AN EARMOLD

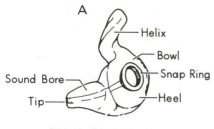

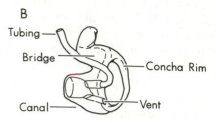

FIGURE 8.5.   Parts of an earmold. The standard earmold with a snap ring attaches to the nubbin of an external receiver used with a body aid. Since nubbin sizes differ, the size should be specified in ordering the snap ring. This earmold fills the concha to provide (1) sufficient support for the receiver and (2) a good seal when high gain is used. A skeleton earmold attaches to a behind-the-ear or eyeglass aid with tubing. Much of the bulk of this earmold has been removed to make it more comfortable and less visible; this provides sufficient acoustic seal for mild or moderate hearing losses. The helix, bridge, bowl, heel, concha rim, and canal are all parts of the body of the earmold. Except for the canal, these parts of the earmold can be made smaller or eliminated without affecting the amplified sound, provided a good acoustic seal is maintained. From W. R. Hodgson and P. H. Skinner 1981. *Hearing Aid Assessment and Use in Audiologic Habilitation*, 2nd ed. Adapted from figure 5.4 in "Earmolds: Acoustic and structural considerations" by R. Leavitt. Copyright 1981, Williams and Wilkins Co., Baltimore. Reproduced with permission of the authors and publisher.

whose internal diameter is constant and small. With this type of earmold the length of the canal can be made shorter or longer, the diameter of the sound bore can be made large (as shown on the skeleton mold in this figure) or belled as it reaches the tip, and a vent can be placed parallel to the sound bore.

The skeleton mold in this figure has standard tubing of constant diameter, which opens into a large, hollowed-out sound bore. The canal is short. A medium-size (for example, 1.5 mm) vent that runs *parallel* to the tubing also opens into the sound bore. A skeleton mold can be made with tubing of a constant internal diameter that ends at the tip of the mold (see figure 8.6A) or with a stepped-bore internal diameter such as the Libby horn (see figure 8.6B). The earmold tip can be long (14.2 mm), medium (8.8 mm), or short (4.4 mm) (Lybarger 1985a), and the length and internal diameter of the venting can be varied. The body of the skeleton earmold (see figure 8.5B) has less bulk than the standard earmold and more than the open earmold shown in figure 8.7A. When more bulk is required to get a good acoustic seal with high-gain, behind-the-ear or eyeglass aids, a shell mold is used (see figure 8.7B). When an open earmold is used, the body of the mold is intended to hold the tube in the earcanal and to preserve the open air space between the outside of the tubing and the walls of the earcanal.

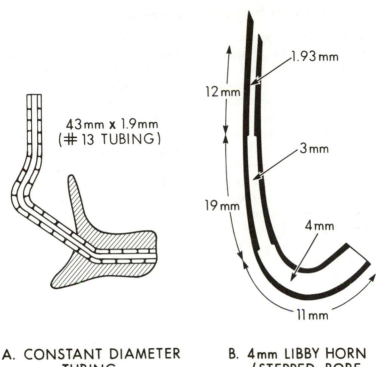

43mm x 1.9mm
(# 13 TUBING)

1.93 mm

12 mm

3 mm

19 mm

4 mm

11 mm

A. CONSTANT DIAMETER
TUBING

B. 4mm LIBBY HORN
(STEPPED-BORE
INTERNAL DIAMETER)

FIGURE 8.6.   Types of earmold tubing **(A)** Standard number-13 tubing of constant diameter. From M. C. Killion 1981. "Earmold options for wide band hearing aids." *Journal of Speech and Hearing Disorders* 46:10-20. Copyright 1981, American Speech-Language-Hearing Association, Rockville, Md. Reproduced with permission of the author and publisher. **(B)** Libby horn, which is a one-piece stepped-bore horn. From E. R. Libby, J. H. Johnson, and T. P. Longwell 198l. *Innovative Earmold Coupling Systems: Rationale, Design, Clinical Applications*. Chicago: Zenetron. Reproduced with permission of the author and the publisher.

A

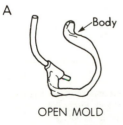

Body

OPEN MOLD

B

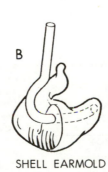

SHELL EARMOLD

FIGURE 8.7.
(A) Open earmold. **(B)** Shell earmold. From W. R. Hodgson and P. H. Skinner 1981. *Hearing Aid Assessment and Use in Audiologic Habilitation*, 2nd ed. Adapted from figure 5.4 in "Earmolds: Acoustic and structural considerations" by R. Leavitt. Copyright 1981, Williams and Wilkins Co., Baltimore. Reproduced with permission of the authors and publisher.

Modifying Acoustic Output with the Earmold

Damping resonant peaks.   The tubing resonances and a Helmholz resonance (produced by the acoustic compliance of the air cavity in front of the hearing aid earphone) cause a sharp peak around 1000 Hz in the output of behind-the-ear hearing aids measured in 2-cc couplers (see figure 4.25). The resonant peaks of in-the-ear hearing aids are around 2000 Hz or higher. These peaks can be reduced with internal damping in the hearing aid, or fused-mesh *acoustic damper* in the earhook or earmold tubing, or a spring damper in the tubing of an in-the-ear aid. The effect of a pair of acoustic dampers on the output is shown in figure 4.26. Some manufacturers and clinicians use a single 680- or 1500- or 2200-ohm acoustic damper in the earhook rather than near the earcanal, because moisture from the earcanal can clog the damper and cut off the sound. When the damper is placed at the tip of the earhook, there is little effect on the resonant peak at 2000 Hz because of the damper's location at a quarter-wavelength node (Lybarger 1985a). The larger the acoustic resistance value of the dampers, the larger the decrease in acoustic output at the resonant peaks.

In a recent study Cox and Gilmore (1986) found that eight out of ten hearing-impaired listeners found that hearing aids without dampers produced slightly clearer, more pleasant-sounding speech than those with dampers. Although further research is needed, these results suggest that acoustic dampers do not necessarily improve sound quality.

Amount of high-frequency gain.   The real-ear gain above 1000 Hz is affected by the dimension of the sound channel from the output of the hearing aid to the earcanal and the volume of air between the earmold tip and the eardrum. The diameter of the sound channel is very important; the smaller the diameter, the less high-frequency gain is delivered to the eardrum. Since most hearing-impaired individuals have more hearing loss in the high frequencies than in the low, *and* occluding earmolds destroy the normal concha and earcanal resonance (see figure 8.8), earmolds can be used to partially compensate for this loss of resonance and preserve high-frequency gain. One way to accomplish this is with tubing whose internal diameter increases from the earhook to the earmold tip; this is called a *horn* earmold (for example, see the Libby horn in figure 8.6B). A 4-mm Libby

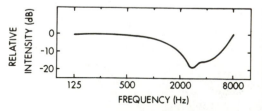

FIGURE 8.8.
Loss of natural resonance by occluding the earcanal with an earmold. From S. F. Lybarger 1978. "Selective amplification: A review and evaluation." *Journal of the American Audiological Society* 3: 258-66. Copyright 1978, Williams and Wilkins Co., Baltimore. Reproduced with permission of the author and publisher.

TABLE 8.4. Average Effect (dB) of Earmold Configuration on the Output of a Hearing Aid Measured in a 2-cc Coupler (HA-2). The Values in This Table Should Be *Added* to the Hearing Aid Output (dB SPL)

EARMOLD	FREQUENCY (Hz)						
	250	500	1000	2000	3000	4000	6000
HA-2 Coupler Snap-ring earmold with 18-mm-long sound bore with internal diameter (i.d.) of 3 mm; or earmold with #13 tubing that is cemented into a sound bore 18 mm long, 3 mm i.d. (almost same as 3-mm Libby horn)	0	0	0	0	0	0	0
Libby Horn (4 mm)[1]	0	0	0	0	6	3	3
Constant-Diameter Sound Channel Snap-ring earmold with 1.5 mm i.d. sound bore[2]	0	0	2	−5	−10	−12	−12
Earmold with #13 Tubing (1.93 mm i.d.) to tip of earmold (most common model)[3]	0	0	0	0	−6	−7	−6
Open mold (IROS) #13 tubing[4]	−36	−24	−12	0	−2	−7	−6
Libby Horn (4 mm)[5]	−36	−24	−10	0	10	3	3
Vented earmold Earmold with #13 tubing, short hollowed-out bore, and positive venting valve (PVV) with largest hole[6]	−24	−2	4	0	0	0	0

[1]Killion 1985.
[2]Lybarger 1978a; Killion 1985.
[3]Killion 1981, 1985 (negative values at 3−6 kHz are due to #13 tubing).
[4]Lybarger 1979.
[5]Mueller, Schwartz, and Surr 1981.
[6]Lybarger, 1979.

horn earmold provides approximately 10 dB more gain between 3000 and 6000 Hz than one with number-13 constant-diameter tubing (see table 8.4), *if* the hearing aid has a wide-band earphone and provides substantial gain in this frequency region. The horn earmold provides more high-frequency gain because the sound channel provides a better match between the high acoustic immittance at the hearing aid receiver and the low acoustic immittance of the air between the earmold tip and the eardrum. In small children

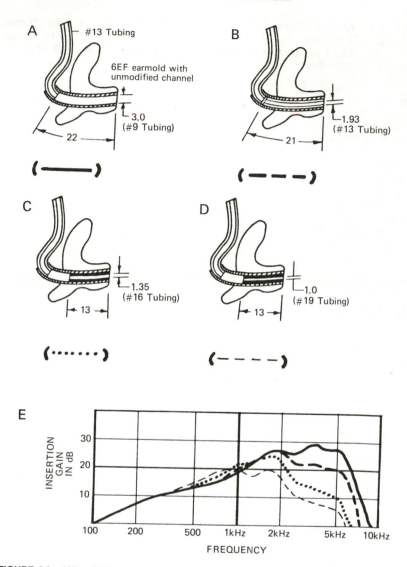

FIGURE 8.9.   Killion 6EF earmold. **(A)** Unmodified channel. **(B)** With constant diameter #13 tubing. **(C)** Insert of #16 tubing. **(D)** Insert of #19 tubing. **(E)** Insertion gain of a hearing aid with 6EF earmold unmodified and with three sizes of tubing inserts. From M. C. Killion 1984. "Recent earmolds for wide band OTE and ITE hearing aids." *The Hearing Journal* 37(8): 15-18, 20-22. Reproduced with permission of the author and publisher.

and some adults who do not have large enough earcanals for a horn earmold, number-13 tubing can be cemented 3 mm into the earmold and the diameter of the bore enlarged. If additional high-frequency gain is needed, it must be provided by the hearing aid.

When the sound channel is short, such as in an infant's earmold, in a standard, snap-ring earmold, or in canal or in-the-ear aids, it is not possible to create the same horn effects as with the long sound channels described above. However, if preserving high-frequency gain is important, the internal diameter of the tubing or bore should be as large as feasible. In standard, snap-ring earmolds, the internal diameter of the sound bore should be 3 mm at the ring and at least this wide at the tip, to preserve the high-frequency gain measured with an HA-2 coupler; if a smaller-diameter bore is used, this gain will be lower.

The same is true for closed earmolds with tubing; that is, the number-13 tubing (internal diameter 1.93 mm) should be cemented to a 3-mm sound bore in the earmold to deliver the amount of high-frequency gain measured in the HA-2 coupler. If constant-diameter tubing (number 13) is used, the gain in the high frequencies will be lower. In canal and in-the-ear aids the sound channel is very short. Furthermore, ear wax must be prevented from working up into the receiver. For this reason, a narrow sound channel is used, and the high-frequency gain must be provided by the hearing aid.

Sometimes it is necessary to decrease the amount of high-frequency gain with the earmold. As shown in figure 8.9 C, D, and E, this can be done by inserting smaller-diameter tubing (of the length noted in the figure) into the Killion 6EF earmold. These inserts are useful for people who need less gain above 1000 Hz than at lower frequencies and for people who find the sound quality of an aid with the prescribed high-frequency gain unpleasant. For this latter group, substantially less high-frequency gain can be given initially and then more added in successive steps as they become used to it. This is possible because the tubing inserts are relatively easy to replace.

The length of the earmold canal also affects the amount of high-frequency gain; that is, the SPL will decrease about 2 dB in the low- to mid-frequencies with short canals compared to medium-length canals, and increase about 2 dB with long canals. This change in gain is due to the change in volume of air between the earmold tip and the eardrum. In addition to the change in gain as a function of frequency, there is also an increase in overall gain with the longer earmold canal.

A *side-branch vent* (see figure 8.10A) may cause 10 dB or more decrease in the gain above 1000 Hz, if the vent is large enough and it intersects the sound bore close to the outside of the mold. To preserve high-frequency gain, parallel vents (for example, see figure 8.10B) are recommended unless there is too little room in the canal (as in a small child's earmold). In this case the side-branch vent should intersect the sound bore as close to the tip as possible, and the bore medial to the intersection should be belled.

As described in chapter 4 and shown in figure 4.7B, there is a smaller residual volume of air between the earmold tip and eardrum in females than in males. This smaller residual volume is associated with SPL at the eardrum that is approximately 5 dB higher between 1500 and 8000 Hz in females (Sachs and Burkhard 1972). Infants, who have an even smaller residual volume than females, will have an even higher SPL in the high frequencies.

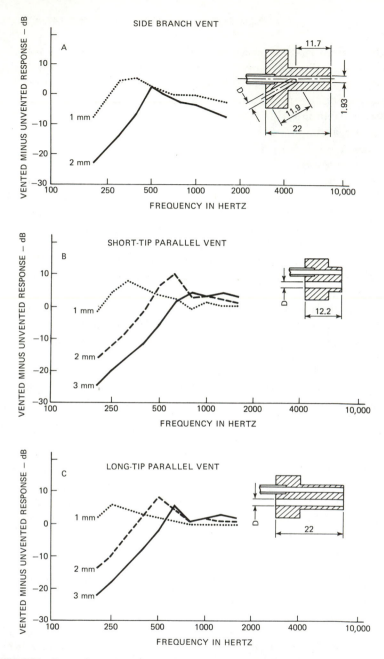

FIGURE 8.10. Types of earmold vents. **(A)** Side-branch vent and the acoustic effect of 1- and 2-mm-diameter vents. Note enhancement of sound around 300 to 400 Hz with 1-mm vent and loss of low- *and* high-frequency energy with 2-mm vent. **(B)** Parallel vent with short canal. Note enhancement of low-frequency energy with vents of 1- and 2-mm internal diameter & decrease in low-frequency energy with 2- and 3-mm vents. **(C)** Parallel vent with long canal. Note enhancement of low-frequency energy is approximately 100 Hz lower than for short canal. From S. F. Lybarger 1979a. "Controlling hearing aid performance by earmold design." In *Auditory and Hearing Prosthetics Research*. Ed. V. D. Larson, D. P. Egolf, R. L. Kirlin, and S. W. Stile. Reproduced with permission of Grune & Stratton, Inc. and the author.

Amount of low-frequency gain.   Vents can be used to increase and/or decrease gain between about 200 and 700 Hz, if sound escaping through the vent does not cause feedback. The increase in gain occurs when the internal diameter of the vent is between approximately 1 and 3 mm. The frequency region at which it occurs depends on the diameter, the length of the vent, and the remaining earcanal volume; that is, the smaller the diameter and the longer the vent, the lower the frequency at which this increase occurs (see figure 8.10B and C). A decrease in low-frequency gain (mainly below 500 Hz) occurs only when the vent diameter is greater than 1 mm; as the diameter increases, the low-frequency gain decreases. This decrease can be as much as 20 dB or more at 250 Hz.

A vent can be drilled a certain diameter and size by either the earmold manufacturer or the clinician. However, this may not result in the desired effect. Vents with adjustable diameters, which can be changed by inserting plugs with different-size holes, are available. The configuration of one of these systems coupled with a hollowed-out bore, and its effect on the low-frequency output of a hearing aid, are shown in figure 8.11A and B. If a long bore is used instead of a hollowed-out short bore, changing the insert hole size will not affect the output because the acoustic effect of the long bore will dominate (see figure 8.11C; #1 and #4 refer to the size of the hole in the insert, and the top two curves refer to the long bore).

In recent years it has been popular to use vents 2 to 3 mm in diameter in earmolds and in-the-ear aids for three reasons. First, they provide attenuation of amplified sound between 250 and 400 Hz, and this may make it a little easier to listen to speech in noisy situations. Second, a vented earmold or aid is more comfortable to wear than a closed one because it allows air to circulate freely between the earcanal and the outside world. Third, vents help prevent the occlusion effect that makes the bone-conducted sound of the person's own voice seem loud and hollow.

The major limiting factor in using vents to control low-frequency gain is acoustic feedback. As described in chapter 4 (see figure 4.24), acoustic feedback starts when the amplified sound is 5 to 10 dB below the level at which it becomes barely audible. This subaudible feedback causes distortion of the amplified sound, and it is assumed that this will make speech less intelligible and sound quality less acceptable. Although the amount of real-ear gain that is possible before audible (and subaudible) feedback occurs varies with the vent size, the individual, and the aid, it is substantially lower than can be achieved with a closed earmold and capillary vent (such as a vent that has an internal diameter of 0.64 mm and allows the air between earmold tip and eardrum to reach atmospheric pressure).

Open earmolds are used primarily in CROS (contralateral routing of signals) and IROS (ipsilateral routing of signals) fittings that are described in the next section. In an open earmold the "vent" is formed by the outside of the tubing and the person's earcanal. If this space is large, the low-frequency

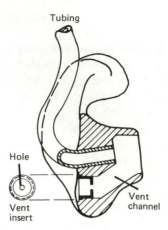

A   POSITIVE VENTING VALVE

Tubing

Hole

Vent
insert

Vent
channel

B   PVV VENTS, S–H TIP

VENTED MINUS UNVENTED RESPONSE – dB

VENT #
5

4

3
2
1

4.6

FREQUENCY IN HERTZ

C   CHANNEL SIZE

VENTED MINUS UNVENTED RESPONSE – dB

† #4
† #1
* #4

* #1

*   4.6

†   20.2

1.5

FREQUENCY IN HERTZ

FIGURE 8.11.   Type of adjustable vent: Positive Venting Valve (PVV). **(A)** Diagram of earmold with PVV. **(B)** Acoustic effect of changing the hole size in the vent insert (1 is the largest hole, and 5 is smallest). **(C)** The hole size on the insert is effective in changing the low-frequency gain with the earmold that has a short, hollowed-out bore, but with the long canal and 1.5 vent, the insert hole size is not effective. From S. F. Lybarger 1979a. "Controlling hearing aid performance by earmold design." In *Auditory and Hearing Prosthetics Research*. Ed. V. D. Larson, D. P. Egolf, R. L. Kirlin, and S. W. Stile. Reproduced with permission of Grune & Stratton, Inc. and the author.

attenuation will be greater than if it is small. If a small amount of gain is desired only around 2000 to 3000 Hz, number-13 tubing (or smaller) can be used. If greater gain is desired in this and adjacent frequency regions, a Libby horn should be used. For an open earmold fit on the same side of the head as the hearing aid microphone (IROS fitting), the maximum real-ear gain that can be obtained before subaudible feedback occurs is about 17 dB; this is 5 dB below the point of audible feedback.[2] If the microphone is on the opposite side of the head from the open earmold (CROS fitting), then approximately 32 dB functional gain can be obtained at 5 dB below the point of audible feedback.

When an individual cannot get sufficient real-ear gain to make sound between 200 and 6000 Hz comfortably loud because the vents or open earmold cause acoustic feedback, then an acoustic damper placed in the earhook or a closed earmold with or without a capillary vent should be used. Adjustment in the low-frequency gain will have to be made by adjusting the tone control of the hearing aid.

Average corrections in hearing aid output for earmold modifications.   The standard procedure for measuring the output of a behind-the-ear or eyeglass hearing aid is with 25 mm of number-13 tubing between the aid and the HA-2 coupler. The tubing is attached to a sound bore in the coupler that is 18-mm long and 3-mm in diameter. (*This "HA-2-coupler" earmold has essentially the same acoustic characteristics as a Libby horn [3 mm] in a closed earmold.*) The internal diameter of the tubing plus sound bore is not the same as that of the number-13 tubing (see figure 8.6A) that earmold manufacturers supply with earmolds unless other configurations are specially requested. For body hearing aids the standard measurement procedure is to snap the insert receiver onto the HA-2 coupler so the acoustic output goes directly into the sound bore described above. Standard, snap-ring earmolds are often manufactured with smaller sound bores than the standard 3-mm diameter; this decreases the amount of high-frequency gain.

When an earmold is selected that has acoustic dampers, venting, an open mold, and/or a sound channel other than the standard HA-2 coupler configuration for an earmold (described above), then the output of the hearing aid will differ from the HA-2 coupler measurements by approximately the amounts shown in table 8.4. The effects of these earmolds on the output of a hearing aid are considered when selecting the aid and earmold for an individual.

Lybarger (1985a) has written an excellent review of how earmolds can be used to modify the acoustic output of hearing aids. A detailed description of the acoustical physics of hearing aid/earmold coupling is given by Cox (1979).

[2]The rationale for 17 dB being the upper limit of real-ear gain that can be delivered to the eardrum with an open earmold is given in Killion (1982).

Ways To Prevent Acoustic Feedback

Acoustic feedback occurs when amplified sound reaches the hearing aid microphone and is amplified again, resulting in the familiar squeal. Within certain limits acoustic feedback can be prevented by (1) reducing the size of or eliminating vents, (2) damping resonant peaks, (3) reducing the high-frequency response, (4) notch filters (Macrae 1982), (5) using soft instead of hard material for the earmold (or using a soft canal with a hard body in the earmold), (6) using dental liner material around the earcanal and concha surfaces of a lucite earmold (described on page 270 in chapter 9), (7) increasing the length of the canal, (8) improving the fit of the earmold, particularly in the region of the tragus, (9) using thick-walled tubing, and (10) using the three-stage ear-impression technique developed by Fifield.[3]

CROS FITTINGS

As mentioned, the acronym CROS means "contralateral routing of signals." In a CROS fitting a microphone picks up sound on one side of the head and delivers it to the other side. This differs from the traditional arrangement in which the microphone and receiver are on the same side of the head.

A number of different arrangements of CROS fittings have been used in the last twenty years. The ones that are used often are described according to their purpose and arrangement in table 8.5. The CROS and BICROS (bilateral CROS) both prevent the head-shadow effect by picking up sound at the unaidable ear and delivering it, along with sound from the other side of the head, to the "aided" ear. The BICROS hearing aid amplifies the sound received from microphones near both ears and delivers the sound to the ear with some residual hearing. The POWERCROS is a CROS arrangement for someone with severe or profound hearing impairment. The microphone of a high-gain, ear-level aid is placed on one side of the head and the receiver delivers sound through a tightly fitting earmold to the ear on the other side. This separation of microphone and receiver is designed to provide higher SPL output before acoustic feedback occurs. The CRISCROS is a POWERCROS fit binaurally. BICROS, POWERCROS, and CRISCROS hearing aids are special-order items. The IROS is not really a CROS hearing aid; it is merely a description of a hearing aid with an open earmold.

[3]This technique was developed by Fifield (1979) at the National Acoustic Laboratories in Australia for making earmolds for those with profound hearing loss. Three different impression materials are used. An earmold impression is made with the first material, which hardens into a firm replica of the concha and earcanal. This impression is trimmed to remove any flare at the end of the canal and to remove excess material around the edge of the mold. Then the impression is coated with a more fluid material, and the impression is reinserted in the ear after lubricating the earcanal and concha with oil. The third step is to syringe an even more fluid material into the earcanal (into which a cotton block has been placed) and the concha, and the earmold impression (consisting of the first and second materials) is gently inserted to its original position. After the third material hardens the earmold impression is removed and the canal portion trimmed. This impression is then sent to the earmold manufacturer.

TABLE 8.5.   Purpose and Arrangement of the Major Types of CROS and IROS Hearing Aids.

NAME	PURPOSE	ARRANGEMENT
CROS	Prevent head-shadow effect caused by severe or profound hearing loss at one ear, when the other ear has near normal hearing.	Microphone placed near ear with hearing loss and signal transmitted by wire or radiofrequency to hearing aid at other, near normal ear. Sound from the aid is delivered through tube in an open earmold so that the naturally occurring sound and the sound from the aid are both received by the near normal ear.
BICROS	Prevent head-shadow effect caused by profound hearing loss at one ear, when there is a significant hearing loss at the other ear. Provides amplification for the aidable ear.	The hearing aid is placed at the aidable ear, and microphones are placed near both ears. The sound from both microphones is processed by the aid and delivered to the aidable ear through tubing and a closed earmold or one with a small diameter vent (1 mm or less).
POWERCROS	Prevent feedback when using high gain with an ear-level hearing aid for a severe hearing loss.	Microphone is placed on one side of the head and the hearing aid is placed on the other side of the head. The amplified sound is delivered via a closed earmold to the ear to be aided.
CRISCROS	Prevent feedback when using high gain with an ear-level hearing aid for a severe hearing loss bilaterally.	Same arrangement as POWERCROS but fit binaurally.
IROS	Provide no low-frequency gain and small amount of high-frequency gain to one ear.	Microphone, hearing aid, and open earmold are all at the same ear. IROS stands for "ipsilateral routing of signals." BIROS is the binaural application of this arrangement.

Two examples of CROS hearing aids using a wire between the microphone and the hearing aid are shown in figure 8.12A and B. There are also models in which the sound is transmitted by radio frequency from the microphone and radio transmitter in the hearing aid case on one side of the head to the radio receiver and hearing aid on the opposite side of the head. In a CROS hearing aid, the gain is minimal and an open earmold is used. This fitting is most successful when there is some hearing loss in the high frequencies in the "normal" ear. If a BICROS aid (see figure 8.12C) is used, a microphone is placed on both sides of the head and the output from them is mixed, amplified, and delivered to the aidable ear; the other ear is considered unaidable. Many people with profound hearing losses at one ear who

CROS HEARING AIDS

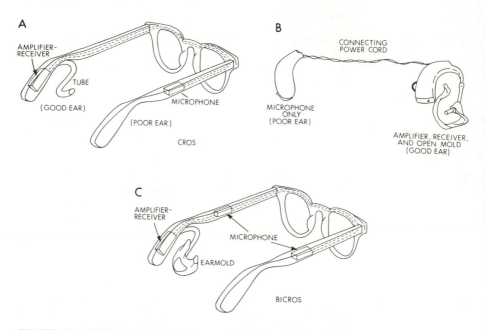

FIGURE 8.12. CROS hearing aids. **(A)** Diagram of a CROS eyeglass hearing aid with wiring from microphone on one side of head to amplifier and receiver on other side. **(B)** CROS hearing with connecting cord between two cases for behind-the-ear aid. **(C)** BICROS eyeglass aid with two microphones and one amplifier-receiver housed in eyeglasses. **(A)** and **(C)** from E. L. R. Corliss 1971. *Facts About Hearing Aids.* National Bureau of Standards, U.S. Department of Commerce. Reproduced with permission of the author. **(B)** from W. R. Hodgson 1986. *Hearing Aid Assessment and Use in Audiologic Habilitation*, 3rd ed. From figure 9.5 in "Special cases of hearing aid assessment" by W. R. Hodgson. Copyright 1986, Williams and Wilkins Co., Baltimore. Reproduced with permission of the author and the publisher.

have tried the CROS or BICROS fitting are pleased with the benefit that these aids provide.

The POWERCROS and CRISCROS aids have been used by some clinicians ever since ear-level hearing aids have been available. Those who wear them learn to localize the source of sound accurately within a number of hours, even though each ear receives sound from the opposite side of the head.

BINAURAL VERSUS MONAURAL FITTING

Advantages of Normal Binaural Condition

Normal-hearing people listen to sound with both ears; this is the binaural listening condition. There are a number of advantages to being able to hear with both ears. One is the ability to localize the source of a sound to identify it and decide whether to pay attention to it. If someone is talking, one can quickly look at the person and focus both auditory and visual attention on what s/he is saying. This attention enables one to comprehend the first few words that are said, which is often important for understanding the whole message, particularly in difficult listening situations.

Another benefit of binaural listening is the ability to hear equally well sounds that originate on both sides of the head. This involves less strain and tension because what is missed with one ear can be picked up with the other. With only one ear functioning the head creates a shadow for the sound originating on the side of the nonfunctioning ear; this effect is described in chapter 4 and shown in figures 4.15 and 4.16. Hearing with both ears also enables one to perceive sound in a three-dimensional space; this gives more information and is more satisfying than hearing with only one ear.

Binaural hearing provides the sensory input for the central auditory system to compare and summate so that very soft sounds can be heard at a slightly lower level than with one ear, and speech can be heard better in the midst of background noise. (The ability to hear speech in noise better binaurally than monaurally is often called the squelch effect.)

Advantages of Binaural Hearing Aid Fitting

Many hearing-impaired individuals can benefit from binaural hearing, either when both ears are fitted with hearing aids or when one ear is fitted and the other is normal. In a study of ninety-nine hearing-impaired adults who had worn one hearing aid for at least two years and who had started to wear two aids two months earlier, the majority found that the binaural fitting was better than the monaural fitting for all situations except hearing speech in high noise levels (see table 8.6). Other hearing-impaired people who wear binaural hearing aids have noted more natural sound quality, a sensation of sound in a three-dimensional space, and being able to set the volume wheels at lower settings (approximately 5 dB; Byrne 1981). The lower volume-wheel settings occur because of binaural summation of loudness. With this lower setting the overall SPL at the cochlea is lower, and there is less chance for distortion and auditory fatigue.

Monaural Instead of Binaural Fitting

Some hearing-impaired individuals hear better with one ear than with two. One possible cause is dysfunction in the central auditory nervous system that prevents the sound coming from the two ears from being processed normally. If there are no other neurological disorders (such as multiple sclerosis or space-occupying lesions), it is often difficult to detect whether a person will do better with one hearing aid rather than two, except by trying both types of fitting. Adults can tell you whether one hearing aid or two gives them better hearing. With small children, only through careful observation by parents and teachers can one detect which is best. Observations should

TABLE 8.6. **Comparison of Benefit of Monaural Versus Binaural Hearing Aids for a Number of Listening Situations as Judged by Ninety-Nine Hearing-Impaired Adults Who Had Worn One Hearing Aid for at Least Two Years and Then Switched to Two Hearing Aids for Two Months. Modified from D. Byrne 1980. "Binaural Hearing Aid Fitting: Research Findings and Clinical Application." In *Binaural Hearing and Amplification*, Vol. II. Ed. E.R. Libby. Chicago: Zenetron. Reprinted with Permission of the Author and the Publisher.**

LISTENING SITUATION	BINAURAL BETTER (%)	MONAURAL BETTER (%)	NO DIFFERENCE (%)
Hearing TV, radio, or records	80	6	9
Listening with comfort	77	12	5
Hearing speech in quiet conditions (1 or 2 persons)	76	4	17
Group conversations (3 or more persons)	66	8	16
Hearing conversation from a distance (over 20 feet)	64	4	13
Locating sounds	56	4	26
Hearing conversation from behind	51	2	22
Recognizing sounds	43	7	35
Meetings, church, theater	48	5	15
Hearing speech in noisy conditions	40	42	15

Note: some people could not answer some questions; consequently, the percentages often do not add to 100 percent.

include the child's (1) ability to localize sound in space with two aids, (2) response to sound (particularly speech) amplified by each aid alone compared to the aids worn simultaneously, and (3) progress in learning language and speech.

A second reason a person may find one hearing aid better than two is that two aids seem to provide too much sound for the person to tolerate. Whether this is related to central-auditory-nervous-system functioning or personal preference is unknown. In either case, it is appropriate to fit such a person with one hearing aid.

Creating a Binaural Listening Condition

Since normal-hearing and most hearing-impaired individuals are able to function better with binaural than with monaural hearing, it should be helpful to create a binaural listening situation. For people with normal hearing (or a very mild hearing loss) in one ear and a mild, moderate, or severe loss in the other ear, a hearing aid at the impaired ear will give binaural hearing. If there is a profound loss in the impaired ear, or if there is little or no ability to recognize sound with that ear, a hearing aid may not be beneficial. In this case a CROS hearing aid (see figure 8.12) may be particularly helpful to an individual who spends a lot of time conversing with other people, even though it does not create true binaural hearing.

Most clinicians report that binaural hearing aid fittings are most successful with people who have the same audiometric configuration and degree of hearing loss at the two ears, that is, a bilaterally symmetrical hearing loss. Those with moderate or severe hearing losses seem to derive greater benefit from binaural hearing aids than those with profound hearing losses. Although this experience with hearing-impaired individuals is useful, individuals with a bilateral hearing loss should have an opportunity to try binaural amplification. Many people who do not fit into the categories described above have derived much benefit and satisfaction from two hearing aids.

When To Fit a Second Hearing Aid

There are two approaches to fitting hearing aids binaurally. One is to fit one aid first, to let the person become accustomed to wearing a hearing aid, and then fit the second aid a month or several months later. By this time the person will have learned to adjust the controls and listen to sound with the aid. Many adults will have developed criteria by which to judge whether the second aid provides enough added benefit to warrant purchase. With children, parents and teachers can observe whether the second aid is beneficial (that is, are the children able to localize sound more readily, hear speech more accurately, and progress in language and speech development more rapidly with two aids than one?).

The second approach is to fit both aids at the same time. During the trial period the individual can either wear both of them all the time or experiment with wearing an aid at the right ear, at the left ear, and binaurally. One argument in favor of the second approach is that some individuals with certain configurations of hearing loss (such as bilateral, steeply falling audiograms from 1000 to 2000 Hz) will find wearing binaural hearing aids more satisfying—and wear them more readily—than when only one hearing aid, with its fewer benefits, is fitted. Another argument is that after wearing a hearing aid at one ear for some time, an individual may not be willing to adjust to listening to sound through two hearing aids.

Criteria for Gain and SSPL90 for Binaural Fitting

When hearing aids are fitted to both ears, criteria for fitting each ear separately can be used and then reduce the SSPL90 by approximately 3 dB and the overall gain by about 5 dB. These reductions compensate for binaural summation of loudness.

NONACOUSTIC NEEDS OF THE INDIVIDUAL

Interpersonal Communication

People vary widely in the amount of time they spend talking with or listening to other people either in person or on the telephone. Some people live alone, work in jobs that require little contact with other people, and/or choose to live rather solitary lives. Some people live with a number of other people and/or spend many hours in meetings, classes, or discussions. For the latter group there are many demands on their ability to hear and understand what is said.

Infants and small children need to hear more of the acoustic cues of speech to recognize what is being said than do adults. For children who have a hearing loss, it is particularly important to amplify speech and other environmental sounds so that they are comfortably loud. This is necessary for normal language and speech development.

Sound Environment

If an individual lives or works in an environment where people talk very softly, such as in a library, amplification will be needed with a milder hearing loss than if key people talk at a normal level. When someone works in a very noisy environment, such as around airplanes or punch presses, a hearing aid will provide little benefit. However, at home or in social situations, such a person may get significant benefit from an aid.

For many people the most important sound is speech, particularly that spoken when they are looking directly at the person. But it is also important for them to hear sounds all around them, including speech and other environmental sounds such as the telephone, doorbell, water running, motors turning on and off, wind blowing, a dog barking, etc.

Physical Limitations

The size and shape of a person's auricle and earcanal may limit the type of hearing aid and/or earmold that a person can wear. If the person has congenital aural atresia (lack of formation of the auricle and earcanal) of both ears, a bone-conduction hearing aid is the only type that can be used (see figure 8.1). If the auricle is small, as it is in a child, then it may not support an ear-level hearing aid (see figure 8.1); in this case, toupe or double-sided tape can be used to attach it to the head. If the earcanal is small and/or tortuous, an in-the-ear or canal hearing aid may not fit, nor will an earmold with large tubing and/or venting.

Some people cannot move an arm, a hand, and/or fingers normally. For example, someone with cerebral palsy may not be able to reach up to put in an earmold or move the controls of an ear-level hearing aid. In such a case, a body hearing aid would allow the individual to control the volume and switches (on/off and microphone/telephone) even though the earmold would have to be put in by someone else. Some people have difficulty moving their fingers, and they may have less sensation of touch in their fingertips than normal; consequently, they need control knobs on the hearing aid that are large enough for them to move.

Cosmetic Appearance

Most adults and older children who have to wear aids prefer to wear ear-level hearing aids instead of body aids. Body hearing aids, with their cords and snap-on receivers, are much more visible than ear-level aids. They may be particularly noticeable in the summer, if one wears lightweight clothing.

Within the category of ear-level hearing aids, most people prefer to have the smallest, least visible hearing aid; this is the canal aid. Many people believe that the in-the-ear aid is less visible than the behind-the-ear aid. This is true for those people who do not have sufficient hair to cover the back of the auricle; however, when there is sufficient hair to cover a behind-the-ear hearing aid, a skeleton earmold is less visible than an in-the-ear aid.

Financial Limitations

The initial cost, the cost of batteries and other accessories, the cost of repairs, and the expected lifespan of the aid are important considerations for anyone who is buying a hearing aid. All hearing aid wearers want an aid that will need few repairs, will have a long warranty as well as lifespan, and will meet their needs for the lowest cost.

PRESELECTION OF A HEARING AID AND EARMOLD

The preselection of a hearing aid or aids and earmold depends on the acoustic and nonacoustic needs of the individual. The flow chart shown in figure 8.13 summarizes the audiologic information to be obtained and the steps to be followed in selecting and adjusting a hearing aid and earmold.

Prescribe Real-Ear Gain

Obtain thresholds. The first step is to obtain unaided sound-field thresholds for warble tones between 250 and 6000 Hz. If the person's attention span is limited, use only 500, 1000, 2000, and 4000 Hz. Thresholds should be expressed in dB HL (see chapter 4 for a description of this

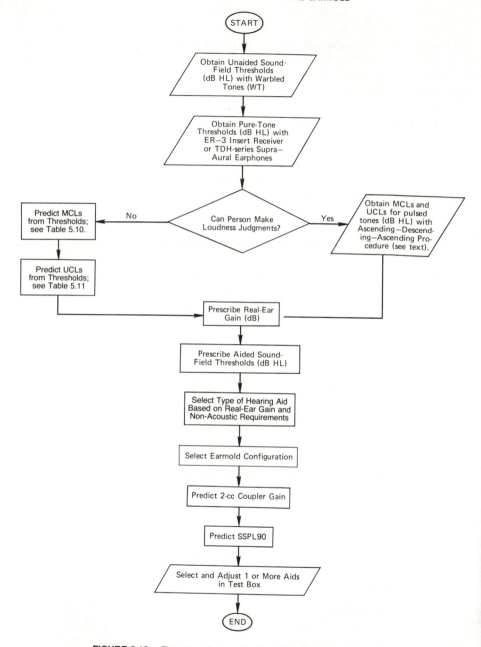

FIGURE 8.13. Flow chart for preselection of hearing aid and earmold.

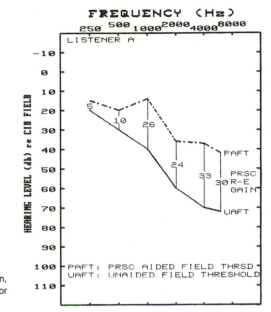

FIGURE 8.14.
Unaided sound-field thresholds, real-ear gain, and prescribed aided sound-field thresholds for listener A.

calibration). The nontest ear needs to be plugged and muffed to prevent it from hearing the sounds. If the thresholds in the nontest ear are 25 to 30 dB better than those in the test ear, it is likely that plugging and muffing will not be sufficient. In this case, the nontest ear should be masked. If the unaided thresholds are above 90 dB HL, it may not be possible to obtain sound-field thresholds because of equipment limitations. Plot the thresholds on an audiogram as shown in figure 8.14; these will be used in calculating the prescribed aided thresholds described below.

The second step is to obtain thresholds for pulsed, pure tones (dB HL) with an ER-3A insert receiver (see figure 3.14). This receiver has been designed to give the same output and frequency response as TDH-39 earphones and can be plugged into the earphone jack of an audiometer designed to accept 10- or 50-ohm loads. If this receiver is not available, use TDH-series supra-aural earphones. Plot these thresholds on an audiogram such as that shown in figure 8.15A.

Although it is beyond the scope of this book to describe the procedures used to estimate threshold, particularly for infants and small children, the following is a brief summary of the types of information that are needed. When a person cannot give reliable, conditioned responses to sound, then the auditory brainstem response (ABR) can provide valuable information about hearing sensitivity when interpreted in conjunction with results of acoustic immittance testing, observation of the person's response to sounds, the case history, and the medical examination. What is needed for prescribing the real-ear gain for a hearing aid are frequency-specific estimates of

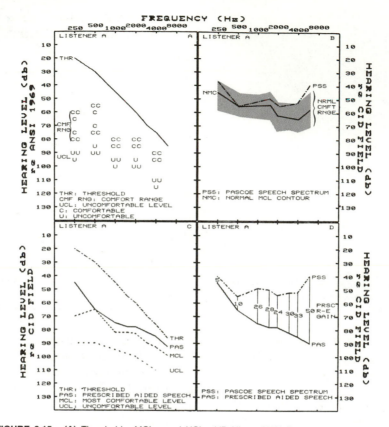

FIGURE 8.15. **(A)** Thresholds, MCLs, and UCLs (dB HL re ANSI S3.6-1969) for listener A obtained with TDH-49 earphones. **(B)** Pascoe average speech spectrum (unaided speech), normal comfort range, and MCL contour for normal-hearing individuals. **(C)** Aided speech levels plotted on audiogram with thresholds, MCL contour, and UCL contour for listener A. **(D)** Unaided and aided speech levels for listener A; real-ear gain, denoted by the numbers on the vertical lines, is the aided minus the unaided speech level at each audiometric frequency.

threshold, and knowledge of whether the hearing impairment is sensorineural, conductive, or mixed. In addition, it is important to know the limits within which the thresholds can be estimated. That is, what is the range of levels (dBnHL) within which the true threshold will fall for a flat audiogram, and what inaccuracy will there be in estimating the thresholds at 500 and 1000 Hz for someone with a sloping audiogram, with worse hearing in the high frequencies?

Obtain or predict MCLs and UCLs. If the person can make consistent judgments of loudness, pulsed, pure tones (dB HL) can be presented through the insert receiver or supra-aural earphone in an ascending-descending-ascending series. Ask the person to rate the loudness on a continuum from "very soft" to "too loud" as described in chapter 5 (see figure 5.4 for those who can read; for those who cannot read, see the pictures in figure 5.5). As the person rates the loudness, mark it down on the same audiogram as the threshold data; an example of this is shown for listener A in figure 8.15A. The MCL for each tone is defined as the midpoint of the comfortable range (numbers 5 to 7). The UCL is that which is consistently judged too loud.

When a person cannot make loudness judgments the thresholds can be used to estimate the MCLs and UCLs. As noted in chapter 5 (for data from people with sensorineural hearing losses), these estimates may differ by as much as 15 dB from the actual value, if they were measured directly. The MCL and UCL estimates shown in tables 5.10 and 5.11 are for people with sensorineural heaing losses. If someone has a conductive hearing loss, one-quarter the air-bone gap (dB) (but no more than 15 dB) should be added to the MCL and UCL estimates shown in the tables (see pp. 146–147 in chapter 5). The MCL and UCL values at each frequency should be plotted on the same audiogram as the thresholds.

Select criteria for prescribing real-ear gain. As described in chapter 6, there are a number of procedures for prescribing real-ear gain. Procedures based on MCL judgments (for example, the Cox and Pascoe procedures) take into account the magnitude and type of hearing loss as well as the growth of loudness above threshold, and consequently are applicable to all hearing-impaired individuals who can make reliable MCL judgments. Estimates of MCL can be made from thresholds for those who cannot make MCL judgments. Of the threshold procedures described in chapter 6, POGO or the Byrne and Dillon procedures provide better predictions of real-ear gain than the Berger and the Byrne and Tonisson procedures. These procedures are intended for people with sensorineural hearing losses, and corrections have to be made for those with conductive and mixed hearing losses as well as those with profound losses. There are a number of other prescriptive procedures, some of which are cited in chapter 6. After considering the benefits and limitations of the available prescriptive procedures, one should be selected that meets the needs of hearing-impaired individuals best.

The prescription of real-ear gain for infants and small children is based on less exact estimates of threshold and dynamic range than is the prescription for older children and adults. For this reason, most clinicians will select characteristics that are conservative. That is, they will select less gain and lower SSPL90 for a given threshold estimate and type of hearing impairment than they would for an adult who gives reliable threshold responses. Two recent articles (Seewald, Ross, and Spiro 1985; Stelmachowicz et al.

1985) describe information that should be considered in selecting hearing aid characteristics for young children.

If the Pascoe procedure is chosen, figure 8.15B can be used as a template to approximate where the aided speech should fall in relation to the individual's MCL contour and still keep it above threshold. The data for listener A have been replotted on the audiogram in figure 8.15C, and levels chosen for the aided speech are shown by the solid line. The real-ear gain is the difference between these aided speech levels and the unaided levels as shown in figure 8.15D. If the unaided speech levels are printed on the audiogram, the real-ear gain can be quickly counted with the graph; in this case, the gain is shown by the numbers within the vertical lines. If a computer program (Popelka 1982; Hewlett-Packard version) is used, the prescribed real-ear gain is computed according to the steps shown in figure 6.18.

Some modification of the prescribed real-ear gain may be needed, as described in chapter 6. This modification may be to: (1) smooth the frequency response (see figure 6.26); (2) reduce the prescribed real-ear gain at 3000 to 6000 Hz if it is much greater (for example, 15 to 30 dB) than at lower frequencies (see figure 6.26); (3) reduce the difference in real-ear gain between 500 and 2000 Hz to less than or equal to 35 dB (see figure 6.27); (4) reduce the gain at 500 Hz; (5) adjust the overall gain so that moderate sound levels are comfortably loud (to account for loudness summation effects); and (6) adjust the prescribed real-ear gain for those with severe to profound hearing losses so that speech is audible but not markedly distorted by limiting (see figure 6.28). In the case of listener A the real-ear gain at 6000 Hz needs to be reduced from 50 to about 30 dB; this will allow only the peak levels at that frequency to be heard.

Prescribe Aided Sound-Field Thresholds

Prescribe the aided sound-field thresholds by subtracting the prescribed real-ear gain from the unaided sound-field thresholds (see figure 8.14). If sound-field thresholds cannot be obtained, earphone thresholds can be used to estimate them between 500 and 4000 Hz. The calculation of the prescribed aided thresholds can be done quickly if they are plotted on the same graph as the unaided thresholds. This graph is used later for plotting actual aided thresholds, so that a visual comparison can be made with the prescribed aided thresholds to verify whether the hearing aid is providing the prescribed real-ear gain.

Select Type of Hearing Aid

Select the type of hearing aid that will meet the acoustic and non-acoustic needs of the person being evaluated. Weigh and balance the advantages and disadvantages of each type shown in tables 8.2 and 8.3 and consider the amount of real-ear gain needed.

Select Earmold

Selection of the earmold configuration and material will depend on the type of hearing aid chosen and the degree of hearing loss. The type of earmold, the earmold material, the length of the canal, and the type of venting suggested as an initial choice are listed in table 8.7. If the prescribed real-ear gain at 500 Hz is less than or the same as it is at 2000 Hz, a horn earmold is recommended. Stepped-bore tubing, and/or tubing glued to a

TABLE 8.7. **Suggested Initial Choice of Earmold Material, Type, and Venting for an Individual. The Sound Channel Dimensions (That Is, Tubing and Sound Bore) Should Be Selected in Conjunction with the Frequency Response and Gain of the Hearing Aid (See Table 8.4 for Earmold Effects). As an Alternative, the Earmold Prescription Guide, Developed by Cox and Risberg (1986) and Based on Categorization of Low- and High-Frequency Hearing Loss, Can Be Used.**

	HEARING AID			
DEGREE OF HEARING LOSS	CANAL	IN-THE-EAR	BEHIND-THE-EAR EYEGLASS	BODY
Mild	Hard acrylic, capillary vent	Hard acrylic, capillary or 2–3-mm vent	Hard acrylic, capillary or 2–3-mm vent, short canal, skeleton, regular thickness tubing	Hard acrylic, capillary vent, short canal, snap-ring
Moderate	Hard acrylic, no vent	Hard acrylic or soft canal, capillary vent, medium canal	Hard acrylic, capillary vent, medium canal, skeleton, regular thickness tubing	Hard acrylic, no vent, medium canal, snap-ring
Severe to profound			Flexible acrylic, no vent, long canal, shell, thick tubing	Flexible acrylic, no vent, long canal, snap-ring
Low frequencies— normal MCLs; High frequencies— moderate HTLs		Hard acrylic, 3-mm vent, short canal	Hard acrylic, 3-mm vent with short canal or open earmold	

sound bore that has a larger internal diameter (3 to 4 mm preferably) can be used with behind-the-ear or eyeglass aids. For body aids, the sound bore should be a constant 3 mm (internal diameter) from the snap ring to the tip (or belled to an even wider diameter at the tip) to preserve high-frequency gain. If the prescribed real-ear gain is less at 2000 Hz than at 500 Hz, the sound channel should have a smaller diameter to reduce the high-frequency energy. For behind-the-ear and eyeglass aids, a constant-diameter tubing that has an internal diameter of 1.93 mm (#13) to the tip of the earmold is recommended. For body aids the sound bore should have a constant diameter of approximately 1.5 to 1.9 mm. A reverse horn, such as Killion's 6EF earmolds with number-16 or number-19 tubing as shown in figure 8.9, can be used when even less gain is needed at 2000 Hz.

Predict 2-cc Coupler Gain

It is *impossible* to predict exactly what the 2-cc coupler gain of a hearing aid should be to give the prescribed real-ear gain for an individual. It can be predicted *approximately* based on average values for several factors including the difference between the SPL in the 2-cc coupler and that at the human eardrum, the position of the hearing aid microphone on the body (taking into account body-baffle or head-diffraction effects), the effect of blocking the external earcanal with an earmold or hearing aid (losing the normal earcanal resonance), and the coupling of the hearing aid to the ear. These factors have been considered in estimating values of hearing aid gain (dB) measured with an HA-2 coupler to provide the prescribed real-ear gain for a behind-the-ear aid with a front-facing microphone and an unvented earmold, as shown in table 8.8. Estimates for a body hearing aid are shown in table 8.9. It is important to note that these values represent use-gain values and *not* full-on-gain values. Consequently, *at least 10 dB should be added to get the approximate full-on gain value.*

If earmolds other than the ones in tables 8.8 and 8.9 are used, corrections in the HA-2 coupler values (in these tables) should be made. Estimates of the acoustic effect of earmolds on hearing aid output are given in table 8.4. When the values in table 8.4 are used to calculate the correction factors in tables 8.8 and 8.9 for earmolds other than the HA-2-coupler earmold, the sign of the values needs to be changed (that is − becomes + , as shown for the earmold with number-13 tubing in table 8.8).

If the output of a behind-the-ear eyeglass or body hearing aid attached to an unvented earmold is measured with an HA-1 coupler, then use the values for the HA-2-coupler earmold (3-mm bore in canal) in tables 8.8 or 8.9 to determine whether the measured values approximate the prescribed real-ear gain. If an in-the-ear or canal aid is used, the correction factors for microphone placement have to be subtracted from the HA-2 coupler ear-

TABLE 8.8. Estimates of 2-cc-Coupler Gain (dB; HA-2) To Provide Prescribed Real-Ear Gain for a Behind-The-Ear Hearing Aid with a Front-Facing Microphone and an Unvented Earmold That Has Either a 3-mm Libby Horn, Which Is Essentially the Same as an HA-2-Coupler Earmold (See A Below) or Number-13 Tubing with a Constant Internal Diameter of 1.93 mm to the Tip (See B Below). The Estimates in This Table Are for Use Gain; at Least 10 dB Should Added to Estimate Full-On Gain.

PRESCRIBED REAL-EAR GAIN	FREQUENCY (Hz)									
	250	500	1000	2000	3000		4000		6000	
	HA-2/#13	HA-2/#13	HA-2/#13	HA-2/#13	HA-2	#13	HA-2	#13	HA-2	#13
0	-3	-3	-2	2	5	11	2	9	-9	-3
5	2	2	3	7	10	16	7	14	-4	2
10	7	7	8	12	15	21	12	19	1	7
15	12	12	13	17	20	26	17	24	6	12
20	17	17	18	22	25	31	22	29	11	17
25	22	22	23	27	30	36	27	34	16	22
30	27	27	28	32	35	41	32	39	21	27
35	32	32	33	37	40	46	37	44	26	32
40	37	37	38	42	45	51	42	49	31	37
45	42	42	43	47	50	56	47	54	36	42
50	47	47	48	52	55	61	52	59	41	47
55	52	52	53	57	60	66	57	64	46	52
60	57	57	58	62	65	71	62	69	51	57
65	62	62	63	67	70	76	67	74	56	62
70	67	67	68	72	75	81	72	79	61	67

(continued)

TABLE 8.8. (Continued)

	FREQUENCY (Hz)						
	250	500	1000	2000	3000	4000	6000
PRESCRIBED REAL-EAR GAIN	HA-2/#13	HA-2/#13	HA-2/#13	HA-2/#13	HA-2/#13	HA-2/#13	HA-2/#13

A. Calculations based on *adding* the following correction factors to the prescribed real-ear gain to estimate the needed HA-2-coupler gain when using an *HA-2-coupler earmold* (3-mm Libby horn).

	FREQUENCY (Hz)						
	250	500	1000	2000	3000	4000	6000
Difference: 2-cc coupler/eardrum[1]	-3	-4	-5	-8	-10	-12	-14
Hearing aid microphone position[2]	0	-1	1	-2	0	0	0
Earcanal resonance loss[3]	0	2	2	12	15	14	5
Correction for HA-2-coupler earmold (3-mm Libby horn)[4]	-3	-3	-2	2	5	2	-9

B. Calculation of correction factors for an unvented earmold other than the HA-2-coupler earmold (an earmold with #13 tubing of constant internal diameter to the tip).

	FREQUENCY (Hz)						
	250	500	1000	2000	3000	4000	6000
HA-2-coupler correction	-3	-3	-2	2	5	2	-9
Earmold: #13 tubing[5]	0	0	0	0	6	7	6
Correction for #13 tubing earmold instead of HA-2-coupler earmold	-3	-3	-2	2	11	9	-3

[1]Sachs and Burkhard 1972.
[2]Studebaker, Cox, and Formby 1980.
[3]Shaw 1976.
[4]These values agree reasonably well with Killion's (1986) estimates of the 2-cc-coupler response for flat insertion gain for behind-the-ear hearing aids with

TABLE 8.9. Estimates of 2-cc-Coupler Gain (dB; HA-2) to Provide Prescribed Real-Ear Gain for Body Hearing Aid with Unvented, Snap-Ring Earmold and (1) 3-mm Sound Bore of Constant Diameter (This Is the Same as an HA-2-Coupler Earmold) (See A Below) or (2) a 1.5-mm Sound Bore of Constant Diameter (See B Below). The Estimates in This Table Are for *Use Gain*; at Least 10 dB Should Be Added To Estimate *Full-On Gain*.

PRESCRIBED REAL-EAR GAIN	FREQUENCY (Hz)												
	250	500	1000		2000		3000		4000		6000	
			3mm	1.5mm	3mm	1.5mm	3mm	1.5mm	3mm	1.5mm	3mm	1.5mm
0	-6	-6	-3	-5	8	13	5	15	2	14	-9	3
5	-1	-1	2	0	13	18	10	20	7	19	-4	8
10	4	4	7	5	18	23	15	25	12	24	1	13
15	9	9	12	10	23	28	20	30	17	29	6	18
20	14	14	17	15	28	33	25	35	22	34	11	23
25	19	19	22	20	33	38	30	40	27	39	16	28
30	24	24	27	25	38	43	35	45	32	44	21	33
35	29	29	32	30	43	48	40	50	37	49	26	38
40	34	34	37	35	48	53	45	55	42	54	31	43
45	39	39	42	40	53	58	50	60	47	59	36	48
50	44	44	47	45	58	63	55	65	52	64	41	53
55	49	49	52	50	63	68	60	70	57	69	46	58
60	54	54	57	55	68	73	65	75	62	74	51	63
65	59	59	62	60	73	78	70	80	67	79	56	68
70	64	64	67	65	78	83	75	85	72	84	61	73
75	69	69	72	70	83	88	80	90	77	89	66	78

(continued)

TABLE 8.9. (Continued)

	FREQUENCY (Hz)						
PRESCRIBED REAL-EAR GAIN	250	500	1000	2000	3000	4000	6000
	HA-2/#13	HA-2/#13	HA-2/#13	HA-2/#13	HA-2/#13	HA-2/#13	HA-2/#13

A. Calculations based on adding the following correction factors to the prescribed real-ear gain to derive the estimated HA-2-coupler gain when an unvented, snap-ring earmold with a 3-mm sound bore of constant diameter will be used (this is the same as an HA-2-coupler earmold).

	FREQUENCY (Hz)						
CORRECTION	250	500	1000	2000	3000	4000	6000
Difference: 2-cc-coupler/eardrum[1]	-3	-4	-5	-8	-10	-12	-14
Hearing aid microphone position[2]	-3	-4	0	+4	0	0	0
Ear-canal resonance loss[3]	0	2	2	12	15	14	5
Correction for HA-2-coupler earmold	-6	-6	-3	8	5	2	-9

B. Calculation of correction factors for an unvented earmold other than the HA-2-coupler earmold (an unvented, snap-ring earmold with a 1.5-mm sound bore of constant diameter).

	FREQUENCY (Hz)						
	250	500	1000	2000	3000	4000	6000
Correction for HA-2-coupler earmold	-6	-6	-3	8	5	2	-9
Earmold: 1.5-mm sound bore[4]	0	0	-2	5	10	12	12
Correction for earmold with 1.5 mm bore	-6	-6	-5	13	15	14	3

[1]Sachs and Burkhard 1972.
[2]Lybarger 1983 in Kuhn and Guernsey 1983.
[3]Shaw 1976.
[4]Lybarger 1978a.

mold values shown in table 8.8 to yield the HA-1 coupler values associated with the prescribed real-ear gain.

The values in table 8.8 and 8.9 are for older children and adults. For infants less than two years of age, approximately 6 dB should be *subtracted* from the HA-2-coupler estimates, and for those from two to five, approximately 3 dB should be subtracted. The reason is that infants and young children have a smaller cavity between the earmold tip and the eardrum, and for a given level of hearing aid output in the standard coupler, the actual SPL in the earcanal, particularly in the high frequencies, will be higher than for adults. If hearing aids are fit binaurally, the overall gain may need to be reduced 5 dB for one or both aids.

Manufacturers may give hearing aid specifications in reference to the Zwislocki ear-simulator coupler or in situ response on KEMAR, or in terms of insertion gain. All these specifications differ from the 2-cc-coupler values and cannot be used in conjunction with tables 8.8 and 8.9.

Predict SSPL90

The prediction of the SSPL90 is based on the individual's UCL at each frequency. Estimates of the SSPL90 (dB SPL) associated with UCLs (dB HL) are shown in table 7.2. As described in chapter 7, the conversion from dB HL (for UCLs) to dB SPL (for SSPL90) takes into account the minimum audible pressure (MAP) at the eardrum of normal-hearing people and the difference between eardrum and 2-cc-coupler measurements. If the UCLs were obtained with TDH-series supra-aural earphones, the SSPL90 should be measured with an HA-1 coupler and the person's own earmold. If the UCLs are obtained with the patient's own earmold and an insert earphone (calibrated with an HA-2 coupler), then the earmold effects have already been included in the UCL measurement and the SSPL90 of the hearing aid should be measured with an HA-2 coupler. The calibration values (dB SPL) for the insert earphone associated with a given UCL value (dB HL) at each of the audiometric frequencies should be made into a table like table 7.2. If the insert earphone is calibrated in an HA-1 coupler with the tubing used for obtaining UCLs, then SSPL90 should be measured with an HA-1 coupler and the person's own earmold. Adjusting the SSPL90 of the hearing aid according to results with an insert earphone and the person's own earmold should yield more exact results than using the supra-aural earphone.

The estimates in table 7.2 are for older children and adults. Just as for the hearing aid gain, the SPL at an infant's or small child's eardrum will be higher than for an adult for the same coupler level. Consequently, the 6 dB should be *subtracted* from the SSPL90 for infants (up to two years of age), and 3 dB should be subtracted for children two to five years of age. For binaural hearing aids, 3 dB can be subtracted from the SSPL90 of each aid.

Select Specific Hearing Aid and Adjust It in the Test Box

The initial choice of a hearing aid should have a frequency response (measured in the 2-cc coupler) without marked resonant peaks. If a body aid is chosen, a receiver with a smooth response can be used, if it gives sufficient gain.

Consider the hearing aid options described earlier in this chapter. If it is financially feasible, select a model with the options that are important for the individual. If the person has a dynamic range less than 30 dB at several frequencies, consider an aid with compression (preferably adjustable). For testing purposes, it is important to choose an aid that has tone and SSPL90 controls.

Select one or several models that will give approximately the 2-cc-coupler gain (appropriate for the earmold configuration that is chosen) and SSPL90 that have been prescribed for the individual. As an example, the relevant information for listener A is shown in table 8.11. The frequency response of the hearing aid should be adjusted in the following way. Attach the hearing aid to the HA-2 coupler and place the hearing aid microphone over the sound source; with the lid open set the hearing aid test box to produce 2000 Hz at 60 dB SPL. Adjust the volume wheel until the gain (SPL output minus 60 dB) is the same as the estimated 2-cc-coupler gain at that frequency; ideally, the volume wheel should be set at approximately half gain. Since this is the use gain, there should be at least 10 dB more gain available (test for this by increasing the volume-wheel setting). Then set 500 Hz at 60 dB SPL and adjust the tone control of the hearing aid until the gain is within a few dB of the estimated 2-cc-coupler gain; check this measurement with the lid of the test box closed and readjust the tone control if necessary. With the volume wheel left in this position, check the gain at the other frequencies for a 60-dB input. Since commercial hearing aids are single-channel devices, only the approximate gain will be obtained at each frequency. The goal is to obtain the appropriate balance between low- and high-frequency gain. The SSPL90 should be set at or below the estimates in table 7.2 (or your own table for an insert earphone); at no frequency should the SSPL90 exceed these levels. Use the HA-1 coupler with the earmold if UCLs were obtained with supra-aural earphones (or an insert earphone calibrated with an HA-1 coupler), and the HA-2 coupler if UCLs were obtained with the person's own earmold and an insert earphone calibrated in an HA-2 coupler.

It is important to remember that these settings of the hearing aid are only an approximation of what will give the prescribed real-ear gain and SSPL90 for the individual. Consequently, it is important to choose an aid that is set approximately in the middle of the range of adjustments for high- and low-frequency gain and for SSPL90 so that there will be room to make further adjustments during subsequent testing.

TABLE 8.10. Correction Factors for Microphone Placement That Should Be *Subtracted* from the Output of a Behind-the-Ear Aid and Earmold Measured in an HA-1 Coupler To Specify the Frequency Response/Gain and SSPL90 Characteristics of a *Canal*[1] or an *In-the-Ear*[2] Aid for a Manufacturer. These Correction Factors Are Based on the Mean Difference Between the Microphone Position for a Behind-the-Ear and the Canal or In-the-Ear Aid.

	FREQUENCY (Hz)							
	250	500	1000	1500	2000	3000	4000	6000
Canal aid	0	0	0	0	2	4	6	5
In-the-ear aid	0	0	2	−1	0	3	2	2

[1]Killion and Monser 1980; Kuhn 1979.
[2]Killion and Monser 1980; Lybarger 1979b; these values agree within 1 dB of Cox and Risberg (1986) except at 4000 Hz.

In the example described above, the hearing aid was a behind-the-ear aid that is readily available as a stock aid or from a hearing aid distributor. If a custom aid, such as a canal, in-the-ear, or eyeglass aid (with a particular length and color temple), is chosen, it has to be ordered specially. To specify what coupler gain and SSPL90 are actually associated with the prescribed real-ear gain, a behind-the-ear aid can be chosen, adjusted to the estimated coupler gain and SSPL90 (as done for listener A), and attached to an instant earmold with the desired tubing (number-13 tubing for canal or in-the-ear aids) including a vent if this is desired. Test the individual with the aid according to the procedures described in chapter 9. If necessary adjust the aid so that (1) the SSPL90 does not allow amplified sound to become too loud, (2) the aid provides approximately the prescribed real-ear gain, and (3) the sound quality is acceptable. If a canal or in-the-ear aid is chosen, measure the *use gain* and SSPL90 of the aid and earmold with an HA-1 coupler (unvented earmold) or an ear-simulator coupler (vented earmold). Add 10 dB to the use gain to get the full-on gain. To account for the difference between the SPL at the microphone of a behind-the-ear and an in-the-ear or canal aid, *subtract* the correction factors shown in table 8.10 from the full-on gain and SSPL90. These corrected values of the full-on gain and SSPL90 are specified on the order sent to the manufacturer. If an eyeglass aid is chosen, measure the output of the behind-the-ear aid in an HA-2 coupler, choose an appropriate make and model aid to order, and order an earmold with tubing that is the same configuration as that used for the testing.

Selected Cases

As shown in figure 8.14, listener A is an example of someone with a moderate sensorineural hearing loss that is more severe in the high frequencies than in the low. The MCLs and UCLs are close to the averages for people

TABLE 8.11.   Selection of Earmold and Hearing Aid Characteristics for Listener A.

Earmold: Skeleton, hard acrylic, parallel capillary vent (internal diameter 0.64 mm),[1] horn earmold with 4-mm sound bore or tubing near tip (e.g., 4-mm Libby horn).

Hearing Aid: Behind-the-ear, low- and high-frequency tone controls, SSPL90 control, telecoil, directional microphone.

Hearing aid characteristics:

FREQUENCY (Hz)	PRESCRIBED REAL-EAR GAIN (dB)	ESTIMATED COUPLER GAIN (dB; HA-2)	UCL (dB HL) SUPRA-AURAL EARPHONE	ESTIMATED SSPL90 (HA-1 COUPLER WITH EARMOLD)
250	5	2	90	105 (95)[2]
500	10	7	90	98
1000	26	24	95	99
2000	24	26	100	107
3000	30	29	105	111
4000	33	38	110	111
6000	30	18	—	—

[1]Cox and Risberg (1986) recommend using a large parallel vent with inserts for this amount of low-frequency insertion gain.
[2]Since hearing aids do not have frequency responses with greater SSPL90 output at 250 Hz than at 500 Hz, the amount from table 8.8 for 250 Hz has been modified to 95 dB SPL.

with sensorineural hearing losses (see tables 5.10 and 5.11). The prescribed real-ear gain can be obtained with either a behind-the-ear aid or an in-the-ear aid except at 6000 Hz. Since it is not feasible to deliver 50 dB gain at 6000 Hz, this has been reduced to 30 dB in table 8.11. Since some gain is needed at 250 Hz, only a capillary vent is recommended. The estimated SSPL90 has been reduced at 250 Hz. When the aid is set so that the SSPL90 levels at 500 to 3000 Hz are 98 to 111 dB SPL, it is likely that the levels at 250 Hz will be 98 dB SPL or less.

For listener A a behind-the-ear aid with a 4-mm horn earmold has been recommended to give the estimated 2-cc coupler gain. It would also be possible to recommend an in-the-ear aid. The full-on gain and SSPL90 can be specified after testing the individual with a behind-the-ear aid and correcting the coupler output as described above. Then these specifications can be sent to the manufacturer.

Listener B has a moderate sensorineural hearing loss through 2000 Hz, with a mild hearing loss at 4000 and 6000 Hz (see figure 8.16). Despite these mild thresholds, the MCLs are at the same level (dB HL) for all frequencies tested. Consequently, the prescribed real-ear gain is similar at all frequencies. The suggested earmold, type of hearing aid, estimated coupler gain, and estimated SSPL90 are shown in table 8.12. Note that the SSPL90

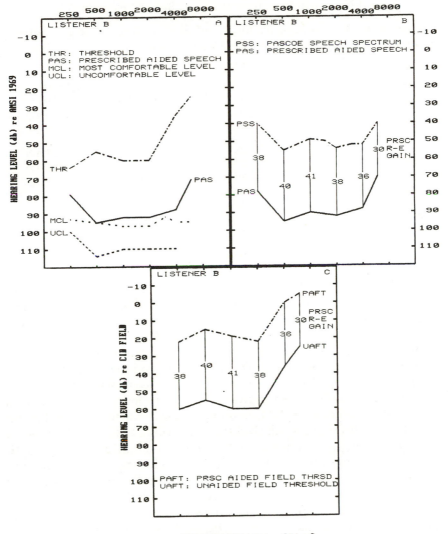

FIGURE 8.16. **(A)** Thresholds, MCLs, and UCLs (dB HL re ANSI S3.6-1969) for listener B. The prescribed aided speech levels are denoted by the solid line. These were determined by using the template in figure 8.15B. **(B)** Unaided and aided speech levels for listener B; real-ear gain is denoted by the numbers on the vertical lines. **(C)** The prescribed aided thresholds are obtained by subtracting the prescribed real-ear gain from the unaided sound-field thresholds.

TABLE 8.12. Selection of Earmold and Hearing Aid Characteristics for Listener B.

Earmold: Skeleton, hard acrylic, parallel capillary vent, horn earmold with 3-mm sound bore or tubing near tip (e.g., 3-mm Libby horn).

Hearing Aid: Behind-the-ear, low- and high-frequency tone controls, SSPL90 control, telecoil, directional microphone.

Hearing aid characteristics:

FREQUENCY (Hz)	PRESCRIBED REAL-EAR GAIN (dB)	ESTIMATED COUPLER GAIN (dB; HA-2)	UCL (dB HL) SUPRA-AURAL EARPHONE	ESTIMATED SSPL90 (HA-1 COUPLER WITH EARMOLD)
250	38	35	100	115 (112)[1]
500	40	37	115	123 (115)[1]
1000	41	39	110	114
2000	38	40	110	117
3000	37	42	110	116
4000	36	38	110	111
6000	25	16	—	—

[1]See text for the reason for modifying the values from table 8.8.

levels at 250 and 500 Hz have been reduced to bring them into closer agreement with those at the higher frequencies. This was done to help prevent auditory fatigue and to bring the recommendation closer to what is actually attainable in commerical hearing aids. The 3-mm sound bore or horn was recommended to give the appropriate gain at 3000 and 4000 Hz. As for listener A, an in-the-ear aid may also provide listener B with the appropriate amplification. A canal aid will not give sufficient gain.

A few hearing-impaired individuals have a moderate sensorineural hearing loss from 125 to 1000 Hz and near normal hearing at 2000 Hz and above. This has been a particularly difficult hearing loss to fit with an aid. A low-frequency-emphasis, open-canal hearing aid that can given up to 30 dB real-ear gain through about 1500 Hz (if the tube is inserted fairly deeply into the external canal) has recently become available; a diagram of this aid and the insertion gain measured on KEMAR is shown in figure 8.17.

Listener C has a severe hearing loss with a narrow dynamic range between threshold and discomfort (see figure 8.18 and table 8.13). The goal is to provide sufficient gain to make speech and other sounds audible and at the same time set the SSPL90 so that the amplified sound does not become too loud. Input or output compression will probably be helpful, if the output level is high enough to be comfortably loud. The estimated SSPL90 was reduced 5 dB at 250 Hz to approximate more closely what is available with commercially available hearing aids.

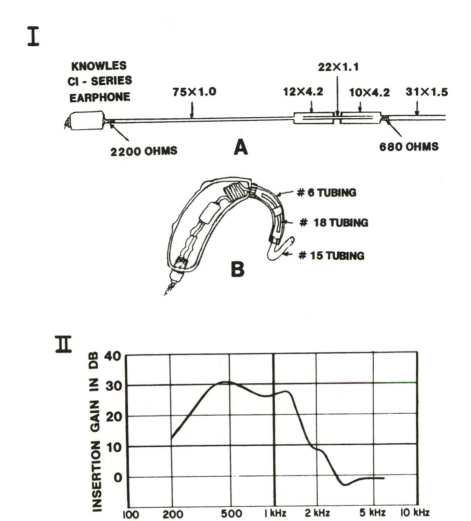

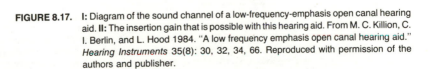

FIGURE 8.17.   I: Diagram of the sound channel of a low-frequency-emphasis open canal hearing aid. II: The insertion gain that is possible with this hearing aid. From M. C. Killion, C. I. Berlin, and L. Hood 1984. "A low frequency emphasis open canal hearing aid." *Hearing Instruments* 35(8): 30, 32, 34, 66. Reproduced with permission of the authors and publisher.

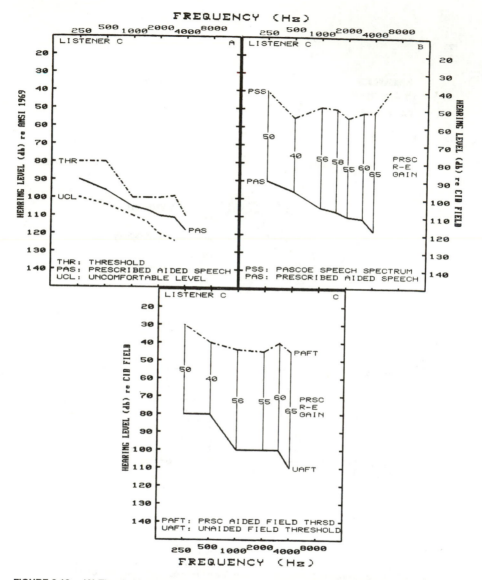

FIGURE 8.18. **(A)** Thresholds, MCLs, and UCLs (dB HL re ANSI S3.6-1969) for listener C. The prescribed aided speech levels are denoted by the solid line. These were determined by placing the prescribed aided speech spectrum halfway between threshold and UCL at each frequency. **(B)** Unaided and aided speech levels for listener C; real-ear gain is denoted by the numbers on the vertical lines. **(C)** The prescribed aided thresholds are obtained by subtracting the prescribed real-ear gain from the unaided sound-field threshold.

TABLE 8.13. Selection of Earmold and Hearing Aid Characteristics for Listener C.

Earmold: Shell, soft acrylic, thick-walled tubing, no vent, horn earmold with 4-mm sound bore or tubing near tip (e.g., 4-mm Libby horn).

Hearing Aid: Behind-the-ear, low- and high-frequency tone controls, compression control, SSPL90 control, telecoil, directional microphone.

Hearing aid characteristics:

FREQUENCY (Hz)	PRESCRIBED REAL-EAR GAIN (dB)	ESTIMATED COUPLER GAIN (dB; HA-2)	UCL (dB HL) SUPRA-AURAL EARPHONE	ESTIMATED SSPL90 (HA-1 COUPLER WITH EARMOLD)
250	50	47	100	115 (110)[1]
500	40	37	105	113
1000	56	54	110	114
2000	55	57	120	127
3000	60	65	125	131
4000	65	70	—	—
6000	—	—	—	—

[1]This value from table 8.8 was reduced so that it was below the SSPL90 value prescribed at 500 Hz.

A soft acrylic shell earmold with thick-walled tubing and no vent is recommended to reduce the possibility of acoustic feedback. The 4-mm Libby horn is recommended to give the estimated coupler gain. A high-gain behind-the-ear or eyeglass aid should meet these specifications; a canal or in-the-ear aid will not give sufficient gain. A body aid should be used only if a behind-the-ear model is not feasible (see tables 8.2 and 8.3) because of the individual's nonacoustic needs.

SUMMARY

Many of the factors that must be considered in preselecting a hearing aid and earmold configuration for an individual have been described in this chapter. These factors include types of hearing aids, options that are available on them, various configurations of earmold coupling of the aid to the ear and acoustic effects of damping, venting, and changing the dimension of the sound channel, CROS hearing aid fittings, binaural versus monaural hearing aid fitting, nonacoustic needs of the individual, and acoustic needs of the individual.

A *prescriptive* procedure should be chosen for specifying the real-ear gain and SSPL90 at specific frequencies between 250 and 6000 Hz. This choice should be based on a consideration of the benefits and limitations of a particular procedure and should be updated according to the most recent research and clinical findings. For examples in this chapter, the real-ear gain and SSPL90 are prescribed by the Pascoe procedure based on MCL and UCL judgments by the individual or estimates made from their thresholds. Tables of these estimates, based on average data, are provided in chapter 5. Sometimes modifications in the prescribed real-ear gain and SSPL90 are indicated, and these are described. Estimates of 2-cc-coupler gain and SSPL90, associated with real-ear gain and UCLs (db HL), are given for behind-the-ear and body hearing aids with several earmold configurations; correction factors for in-the-ear and canal aids are given. These estimates of coupler gain and SSPL90 may give only a rough approximation of the prescribed real-ear gain and maximum acoustic output of the hearing aid. Consequently, it is very important to evaluate the person with the aid, as described in the next chapter, to verify whether it meets the prescribed criteria and whether these criteria need to be modified.

Chapter Nine
MEASURING FOR A SUCCESSFUL FIT

ELECTROACOUSTIC MEASUREMENTS

FIT AND FUNCTION OF THE EARMOLD

SETTING OVERALL GAIN

SETTING SSPL90

DETERMINING ACTUAL REAL-EAR GAIN

Functional Gain

Accuracy

Procedure

Insertion Gain

Probe-Microphone versus Probe-Tube-Microphone Systems

Accuracy

Procedure

ACTUAL SSPL90 VERSUS UNCOMFORTABLE
LOUDNESS LEVEL

ACTUAL AND PRESCRIBED REAL-EAR GAIN

Expression of Results

Analysis of Actual versus Prescribed Real-Ear Gain

ADJUSTMENT OF HEARING AID AND EARMOLD

Electroacoustic Measurements

Selected Cases

COMPARING HEARING AIDS

Historical Perspective

Rationale for Comparing Aids

EVALUATION OF HEARING AID AND EARMOLD WITH
PRESCRIBED CHARACTERISTICS

Comparison of Hearing Aids

Judgments of Sound Quality

Judgments of Speech Intelligibility

Tests of Speech Recognition

Judgments of Nonacoustic Characteristics of the Aids

Basis for Choosing One Aid

Determining the Acceptability of a Hearing Aid
Anecdotal Observation by Individual
Observations of the Person's Response to the Hearing Aid
Readjustment of the Hearing Aid and/or Earmold
FINAL RECOMMENDATION
SUMMARY

The goal in fitting a hearing aid and earmold is to provide the appropriate frequency response, overall gain, and SSPL90 for the individual. The only way this goal can be achieved accurately is to obtain measurements with the person wearing the aid with a custom-fit earmold and by making adjustments if necessary.

The hearing aid and earmold that is evaluated may be the person's own or those which have been preselected according to the procedure outlined in chapter 8. In either case, it is important to determine whether the prescribed real-ear gain has been provided and whether the SSPL90 prevents amplified loud sound from being too loud. If the actual SSPL90 and/or real-ear gain are not the same as the prescribed characteristics, adjustments need to be made to the aid and/or the earmold, or another combination needs to be chosen. If the goal is to select one from among several hearing aids, each should be adjusted to provide the prescribed characteristics. Then they can be compared using ratings of sound quality, judgments of intelligibility of speech and word recognition in quiet and in noise, and the individual's observations.

Although adjusting the aid and earmold to provide the prescribed characteristics is an important step in the fitting process, further adjustments may be necessary to meet the individual's needs. These adjustments may be prompted by anecdotal comments about the fit of the earmold, the sound of the patient's own voice, and the quality or loudness of the sound, or they may be based on a rating scale of sound quality, judgments of speech intelligibility, or word-recognition tests. As the person uses the aid in everyday life, a series of adjustments may be made. The goal is for the hearing aid and earmold to be comfortable, provide acceptable sound quality, and make understanding speech as easy as possible.

A chart summarizing measurements and adjustments to optimize the fit of a hearing aid and earmold for an individual is shown in figure 9.1. Each step in the chart is described in this chapter.

ELECTROACOUSTIC MEASUREMENTS

Before testing a person with a hearing aid, it is important to determine whether it is functioning properly. This is done by using a charged battery and measuring the hearing aid output in either an HA-1 or HA-2 coupler; these couplers and the standard parameters that are measured (such as frequency response, SSPL90, and distortion) are described in chapter 4. The measurements of these parameters should agree with the manufacturer's specifications. In addition, it is important to listen to the output of the hearing aid through a stethoscope or monitor it with a sound-level meter (see figure 3.20). If the output sounds clear and meets the manufacturer's

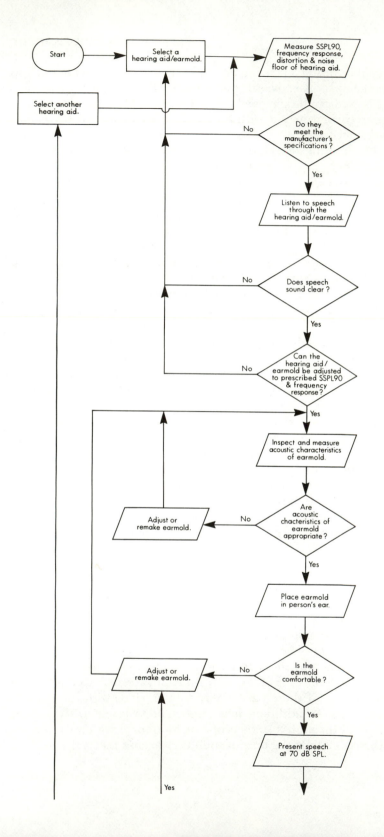

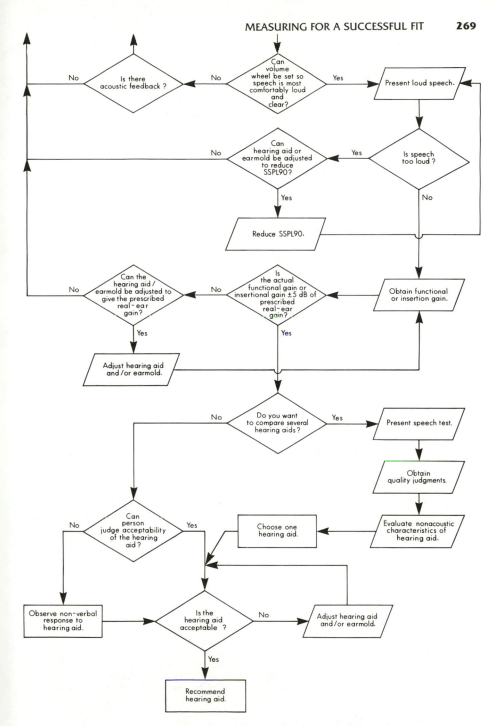

FIGURE 9.1.   Flow chart of measurements and adjustments to optimize the fit of hearing aid and earmold.

specifications, the aid should be evaluated on the person. If the hearing aid is grossly malfunctioning, another aid should be selected and evaluated.

It may be appropriate to evaluate the person's own hearing aid, if it has been worn satisfactorily in the past. However, its output must sound clear and meet the manufacturer's specifications. Electroacoustic measures will indicate whether it provides the prescribed real-ear gain and SSPL90 and, if not, how much it differs from these characteristics. Another alternative is to set the frequency and gain characteristics and SSPL90 to those prescribed, taking into account the earmold acoustics. If the actual and prescribed characteristics are reasonably close, then continue with the evaluation. If the hearing aid and earmold provide very different results from those prescribed (and cannot be adjusted), it may be more efficient to preselect one or several other aids for the evaluation.

If the person does not own a hearing aid or wants to buy a new one, then one or more aids should be preselected and adjusted according to the criteria and procedure described in chapter 8.

FIT AND FUNCTION OF THE EARMOLD

The second step is to assess the physical fit and acoustic function of the earmold in the person's ear and adjust it if necessary. If the person's own earmold is being evaluated, note whether feedback occurs when the person has the gain of the hearing aid turned up to hear sounds at a comfortable level. If so, determine whether the feedback is related to (1) loose fit of the mold in the earcanal, (2) large vents, (3) cracked tubing or earhook, or (4) loose fit of tubing around the earhook. Correct any of these conditions prior to further testing.

A loose fit of the earmold in the canal can be corrected temporarily by coating the canal and pinna portion with a thin layer of petroleum jelly, glycerin, or earmold-impression material and then pushing it carefully into the earcanal. To correct it permanently, feedback sleeves can be placed over the canal portion or the earmold built up with several coats of liquid plastic.[1] If it is a Lucite mold, the surface can be coated with dental liner material that will form to the contour of the person's earcanal when inserted.[2] If these

---

[1]Liquid plastic must dry for twelve hours to allow the toxic ingredients to cure and evaporate; this should prevent irritation of the person's earcanal.

[2]Dental liner material is usually used to hold dentures in the mouth, but it also can be used to help seal an earmold in the earcanal. There are several steps in applying the material to the earmold and molding it. The first step is to dip a cotton swab in baby oil and coat the individual's earcanal and concha. The second step is to roughen the surface of a lucite mold along the earcanal and concha with steel wool and then remove all the steel wool particles (for example in solution an ultrasound cleaner is effective; then dry thoroughly). The third step is to prepare enough material to wrap around the canal portion of the earmold and concha surface. While the material is still soft, insert the earmold into the earcanal. It will take approximately 10 minutes to harden. Then remove the earmold and trim off any excess material. The liner material should maintain its effectiveness for six months to one year.

techniques are not sufficient, then a new earmold should be made. It is difficult, if not impossible, to prevent feedback with any earmold when gains of more than 60 to 65 dB are used.

Feedback that occurs through a large vent can be corrected by plugging the vent temporarily (at the earmold tip) with earmold-impression material and permanently with liquid plastic. If the tubing fits poorly around the earhook or is crushed in the sound bore, it needs to be removed and replaced. If the bore is not large enough for the tubing, it needs to be enlarged. The new tubing, when cemented in place, should not move or allow sound to escape around it.

If a new earmold has been ordered, it should be inspected prior to the person's appointment, to see whether (1) the tubing is the size requested, (2) the tubing is crushed in the sound bore, and (3) the vent is the size, shape, and position requested. If necessary, replace the tubing and/or change the vents. The acoustic characteristics of an earmold without a vent can be determined approximately by (1) measuring the frequency response of a wide-band, linear hearing aid (no compression) in an HA-2 coupler using a 60-dB-SPL input, (2) attaching the earmold to the hearing aid, (3) sealing the earmold onto an HA-1 coupler, and (4) without changing any of the settings, measuring the frequency response again with a 60-dB-SPL input. The difference (dB) between the two frequency responses, as shown in figure 9.2 for an earmold with number-13 tubing, reflects the acoustic characteristic of the earmold. This difference agrees within 1 dB of the values in table 8.4. If an earmold is vented, then ear simulator couplers must be used instead of an HA-2 and HA-1 coupler.

When a new earmold or in-the-ear aid is placed in an individual's ear, it should fit comfortably. Surfaces that cause irritation or discomfort may not be noticed until the earmold has been worn for one or several days. If it causes discomfort, the earmold will need to be cut or ground off and buffed smooth. Sometimes pressure is caused by a surface that is too large on the opposite side of the earmold; consequently, it is important to find out what is actually causing the discomfort. The canal portion of the earmold should be the right

FIGURE 9.2.
Measurement of the acoustic characteristics of an earmold (with #13 tubing to the tip of the earmold) obtained by measuring the output of a broad-band hearing aid in an HA-2 coupler (curve A) and then attaching this aid to the earmold and measuring the output in an HA-1 coupler (curve B). The acoustic characteristics of the earmold are the difference (dB) between these two curves at each frequency as shown by the numbers on the vertical lines.

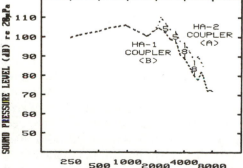

length. If it is too long, it will cause discomfort when the person talks, laughs, or chews; in this case, the canal needs to be cut and buffed smooth. If the canal is too short, it may allow feedback; if this occurs, a new earmold must be made. The tubing of an earmold has to be cut exactly the right length so that it does not pull the hearing aid down tightly against the pinna, cause irritation to the pinna, or allow the aid to flop off. The tubing may need to be shaped by heating it to fit the contour of the pinna.

The earmold should be adjusted so that it is comfortable and prevents feedback before doing any other testing, because the fit of the earmold affects the sound reaching the eardrum. Further adjustments or a new earmold may be needed after testing to prevent feedback, to modify the low- or high-frequency gain, or to relieve pressure in the earcanal.

SETTING OVERALL GAIN

The third step is to set the overall gain with the volume-control wheel so that speech presented at 70 dB SPL (54 dB HL at 0° azimuth; see chapter 4 for calibration procedure) is comfortably loud and as clearly intelligible as possible for the individual. Ideally, a recording of continuous discourse should be presented at this level through a loudspeaker; however, it takes less time for the clinician to talk to the person. *If* the clinician will stand at the same position and speak at approximately 70 dB SPL each time, this will give the desired results. It is important to have the person adjust the volume up and down several times to determine where the best level is. At this position the hearing aid should have in reserve at least 10 to 15 dB more gain, which may be needed for listening to soft sounds or if the hearing loss gets worse. The volume wheel should not be at its lowest setting, because at this setting it cannot be turned down for loud sound.

If the person cannot turn the volume wheel high enough for speech to be most comfortable and clear, there are several probable reasons. The most likely is that there is acoustic feedback, and this is usually remedied by making the earmold (or in-the-ear or canal aid) fit more tightly in the earcanal and/or plugging vents. If this adjustment is successful, the person will be able to turn the volume up higher. A second reason is that the sound is not reaching the eardrum because the tubing is twisted or there is cerumen in the earcanal. A third reason is that there is insufficient gain. Although more gain can sometimes be obtained with another battery (e.g., silver oxide instead of zinc air or mercury oxide), with rotation of a gain potentiometer, an increase in the setting of the AGC control, or a different earmold, usually it is necessary to select another hearing aid. A fourth reason is that the SSPL90 may be set too low and the speech signal is grossly distorted when the gain is turned up. Raising the SSPL90 should remedy this problem. If none of these adjustments allows sufficient gain, then more powerful aids should be selected and adjusted according to the steps described above. However, hearing aids with output in excess of 132 dB SPL should be used only with great caution, because their use may lead to further hearing loss (Binnie 1985).

SETTING SSPL90

The fourth step is to speak in a loud voice (at approximately 80 to 90 dB SPL) to determine whether the amplified sound is uncomfortably loud. If it is, the SSPL90 needs to be reduced. If the amplified loud voice is not too loud but seems very distorted, the SSPL90 may need to be raised and/or compression introduced. It is important to observe whether the person is being too conservative or too cavalier in his or her judgments of uncomfortable loudness. In either of these cases, the SSPL90 should be adjusted according to what seems appropriate to the clinician. If the SSPL90 cannot be reduced either by adjustments on the aid or by a damper in the earhook, another aid should be selected.

If it is important to determine whether the SSPL90 is too high at specific frequencies (particularly near the peak of the frequency response) warble tones can be presented at 80 to 90 dB SPL in the sound field with the hearing aid set where conversational speech is most comfortable and clear. If the amplified sound is uncomfortable, the SSPL90 at that frequency is too high. After testing at all frequencies, return to the ones that were too high, and reduce the SSPL90 until the warble tones at 80 to 90 dB are tolerably loud.

DETERMINING ACTUAL REAL-EAR GAIN

The fifth step is to obtain the actual real-ear gain. Real-ear gain is defined as the actual gain provided to an individual by a hearing aid. *Functional* gain and *insertion* gain provide two ways to estimate real-ear gain. Functional gain is measured behaviorally, and insertion gain is measured electroacoustically.

Functional Gain

Functional gain is measured by subtracting the aided from the unaided sound-field threshold. The measurement of functional gain takes into account (1) all the factors affecting the hearing aid output at the eardrum, (2) the effect of the eardrum and middle ear on the sound energy reaching the inner ear, (3) the way in which this sound energy is transduced to neural energy and transmitted to the brain, and finally (4) how it is perceived by the person.

Accuracy. The accuracy with which the actual real-ear gain can be estimated with functional-gain measurements depends on several factors. First, the person needs to give reliable responses at threshold levels. Second, the sound stimuli need to be frequency specific, as described in chapter 4.

That is, the level of sound at nontest frequencies (one or more octaves away) needs to be at least 30 to 40 dB lower than that at the test frequency. Third, the person needs to hold her or his head in the *same* position in relation to the loudspeaker for all the threshold determinations. Changing head positions can change the level by as much as 4 to 10 dB, and this can seriously affect the accuracy of the functional-gain estimates. Fourth, the amount of ambient noise in the test room may cause the thresholds to be masked thresholds, particularly if the aided thresholds are close to 0 dB HL. (Measurements should be made of the sound in the test room to determine the lowest level at which unmasked thresholds can be obtained; a procedure for doing this is described in chapter 4.) Fifth, the internal noise of the hearing aid may also mask the person's true threshold. A procedure for measuring the internal noise is described in chapter 4. Sixth, the thresholds may be detected in response to sound at the nontest ear, if the nontest ear is not plugged and muffed or if the unaided thresholds at the nontest ear are 20 to 30 dB better than those at the test ear even when the nontest ear is plugged and muffed. Seventh, if the compression of the hearing aid causes nonlinear gain for input sound levels of 50 to 70 dB SPL and the aided thresholds are at lower levels than this, the actual functional gain for average conversational speech may not be sufficient to allow the aid to reach preferred listening levels.

When the adverse effects of the factors mentioned above are minimized, the test-retest reliability of a single threshold is approximately 2.7 dB (standard error of the mean), and the test-retest reliability of the functional gain (two thresholds) is approximately 3.4 dB (standard error of the mean).[3] This degree of accuracy is possible if 2-dB steps are used near threshold and the person is informed when a sound is being presented by turning on a light (and monitor for false responses to make sure the person was responding to the sound and not the light). Hawkins (1986) has found that aided sound-field thresholds need to differ by approximately 15 dB to be significantly different at the 0.05 level of confidence.

Procedure.   The person should be seated so her or his head is at the position previously found to give the smallest changes in sound level for slight head movements (see chapter 4). Ask the person to look directly at the loudspeaker and to keep his or her head and body in the same position for all the tests; then actually look from time to time to make sure the person has done this. (It is very easy for the person to forget to keep her or his head still when concentrating on hearing.) Put an earplug and an earmuff over the nontest ear. Obtain aided sound-field thresholds at the octave frequencies between 250 and 4000 Hz, at 1500 and 6000 Hz, and at 750 and 3000 Hz if there is 15 dB or more difference in the threshold at the two adjacent frequencies. If the dial reading on the audiometer does not correspond to

---

[3]Research with twenty hearing-impaired individuals by Skinner et al. 1986.

TABLE 9.1. **Calculation of Actual Functional Gain (Listener 1) Using Dial Readings, When Calibration of the Sound Level in the Field Cannot Be Made. The Unaided and Aided Thresholds Must Be Obtained in the Sound Field for This Calculation to Be Accurate.**

	FREQUENCY (Hz)							
	250	500	1000	1500	2000	3000	4000	6000
Unaided threshold (dB dial reading)	15	20	25	51	55	58	68	74
Aided Threshold (dB dial reading)	15	12	12	18	25	32	40	45
Actual Functional Gain (dB)	0	8	13	33	30	26	28	29

the level in the sound field (dB HL), then a table of correction factors should be used (see chapter 4). It is useful to have the thresholds expressed in dB HL instead of dB SPL, so that they can be plotted on the audiogram.

If the sound field cannot be calibrated because a sound-level meter is not available, a table of the dial readings can be made for the unaided and aided sound-field thresholds (earphone thresholds cannot be used) and the aided thresholds subtracted from the unaided thresholds at each frequency to determine the actual functional gain. Then these values can be compared with the prescribed functional gain. An example of this is shown in table 9.1.

The unaided sound-field thresholds can be obtained before adjusting the volume wheel and SSPL90 of the hearing aid or after the aided thresholds are obtained. For sound-field thresholds, it is important to make sure the person keeps his or her head and body in the same position for both the aided and the unaided thresholds. If the hearing loss is profound and there is no response at the highest undistorted output level of the loudspeaker, then use the unaided earphone thresholds (dB HL). The unaided thresholds (sound field or earphone) are then plotted on the audiogram where they can be compared with the aided sound-field thresholds and prescribed aided thresholds. The difference between the unaided sound-field and actual aided thresholds is the *actual functional gain,* as shown in figure 9.3A. If earphone thresholds are used, the difference is only an estimate of the functional gain.

If more than one hearing aid is tested at the same ear, only the aided thresholds need to be repeated with the other aids. It is convenient to have the aided thresholds of all the aids plotted on the same audiogram (see figure 9.4), so that they can be compared. If one or more hearing aids are tried at the other ear, unaided and aided thresholds must be obtained with that ear. For clarity, another audiogram should be used for the results for the second ear.

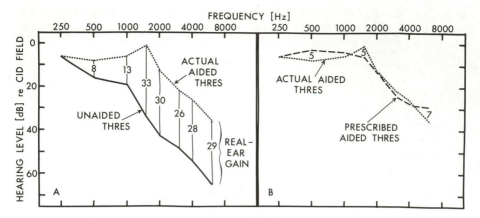

FIGURE 9.3.   (Listener 1): **(A)** Unaided and actual aided thresholds for FM pure tones presented at 0° azimuth in the sound field. Actual real-ear gain (dB), shown by the numbers on the vertical lines, is unaided threshold minus aided threshold at each frequency. **(B)** Actual aided thresholds are plotted on the same graph as prescribed aided thresholds. For this individual the hearing aid/earmold is set to give ±5 dB of the prescribed threshold between 500 and 4000 Hz. From M. W. Skinner 1984. "Recent advances in hearing aid selection and adjustment." *Annals of Otology, Rhinology and Laryngology* 93:569-75. Reproduced with permission of the publisher.

Insertion Gain

Insertion gain is defined as the difference between the SPLs measured in the external earcanal of the individual with and without a hearing aid. The sound is measured with either a probe microphone or a probe tube

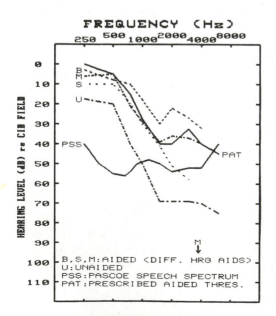

FIGURE 9.4.

(Listener 2): Aided thresholds for three hearing aids (B, M, S) plotted on the same audiogram as prescribed aided thresholds for the left ear (PAT), the unaided thresholds (U) and the unaided speech spectrum (PSS).

(attached to a microphone outside the earcanal), which is placed between the tip of the earmold and the eardrum. If reliable, valid measures of *actual* insertion gain and *actual* functional gain are obtained for the same aided condition, the values of real-ear gain should be the same within the errors of measurement. The major advantages of insertion-gain measurements compared with functional-gain measurements are (1) for a given measurement they take much less time; (2) many more frequencies are sampled; (3) the click stimulus used with Fast Fourier Transform (FFT) analysis gives a realistic measure of a hearing aid's response to transient and broad-band stimuli; (4) the nontest ear does not participate in the results; and (5) an audiometric sound booth is not necessary. The disadvantage of insertion-gain measurements is that they are not based on the person's behavioral response.

Probe-microphone versus probe-tube-microphone systems. Relatively accurate measurements can be made with a probe microphone in adults with large earcanals at frequencies from 250 to 2000 or 3000 Hz; however, the probe-tube microphone can be used in any size earcanal (even with infants) with reasonable accuracy through 4000 Hz. Since a probe-tube-microphone system is applicable in most clinical situations, one that is commercially available is recommended. The following comments that relate to probe-tube placement alongside the earmold (instead of through it) are specific to the commercial system described in chapters 3 and 4.

Accuracy. If the following factors are considered, the accuracy of insertion-gain measurements with the probe-tube microphone can be maximized. First, the sound stimuli being measured need to be frequency specific unless FFT analysis of broad-band stimuli is available. Second, the person needs to hold her or his head in the same position in relation to the loudspeaker for the unaided and aided measurements. Third, the amount of ambient noise needs to be at least 10 dB below the stimulus level in the field at each of the relevant frequencies. Fourth, the linear gain of the hearing aid can be measured only if the input stimulus level is low enough not to cause the output to be limited by the SSPL90 and to be below the threshold of compression. Fifth, the probe-tube tip needs to be in the same position in the earcanal for both the unaided and aided measurements. Sixth, the probe tip is 4 to 5 mm beyond the tip of the earmold and at least 2 to 3 mm away from the eardrum. Seventh, the probe tube cannot be (1) blocked by cerumen, (2) compressed with a tightly fitting earmold so that it is blocked, or (3) blocked due to the tip being pressed against the canal wall.

It is important to minimize as many sources of inaccuracy as possible and to know which ones remain. When these sources are minimized, the test-retest reliability of insertion gain is approximately ±3 dB (±2 standard deviations) from 250 to 4000 Hz.[4] Since the position of the probe tip in the earcanal strongly affects the sound level measured above 4000 Hz, measurements at these frequencies are not reliable for clinical use.

Procedure. Before testing, calibrate the sound level from 125 to 10,000 Hz at the tip of the probe tube, holding the reference microphone at the center of where the person's head will be during testing; enter these calibration data in the computer memory. Then look into the person's earcanal with an otoscope; if there is excess cerumen have it removed by a physician.

Seat the person and ask him or her to look directly at the loudspeaker. During the measurements make sure s/he maintains the same position. Place the probe tube along the side of the earmold with the tube tip extending 4 to 5 mm beyond the earmold tip and set the marker so it is flush with the outside surface of the earmold. Then carefully insert only the probe tube so the marker is flush with the tragus and placed where the outside lateral surface of the earmold would reach. Measure the sound level from 125 to 10,000 Hz (or click) at the tip of the probe tube with the level of the sound at the reference microphone set at 60 or 70 dB SPL if possible (these input levels approximate the level of conversational speech in specific frequency regions). This will give the unaided SPL in the earcanal.

The next step is to insert the earmold (or in-the-ear hearing aid) carefully into the earcanal, making sure that the probe-tube marker stays in the same place. Then have the person adjust the volume wheel so that speech at 70 dB SPL is most comfortable and as clear as possible (described in the section "Method for Setting Overall Gain"). This setting of the volume wheel is called the "use gain" of the hearing aid. For high-gain hearing aids, it may not be possible to turn the gain up high enough without feedback, because the probe tube creates a small space for the amplified sound to leak out. This leak may be eliminated with petroleum jelly or earmold-impression material placed around the canal of the earmold.

The next step is to speak in a loud voice to find out whether the sound is too loud for the person; if it is, the SSPL90 needs to be reduced by adjusting the control on the hearing aid or with an acoustic damper. If it cannot be reduced enough, another hearing aid should be selected.

---

[4]Test-retest reliability measurments made by Mason and Popelka (1986) and Chasin (1985). Mason and Popelka found that the difference between two successive measurements of insertion gain made with twelve hearing-impaired individuals was within ±2 dB between 250 and 4000 Hz. Chasin found that the size of the earmold opening does affect the reliability of two successive measurements of insertion gain using the same probe-tube microphone system that Mason and Popelka used (Rastronics Computer System CCI-10). The reliability was significantly better (at the 0.05 level of confidence) at 3000 and 4000 Hz with a 3.5- to 4.5-mm Libby horn (SD = 1.4 and 1.6 dB respectively) than with a standard 1.9-mm bore (SD = 2.9 and 2.6 dB respectively) or a reverse horn of 1.3 mm (3.4 and 3.1 dB respectively). Chasin made measurements with twenty-five people who had no history of middle- or outer-ear abnormalities. In addition to those studies, Hawkins and Mueller (1986) have analyzed a number of variables that affect the accuracy of probe-tube-microphone measurements.

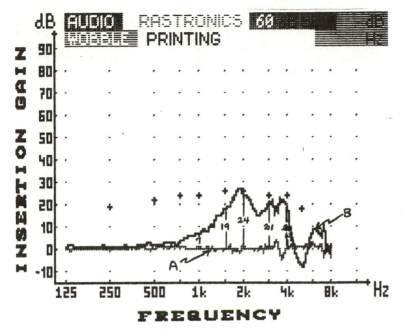

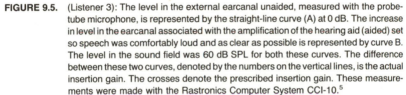

FIGURE 9.5.   (Listener 3): The level in the external earcanal unaided, measured with the probe-tube microphone, is represented by the straight-line curve (A) at 0 dB. The increase in level in the earcanal associated with the amplification of the hearing aid (aided) set so speech was comfortably loud and as clear as possible is represented by curve B. The level in the sound field was 60 dB SPL for both these curves. The difference between these two curves, denoted by the numbers on the vertical lines, is the actual insertion gain. The crosses denote the prescribed insertion gain. These measurements were made with the Rastronics Computer System CCI-10.[5]

With the volume wheel at "use gain," present the sound sweep or click at the same level used for the unaided measurement and the person's head in the same position. The difference between the aided and the unaided output measured with the probe-tube microphone is the insertion gain. This actual insertion gain can be compared with the prescribed real-ear gain, as shown in figure 9.5.

ACTUAL SSPL90 VERSUS UNCOMFORTABLE LOUDNESS LEVEL

The major difficulty in accurately comparing the maximum acoustic output (SSPL90) of a hearing aid with an individual's UCLs at specific frequencies and the person's UCL for broad-band sound is the different reference

[5]This system is available from Rastronics USA, Inc., 1125 Globe Avenue, Mountainside, N.J. 07092 (800-524-1609). It is described in articles by Libby (1985), Birk-Nielson (1985), and Sullivan (1985).

TABLE 9.2.   **Comparison of UCLs with SSPL90 of a Behind-the-Ear Hearing Aid (Listener 4). The UCLs Were Obtained with an Insert Earphone Attached to Standard Tubing and Calibrated with an HA-1 Coupler. The SSPL90 of the Hearing Aid Was Obtained in an HA-1 Coupler. As Shown Here, the SSPL90 Is at Least 3 dB Below the UCL at Every Frequency.**

	FREQUENCY (Hz)						
	250	500	1000	1500	2000	3000	4000
UCLs (dB SPL re HA-1 Coupler)	123	119	123	124	127	133+	126+
SSPL90 (dB SPL re HA-1 Coupler)	112	116	119	118	121	112	113

points at which the sound-generating systems are calibrated. Despite this difficulty the comparison is helpful in adjusting an aid for optimal fit.

There are several ways to compare the SSPL90 at specific frequencies with the individual's UCLs. One clinically efficient way is to obtain UCLs with an insert earphone (see figure 3.14) attached to standard tubing or the

FIGURE 9.6.   (Listener 1): Aided speech spectrum and maximum output (MPO) of the hearing aid are shown in relation to the patient's threshold, MCL, and UCL contours. All data are expressed in dB HL in reference to sound-field calibration. From M. W. Skinner 1984. "Recent advances in hearing aid selection and adjustment." *Annals of Otology, Rhinology and Laryngology* 93: 569-75. Reproduced with permission of the publisher.

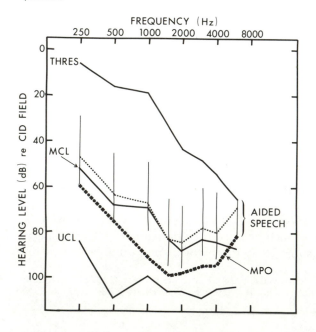

person's own earmold and the output measured with an HA-1 coupler, as described in chapter 7. The SSPL90 of the hearing aid, after it has been set so that loud speech is not uncomfortable, also is measured in the HA-1 coupler with the person's own earmold. These results can be directly compared with the individual's UCLs for all types of air-conduction aids. An example of this comparison is shown in table 9.2.

Another way to make this comparison is to convert the SSPL90 of the hearing aid measured in the coupler to the sound-field reference and compare it with the individual's UCL contour. Measurements of the SSPL90 in the coupler, the coupler gain of the hearing aid, the functional gain of the hearing aid, and the head-baffle effect are inserted into the equation given in chapter 5. This comparison is clinically efficient only if a computer program (such as Popelka 1982) is used to make the calculations and display the data graphically. An example of the graphic display of SSPL90 and UCLs is shown in figure 9.6.

ACTUAL AND PRESCRIBED REAL-EAR GAIN

Expression of Results

There are several ways to compare the actual and prescribed real-ear gain. First, the actual functional gain at each frequency can be calculated by subtracting the aided thresholds from the unaided thresholds, as shown in table 9.1 (note that the values in this table are in dial reading, whereas normally they would be referenced to 0 dB HL), and then compared with the prescribed functional gain. Second, the actual and prescribed aided thresholds can be plotted on the same audiogram, as shown in figure 9.3B, and the difference noted at each frequency. Third, the actual and prescribed insertion gain can be plotted on the same graph, as shown in figure 9.5, and the difference noted. Fourth, the actual functional gain can be added to the average speech spectrum and plotted on the same graph as the individual's threshold, MCL, and UCL contours, as shown in figure 9.6.

Although all these ways are useful, methods one, two, and three take less time than the fourth unless you have a computer program to generate it. However, the graph for the fourth method clearly shows the relation of the amplified speech spectrum to the individual's auditory area, and this information is particularly useful in deciding what compromises are feasible in adjusting the hearing aid to meet the individual's needs.

If the actual and prescribed real-ear gain at the frequencies between 500 and 4000 Hz are within ±5 dB, this is considered good agreement. If there are larger differences between the actual and the prescribed real-ear gain, it is important to determine possible reasons for these differences to decide what adjustments are appropriate and what compromises are acceptable.

Analysis of Actual versus Prescribed Real-Ear Gain

There are a number of reasons for differences between the actual and prescribed real-ear gain. In general, these are related to factors affecting the volume wheel setting chosen by the individual.

Actual functional or insertion gain is obtained with the volume wheel of the hearing aid set at a certain position. The individual's choice of this setting can be affected by (1) resonant peaks in the real-ear frequency response and SSPL90, (2) a value of SSPL90 for the hearing aid that is too high or too low, (3) acoustic feedback occurring at a level below that which makes speech most clear and comfortable, (4) an inappropriate balance between low- and high-frequency gain of the hearing aid, and (5) loudness summation of broad-band sound.

If resonant peaks in the real-ear frequency response and SSPL90 are not damped, the overall gain may be set so that the speech energy in the frequency region of the highest resonant peak is comfortable. However, the speech energy in other frequency regions may be lower than optimal. An example of the actual functional gain of a hearing aid with sharp resonant

FIGURE 9.7. (Listener 5): **(A)** Actual functional gain and prescribed functional gain of a hearing aid with sharp resonant peaks. The overall gain was set too low because of the resonant peak at 1000-2000 Hz. **(B)** Actual functional gain and prescribed functional gain of the same hearing aid set to MCL after inserting an acoustic damper in the earhook. **(C)** Electroacoustic output without the acoustic damper with the hearing aid at use-gain setting. **(D)** Electroacoustic output with the acoustic damper with the hearing aid at use-gain setting.

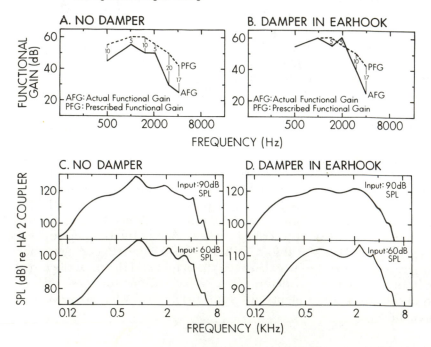

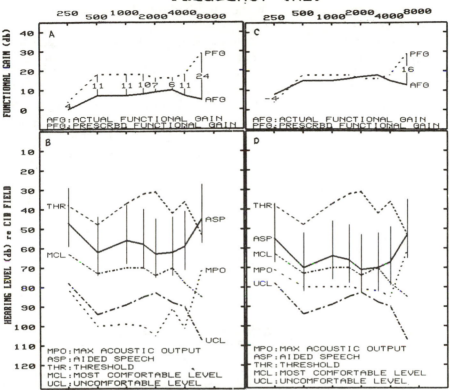

FIGURE 9.8. (Listener 6): **(A)** Actual and prescribed functional gain of a hearing aid with the SSPL90 set too high. **(B)** SSPL90 and amplified speech spectrum plotted in relation to thresholds, MCLs, and UCLs obtained in the sound field (dB HL). **(C)** Actual and prescribed functional gain when SSPL90 of the hearing aid was set below UCLs. **(D)** SSPL90 and amplified speech spectrum plotted in relation to thresholds, MCLs, and UCLs in the sound field after reducing the SSPL90.

peaks is plotted on the same graph as the prescribed functional gain in figure 9.7A (see figure 9.7C for the electroacoustic output). When an acoustic damper was used, the overall gain chosen was higher, and the actual functional gain closely approximated the prescribed functional gain as shown in figure 9.7B.

If the SSPL90 of a hearing aid is set too high, then the occasional peak energy is uncomfortable and the person will set the overall gain of the hearing aid lower to avoid this discomfort. An example of the actual functional gain for a hearing aid with the SSPL90 set too high is shown on the same graph as the prescribed functional gain in figure 9.8A. The SSPL90 and the amplified speech for this hearing aid are shown in relation to the individual's thresholds, MCLs, and UCLs in figure 9.8B. When the SSPL90 was set so that amplified sound did not surpass discomfort, this person set the overall gain higher and the actual functional gain more closely approximated the prescribed functional gain (figure 9.8C). The effect of this change in the SSPL90 and overall gain on the amplified speech spectrum is shown in figure 9.8D.

If the SSPL90 is set too low, the amplified speech will be distorted when the overall gain of the hearing aid is turned up to an appropriate level. Consequently, the person sets the volume wheel at a lower level so the signal is relatively undistorted. The actual and prescribed functional gain for someone wearing an aid with too low an SSPL90 is shown in figure 9.9A. The SSPL90 and amplified speech spectrum are plotted in relation to this person's thresholds, MCLs, and UCLs in figure 9.9B. When the SSPL90 was set higher but not too high, the overall gain chosen was appropriate (see figures 9.9C and D).

Acoustic feedback is an important limiting factor in how high people set the volume wheel. For those with mild and moderate hearing losses, feed-

FIGURE 9.9. (Listener 1): **(A)** Actual and prescribed functional gain for hearing aid with the SSPL90 set too low. **(B)** SSPL90 and amplified speech spectrum plotted in relation to thresholds, MCLs, and UCLs obtained in the sound field (dB HL). **(C)** Actual and prescribed functional gain when the SSPL90 of the hearing aid was set so that the peaks of speech were not clipped. **(D)** SSPL90 and amplified speech spectrum in relation to threshold, MCLs, and UCLs obtained in the sound field after raising the SSPL90.

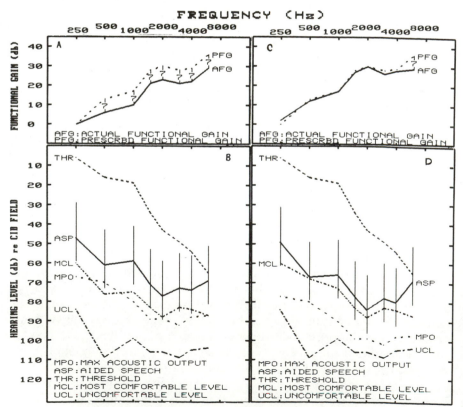

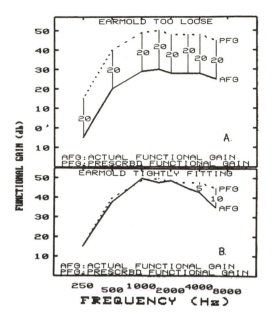

FIGURE 9.10.

(Listener 7): **(A)** Actual and prescribed functional gain obtained with a loosely fitting earmold at the left ear. **(B)** Actual and prescribed functional gain obtained when a well-fitting earmold was used. After Pascoe 1985, with permission.

back is often associated with open-mold fittings or large vents. For those with severe and profound hearing losses, feedback is caused by not getting a tight enough seal between the earcanal and the earmold. For example, when listener 7, who has a moderate sensorineural hearing loss, had an earmold that fit too loosely, he set the overall gain so that there was no audible feedback (see figure 9.10A). At this setting the actual functional gain was 20 dB lower than the prescribed functional gain. With a well-fitting earmold, the volume wheel could be turned up and the actual functional gain was close to the prescribed functional gain between 750 and 4000 Hz (see figure 9.10B). As described in chapters 4 and 8, the overall gain must be at least 10 dB lower than that associated with the audible squeal of feedback to eliminate subaudible oscillation, which can also distort the amplified sound.

If the hearing aid provides too much or too little low-frequency gain in relation to the high-frequency gain, the person will set the volume wheel so that the broad-band speech is most comfortable, but the speech energy in some frequency regions will be either too soft or inaudible. An example of too little gain in both the low- and high-frequency regions (above 2000 Hz) is shown in figure 9.11A. This imbalance was caused by an earhook with no acoustic damper and an earmold that had #13 tubing, an enlarged sound bore, and an open select-a-vent (SAV). When an earhook with a 680-ohm damper and an earmold with a 3-mm Libby horn and a parallel capillary vent were used, the sound quality was much more acceptable. There was better balance between low- and high-frequency gain, and more of the speech spectrum was audible (see figure 9.11B).

An example of too little gain in the high frequencies is shown in figure 9.12. This may be corrected with a high-frequency tone control on the

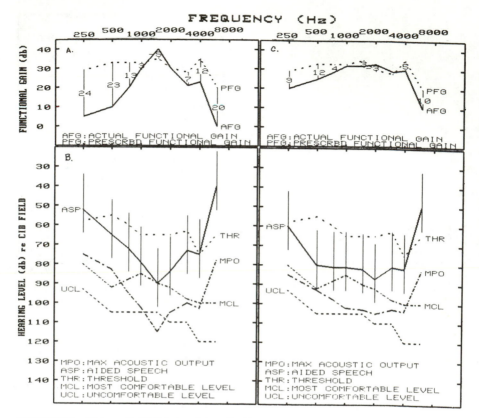

FIGURE 9.11. (Listener 8): **(A)**Actual and prescribed functional gain for behind-the-ear aid coupled to an earmold with #13 tubing, an enlarged sound bore, and an open SAV. **(B)** Amplified speech spectrum and SSPL90 plotted in relation to thresholds, MCLs, and UCLs. **(C)** Actual and prescribed functional gain when an acoustic damper was placed in the earhook of hearing aid and the earmold was changed to one with a 3-mm Libby horn and a capillary vent for air-pressure equalization. **(D)** Amplified speech spectrum and SSPL90 plotted in relation to thresholds, MCLs, and UCLs.

hearing aid, a horn earmold, or both. Otherwise, another hearing aid should be tried. Occasionally, the person's earcanal is too narrow and tortuous to use a horn or belled-bore earmold; it is very difficult to achieve sufficient high-frequency gain in such a case.

Even after all the above factors (damping the resonant peaks, finding the appropriate SSPL90, eliminating acoustic feedback, and obtaining the appropriate frequency response) are optimized, some people may still choose a volume-wheel setting that causes the real-ear gain at all frequencies to be lower than that prescribed (for example, see figure 9.13A and B). This may be due to loudness summation effects and/or particular sensitivity to loud sound such as is found in some patients with Ménière's disease. In cases such as this, no further adjustments are indicated.

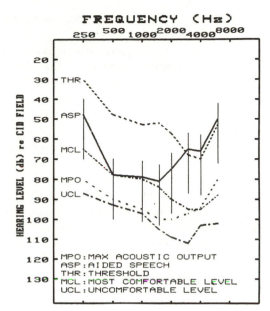

FIGURE 9.12.
(Listener 9): Amplified speech spectrum and SSPL90 plotted in relation to thresholds, MCLs, and UCLs. The aid provides too little gain above 1500 Hz.

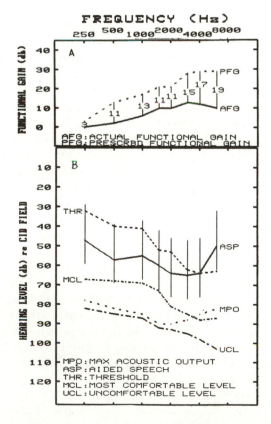

FIGURE 9.13.
(Listener 10): **(A)** Actual and prescribed functional gain for Listener 10, who chose a volume-wheel setting approximately 10 dB lower than that which would have given the prescribed functional gain, even though all other factors were optimized. **(B)** Amplified speech spectrum and SSPL90 plotted in relation to thresholds, MCLs, and UCLs.

ADJUSTMENT OF HEARING AID AND EARMOLD

If the actual real-ear gain differs more than ±5 dB from the prescribed real-ear gain between 500 and 4000 Hz, it is important to consider the possible reasons and decide whether the earmold, the hearing aid, or both should be changed to provide the prescribed real-ear gain and SSPL90. In some cases it may be appropriate to settle for less agreement than ±5 dB since no hearing aid can be adjusted to give the prescribed real-ear gain exactly, whereas in other cases changes should be made. To make these changes, the acoustic characteristics of earmolds and the effect of acoustic dampers described in chapter 8 need to be considered. In addition, it is important to consider the effect of different earhooks and the range of SSPL90, AGC, and tone-control settings on the hearing aid as well as on other aids that may be used instead. It takes time and commitment to acquire the experience to make these adjustments efficiently.

Electroacoustic Measurements

Electroacoustic measurements of the hearing aid and/or earmold output can expedite making the changes that will give the prescribed real-ear gain. If a probe-tube microphone system is used, the original measurement of the actual insertion gain and the marks for the prescribed insertion gain on the screen should be saved. If a change in the gain in the low or high frequencies is needed, switch to the mode with which a single warble tone (for example, 500, 2000, 3000, or 4000 Hz) at 60 dB SPL can be presented. As the tone control is adjusted, the change in insertion gain can be seen on the monitor. In addition, the actual insertion gain can be compared with the prescribed insertion gain at that frequency. The AGC and SSPL90 controls can also be adjusted to see what effect they have on the insertion gain at a particular frequency, or a frequency sweep (or click) can be presented to create a new insertion gain curve on the screen. This curve can be compared with the previous one to see the change in output and with the prescribed insertion gain to see whether the changes are sufficient. A similar frequency sweep and curve can be recorded after modifying or changing the earmold. If modifying the earmold and hearing aid are not sufficient, then another hearing aid can be tried and similar measurements made. One of the advantages of probe-microphone or probe-tube-microphone systems is that the effect of changes can be measured so quickly.

The test box and a 2-cc coupler can be used to measure the changes made in either hearing aid or earmold. An HA-1 coupler can be used with any air-conduction aid and the person's own earmold. If the hearing aid is not a canal or in-the-ear aid, the HA-2 coupler can be used to measure the output of the hearing aid alone. If a change in gain is needed, first measure the coupler gain at all the same settings used originally in obtaining the functional gain. An example of this coupler-gain measurement is shown in figure 9.14B (labeled "actual coupler gain"). For this individual, the needed

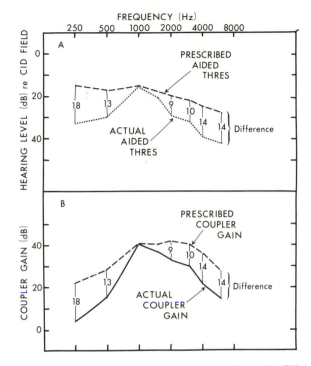

FIGURE 9.14. (Listener 11): **(A)** Actual and prescribed aided thresholds. Difference (dB) is amount by which actual coupler gain needs to be changed to provide prescribed coupler gain if the earmold remains unchanged. **(B)** Actual and prescribed coupler gain. From M. W. Skinner 1984. "Recent advances in hearing aid selection and adjustment." *Annals of Otology, Rhinology and Laryngology* 93: 569-75. Reproduced with permission of the publisher.

change is the *difference* between actual and prescribed aided thresholds (see figure 9.14A). When this difference is added to the actual coupler gain, the coupler gain values are those that will give the prescribed functional gain (see figure 9.14B). If possible, the aid should be adjusted to give the prescribed coupler gain according to the procedure described in chapter 8. If the earmold is modified, aided thresholds must be obtained again and compared with the prescribed aided thresholds to respecify the prescribed coupler gain with the modified earmold. If the SSPL90 needs to be changed, it should be measured before and after adjusting the SSPL90 or changing to an earhook with or without an acoustic damper.

Selected Cases

The following two cases, whose own hearing aids were evaluated and adjusted by Dr. David Pascoe of Central Institute for the Deaf, demonstrate how achieving the best fit with a commercially available aid depends on the clinician's understanding of the composite adjustments needed.

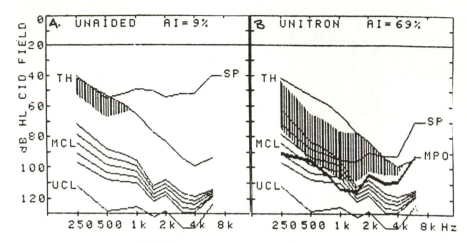

FIGURE 9.15.   (Listener M): **(A)** Unaided sound-field thresholds, MCLs, and UCLs plotted on same graph as the Pascoe speech spectrum (unaided). **(B)** Amplified speech spectrum and SSPL90 plotted on the same graph as thresholds, MCLs, and UCLs. The hearing aid was not readjusted from its original setting for these data. From graph produced by computer program written by Popelka 1982. From Pascoe 1985, with permission.

The first case, listener M, was a sixteen-year-old male with a congenital, bilaterally symmetrical sensorineural hearing loss. His unaided sound-field thresholds, MCLs, and UCLs at the left ear are shown on the same graph as the Pascoe speech spectrum in figure 9.15A. The vertical lines denote the portion of the 30-dB range of speech energy that is above threshold and, therefore, audible. The portion that is above threshold at each of the audiometric frequencies, multiplied by the contribution speech energy makes to intelligibility in the corresponding frequency region, provides an articulation-index (AI) value, as described in chapter 2. If all the speech energy were audible, the AI value would be 100 percent. In this case, the unaided AI value was 9 percent. His hearing aid (Unitron E1P), set at a comfortable listening level, amplified the Pascoe speech spectrum to the levels shown in figure 9.15B, and the SSPL90 (MPO) of his aid fell well below his UCL contour. His aided AI value of 69 percent reflects the fact that his hearing aid/earmold gave too little gain above 1500 Hz. The coupler gain and SSPL90 curves shown in figure 9.16A show a resonant peak at 1000 Hz. When a 680-ohm damper was placed in the earmold tubing and the SSPL90 was raised, the "use gain" that he preferred was higher. This resulted in approximately 5 to 10 dB more gain at all frequencies, except those at the resonant peak. Less low-frequency gain was achieved by using the H setting instead of the N setting of the tone control. The HA-1-coupler measurements showing the effect of this change in tone control are shown in figure 9.16B. The composite effect of these changes is shown in figure 9.17. More of the high-frequency speech energy is audible, and the AI value has increased from 69 to 84 percent as a result of the adjustments to the original setting of the aid.

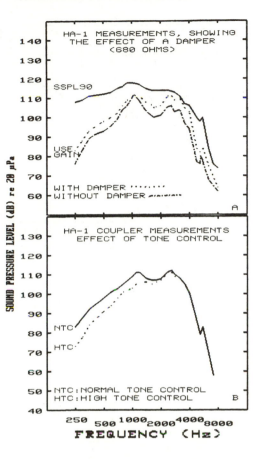

FIGURE 9.16.
(Listener M): **(A)** HA-1—coupler measurements of SSPL90 and the frequency response of his Unitron hearing aid set at the most comfortable listening level (use-gain setting) with and without a 680-ohm acoustic damper. **(B)** HA-1—coupler measurements of the frequency response with the tone control set at N and H. After Pascoe 1985, with permission.

FIGURE 9.17.
(Listener M): Amplified speech spectrum and SSPL90 plotted on the same graph as thresholds, MCLs, and UCLs. These data reflect the composite effect of the adjustments described in the text. From Pascoe 1985 with permission; graph produced by the computer program written by Popelka 1982.

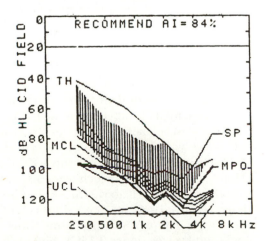

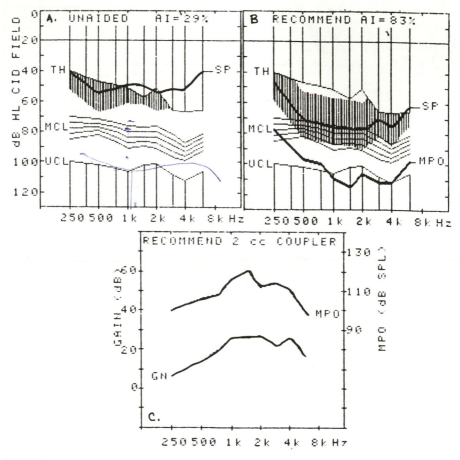

FIGURE 9.18. (Listener N): **(A)** Unaided sound-field thresholds, MCLs, and UCLs plotted on the same graph as the Pascoe speech spectrum (unaided). **(B)** Amplified speech spectrum and SSPL90 of hearing aid plotted on the same graph as thresholds, MCLs, and UCLs. **(C)** Gain and SSPL90 (MPO) of hearing aid measured with an HA-2 coupler. The hearing aid was at its original settings for these data. From Pascoe 1985 with permission; graphs produced by the computer program written by Popelka 1982.

The second case, listener N, is an eighty-one-year-old female with a bilaterally symmetrical sensorineural hearing loss. Her unaided sound-field thresholds, MCLs, and UCLs at the left ear are shown in figure 9.18A along with the Pascoe speech spectrum. Her unaided AI value of 29 percent is consistent with the difficulty she has understanding conversational speech without a hearing aid. When she set the volume wheel of her hearing aid (Maico K-220) so that speech was comfortably loud, much of the amplified speech spectrum fell above threshold and the AI value was 83 percent (see figure 9.18B). However, the SSPL90 (MPO) fell above UCL at 1000 to 3000 Hz and the coupler measurements showed a resonant peak between 1000 and 1500 Hz (see figure 9.18C). The undamped ear hook was changed to a

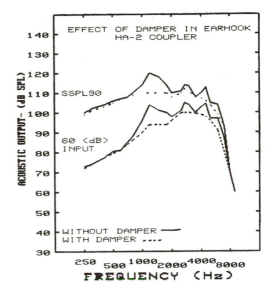

FIGURE 9.19.
(Listener N): Effect of changing the earhook on the output of the hearing aid, which was measured in an HA-2 coupler without (solid curve) and with (dashed curve) an acoustic damper. After Pascoe 1985, with permission.

damped ear hook; the effect of this change is shown in the HA-2-coupler measurements in figure 9.19. In addition, her vented earmold was changed to a closed mold with a 3-mm Libby horn. Then the SSPL90 was lowered so it was below her UCL contour. After these adjustments were made and she set the volume wheel so speech was comfortably loud, more of the amplified speech spectrum was above threshold (AI value was 94 percent instead of 83 percent), the balance between low- and high-frequency gain was better, and the SSPL90 (MPO) more closely approximated her UCL contour (see figure 9.20A) than with the original setting of the aid. The HA-1-coupler mea-

FIGURE 9.20.   (Listener N): **(A)** Amplified speech spectrum and SSPL90 plotted on the same graph as thresholds, MCLs, and UCLs. These data reflect the composite effect of the adjustments described in the text. **(B)** HA-1 – coupler measurements of the use gain and SSPL90 of the hearing aid after the adjustments were made that are described in the text. From Pascoe 1985 with permission; graphs produced by the computer program written by Popelka 1982.

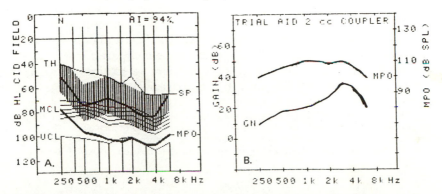

surements of use gain and SSPL90 (MPO) for the adjusted aid and earmold are shown in figure 9.20B.

COMPARING HEARING AIDS

Historical Perspective

The comparison of an individual's performance with several hearing aids has been made by many audiologists in the United States. Carhart (1946a, 1946b) described a procedure developed for veterans with significant hearing losses. While the men were still on active duty, they were assigned to the U.S. Army aural-rehabilitation program for a period of weeks during which they were evaluated with all the commercially available hearing aids that provided sufficient overall gain and a range of frequency/gain characteristics. They wore each of the aids for a period of days during which they listened critically to many sounds in the test rooms and everyday life. Performance with the aids was compared on the following parameters: (1) threshold for speech in quiet (SRT), (2) the maximum noise level in which the person could recognize two-syllable words presented at 50 dB sensation level, (3) recognition of monosyllabic words (at 25 dB sensation level re the aided SRT) in quiet, (4) the ability to distinguish small sound differences, and (5) the tolerance limit for loud sound (continuous discourse). The goal was to select a hearing aid best suited to the individual's needs and to identify special problems. Speech stimuli, rather than frequency-specific sounds, were used to assess the potential value of the aids for communication in everyday life.

When this extensive program was modified to make it feasible for people who personally paid for this clinical service in civilian life, two or three hearing aids were chosen for comparison during a one- to two-hour evaluation. No specific criteria were defined for selecting the hearing aid characteristics because the Harvard Report (Davis et al. 1946) indicated that most people performed best with the same frequency response (a flat or 6-dB-per-octave rising response in the 2-cc coupler between 300 and 4000 Hz). Since the research of Davis and colleagues at Harvard was highly esteemed, no attempt was made to prescribe frequency/gain characteristics to optimize speech intelligibility.[6] Since there was no prescriptive procedure to follow, audiologists used a variety of criteria, based mainly on personal experience, for selecting the hearing aids to be compared.

In the modified Carhart procedure there is no time to wear each hearing aid in everyday life, and the comparison is based on the speech-

---

[6]From the 1920s until 1946, several prescriptive procedures were developed for adjusting hearing aids for individuals, among them the half-gain rule of Lybarger (1944) and the amplification of speech to an equal-loudness contour at a comfortable listening level as recommended by Watson and Knudsen (1940). These continued to be used by hearing aid dispensers after 1946.

reception threshold (SRT), speech discrimination test score for phonetically balanced lists of monosyllables presented in quiet and/or in noise, and the individual's comments about sound quality and acceptability of each of the aids. The aid chosen with this comparative procedure is limited to the aids compared (and the specific settings of tone control, compression, and SSPL90 for each).

Research in the last twenty-five years has shown that the frequency/gain characteristics of a hearing aid are important for optimizing speech intelligibility, particularly for people who have sensorineural hearing losses (most of the people studied in the Harvard Report had conductive hearing losses). In addition, we are now keenly aware of the difference between coupler measurements of hearing aid output and the real-ear gain at specific frequencies that the *individual* obtains with different earmold configurations (see chapter 8). In light of this knowledge, it appears important to prescribe frequency/gain characteristics and verify that they have been obtained with functional-gain or insertion-gain measurements, if the amplification needs of the individual are to be met optimally. For those who want to use the modified Carhart procedure, this specification and verification of the frequency/gain characteristics of two or three hearing aids can serve as the basis for selecting these aids.

Rationale for Comparing Aids

The rationale for comparing several aids in a clinical situation is that there may be significant differences in the amplified signal that these aids provide to the individual and that these differences will result in more or less successful use of the aid in everyday life. Since this comparison needs to be efficient in terms of time and cost, the frequency/gain characteristics of the aids that are chosen should be close to those which will theoretically optimize speech intelligibility. That is, they should all have these characteristics. Even if they meet this goal, they will probably differ slightly in the amount of gain given in specific frequency regions, in the contour of the SSPL90 curve, and in the effect of automatic gain control on the amplified sound.

These small differences in the amplified signal may or may not lead to significant differences in the intelligibility of the speech and sound quality for the individual. Recent research[7] indicates that hearing-impaired indi-

---

[7]Walden et al. (1983) evaluated the assumptions underlying the use of monosyllabic word lists in comparing an individual's performance with three hearing aids as a means for choosing one.

In the first experiment they used three aids with very similar electroacoustic frequency/gain characteristics, and in the second experiment these characteristics were dissimilar. For each aid, pairs of lists (100 words) were presented at 0-dB MCR with speech babble, and for one aid a repeat test was obtained. Those individuals who showed a significant difference between aids wore each aid during the following week, were reevaluated with the initial tests, and were asked to rank order the aids according to their preference. For the aids with similar characteristics, the mean difference in score was 4.5%. For the dissimilar aids, the mean difference in

viduals who listen to monosyllabic word lists (such as the NU-6 or CID W-22 tests) with several electroacoustically similar hearing aids obtain scores with the aids that differ not more than 8 percent (95 percent of the time); when tested with the same aid twice the scores may differ by 8 percent or more in 30 percent of the cases. These score differences are for lists of fifty or one hundred words (in clinical practice many clinicians use only twenty-five words). It is clear from these results that phonetically balanced, monosyllabic word lists, for the number of words that are typically given in a clinical situation, are *not* a reliable indicator of performance differences that may be significant among hearing aids that provide approximately the same real-ear gain and SSPL90 (see table 9.3).[8] Furthermore, if the person was allowed to use all the aids over a period of time, s/he may learn to use each effectively so that the small differences in amplification are no longer significant.

The intelligibility of speech (in noise) may be determined (1) from listeners' judgments or (2) by obtaining the noise level associated with listeners' recognition of 50 percent of the words; these procedures are described in the next section of this chapter. Although the reliability of these measures appears reasonable, specific values for significantly different results are not available. This is also true for rating scales for sound quality.

Even though most, if not all, of our clinical tests are not sufficiently reliable to differentiate among hearing aids that provide approximately the same aided characteristics, they still can play a useful role in a hearing aid evaluation. The process of identifying words and making judgments about the sound quality can sharpen the person's critical listening skills. In addition, this process gives him or her a chance to know how the different aids amplify sound and to participate in deciding which hearing aid s/he will get.

---

score between aids was 14.2%, and the preference rankings agreed with the scores.

In a study by Schwartz and Walden (1980) using the NU-6 lists, the scores with aids with similar electroacoustic characteristics differed no more than 8% in 70% of 164 interaid comparisons. With the same group of subjects, scores on successive tests with the same aids were 8% or more in 54 comparisons. These results support those of Beattie and Edgerton (1976), who found that the score differences between aids had to be 12.4% to be statistically significant for 50-word lists of the NU-6 test with competing noise at 0-dB MCR based on test-retest reliability measures.

Given the test-retest variability of speech recognition scores when using 25- or 50-word lists of monosyllables in clinical testing, this variability may obscure the real differences or may be misinterpreted as a real difference when there is none (Schwartz and Walden 1983).

[8]This table is based on a binomial model that agrees well with actual scores of 4,120 tests with hearing-impaired individuals between twenty and eighty years of age who responded to 50-word lists of the CID W-22 test (original recordings) presented at 40 dB SL wherever possible. This table indicates that for 50-word lists (which take approximately five minutes to present), the two scores need to be different by 4% to 30%, depending on the absolute value of one of the scores, to be statistically significant. If shorter lists are used, even larger differences are needed. Tables of confidence levels for determining the probability of differences between speech-recognition sources are available in Raffin and Thornton (1980). Studebaker (1982) commented that these values agree reasonably well with "real-world outcomes."

TABLE 9.3. Lower and Upper Limits of the 95 Percent Critical Differences for Percentage Scores. Values Within the Range Shown Are not Significantly Different from the Value Shown in the Percentage Score Columns (P>0.05). From A.R. Thornton and M.J.M. Raffin 1978. "Speech-Discrimination Scores Modeled as a Binomial Variable." *Journal of Speech and Hearing Research* 21:507−18. Copyright 1978, American Speech-Language-Hearing Association, Rockville, Md. Reprinted with Permission of the Authors and Publisher.

% SCORE	n = 50	n = 25	n = 10	% SCORE	n = 100*
0	0−4	0−8	0−20	50	37−63
2	0−10			51	38−64
4	0−14	0−20		52	39−65
6	2−18			53	40−66
8	2−22	0−28		54	41−67
10	2−24		0−50	55	42−68
12	4−26	4−32		56	43−69
14	4−30			57	44−70
16	6−32	4−40		58	45−71
18	6−34			59	46−72
20	8−36	4−44	0−60	60	47−73
22	8−40			61	48−74
24	10−42	8−48		62	49−74
26	12−44			63	50−75
28	14−46	8−52		64	51−76
30	14−48		10−70	65	52−77
32	16−50	12−56		66	53−78
34	18−52			67	54−79
36	20−54	16−60		68	55−80
38	22−56			69	56−81
40	22−58	16−64	10−80	70	57−81
42	24−60			71	58−82
44	26−62	20−68		72	59−83
46	28−64			73	60−84
48	30−66	24−72		74	61−85
50	32−68		10−90	75	63−86
52	34−70	28−76		76	64−86
54	36−72			77	65−87
56	38−74	32−80		78	66−88
58	40−76			79	67−89
60	42−78	36−84	20−90	80	68−89
62	44−78			81	69−90
64	46−80	40−84		82	71−91
66	48−82			83	72−92
68	50−84	44−88		84	73−92
70	52−86		30−90	85	74−93
72	54−86	48−92		86	75−94
74	56−88			87	77−94

(continued)

---

*If score is less than 50%, find % Score = 100-observed score and subtract each critical difference limit from 100.

TABLE 9.3. *(Continued)*

% SCORE	n = 50	n = 25	n = 10	% SCORE	n = 100*
76	58–90	52–92		88	78–95
78	60–92			89	79–96
80	64–92	56–96	40–100	90	81–96
82	66–94			91	82–97
84	68–94	60–96		92	83–98
86	70–96			93	85–98
88	74–96	68–96		94	86–99
90	76–98		50–100	95	88–99
92	78–98	72–100		96	89–99
94	82–98			97	91–100
96	86–100	80–100		98	92–100
98	90–100			99	94–100
100	96–100	92–100	80–100	100	97–100

*If score is less than 50%, find % Score = 100-observed score and subtract each critical difference limit from 100.

EVALUATION OF HEARING AID AND EARMOLD WITH PRESCRIBED CHARACTERISTICS

One aid or several can be evaluated. Only one aid is evaluated with young children and some adults who cannot give reliable responses on tests of speech recognition and judgments of speech quality and intelligibility. In addition, one aid is evaluated when it is custom-made, such as an in-the-ear or a canal aid. In other cases, particularly with people who have worn hearing aids before, it may be helpful to evaluate and compare several hearing aids that provide the prescribed real-ear gain and SSPL90, and select one for the second part of the evaluation.

The second part of the evaluation is to determine whether the aid that is chosen has characteristics that are acceptable to the individual. This part of the evaluation should include the clinical testing and the individual's use of the aid in everyday life. During this time further adjustments of the aid or earmold may be needed.

Comparison of Hearing Aids

Judgments of sound quality. Judgments of sound quality can usually be made by older children and adults. These may be spontaneous observations made during other parts of the evaluation, they may be answers to general questions asked by the clinician, or they may be ratings along a number of continua such as those listed in figure 9.21. If ratings are used, each of the sound qualities are judged (on a scale from 1 to 10) after listening to ten to fifteen seconds of a recording of a continuous discourse presented at 70 dB SPL in the field. Listening for all nine qualities takes approximately three minutes for one hearing aid.

FIGURE 9.21.
Eight scales for rating the quality of amplified sound. From Hawkins 1985. "Reflections on amplification: Validation of performance." *Journal of the Academy of Rehabilitative Audiology* 18:42–54. Reproduced with permission of the author and publisher. These sound-quality dimensions are based on work done in Sweden (Gabrielsson and Sjögren 1979).

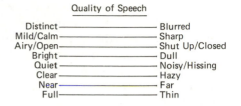

Quality of Speech

Distinct ———————	Blurred
Mild/Calm ———————	Sharp
Airy/Open ———————	Shut Up/Closed
Bright ———————	Dull
Quiet ———————	Noisy/Hissing
Clear ———————	Hazy
Near ———————	Far
Full ———————	Thin

The spontaneous observations, general comments, and ratings provide important information about the individual's perception of the amplified sound. Spontaneous observations indicate the aspects that are the most meaningful to the individual and the degree to which changes are needed. The general comments in response to questions may give the clinician a better understanding of how the amplified sound is perceived, and the rating scale encourages the hearing-impaired individual to listen critically to what is being heard. The rating scale is particularly useful in comparing the results from several different hearing aids.

Judgments of speech intelligibility.   Many older children and adults can judge what percentage of a recording of continuous discourse they can understand (0 percent to 100 percent, in 10-percent steps). For this test speech is presented at 70 dB SPL, and the volume wheel of the hearing aid is set so the speech is most comfortable and clear. If the person has great difficulty understanding speech, then it is presented in quiet. If s/he has less difficulty understanding speech, it is presented in a background of speech babble. In the latter case the level of the speech babble may be set close to a 0-dB signal-to-babble ratio, or it may be varied. If two or three hearing aids are being compared, the same procedure should be used for all the aids. Usually three judgments of intelligibility are obtained for each aid, and the score (for a given speech-to-babble ratio) is the average of the three judgments. The aids are ranked based on this average score. If three aids and thirty-second passages of the speech are used, this test usually takes ten minutes.[9]

Tests of speech recognition.   Many different tests of speech recognition can be used in evaluating hearing aids (see chapter 3 for a description of various materials). Either the ability to recognize spondees at threshold or the ability to recognize single-syllable words (or sentences, spondees, or nonsense syllables) presented at a normal conversational level in quiet or noise can be evaluated, for one or several hearing aids.

The material chosen should depend on the language skills of the individual, the degree of hearing impairment, and the frequency range

---

[9]The validity and sensitivity of this procedure for differentiating between hearing aids of fairly similar frequency/gain characteristics is described by Cox and McDaniel (1984).

being amplified. If a young child is tested, the words should be within her or his vocabulary, and often these are presented live voice. If a person has a mild hearing loss, the test material should be difficult enough to make him or her get less than a perfect score; this can be achieved with a talker, such as Rush Hughes, who spoke rapidly and did not fully articulate word endings, or with a competing sound. If a person has a profound hearing loss, a recording of well-articulated words or sentences, presented at a sufficiently slow rate, may allow her or him to recognize some phonemes or words. If the person has a hearing loss only above 1000 Hz, then a test such as the California Consonant Test, which requires discrimination of consonants with high-frequency acoustic cues, usually reveals the effects of different amounts of high-frequency amplification. Tests without a preponderance of high-frequency cues often do not reveal these differences.

Competing stimuli may be white noise, noise shaped according to the speech spectrum, multitalker babble, cafeteria noise, or another speech signal. If a competing signal is used, it can be presented from the same loudspeaker as the test words or from another loudspeaker that may be at any azimuth in relation to the person being tested. It is most realistic for test words to be presented at 0° azimuth (as described in chapter 4), and the competition from another sound source and azimuth, since in everyday life one usually looks directly at the person who is talking and the competition often comes from a different direction. It is particularly effective to test a person with CROS hearing aids when the speech and competing sound are coming from different directions.[10]

There are a number of different test procedures to assess speech recognition. One is the search for threshold (50 percent correct recognition of spondees, SRT) in the quiet. The test-retest reliability of this test is ±5 dB (total range) for adult subjects.[11] When comparing several hearing aids, the SRT is often not obtained, because it does not give much information for the time spent. However, it may be useful for young children or hard-to-test adults. The goal is to obtain aided SRTs between 15 and 20 dB HL. Higher SRTs may be appropriate for those with severe or profound hearing losses, but soft speech will be inaudible to them. Lower SRTs may be obtained by those with normal hearing in the frequencies below 1000 Hz, but they

[10]In the procedure described by Jerger and Hayes (1976), the sentences from the Synthetic Sentence Identification Test (SSI) are presented from one loudspeaker and the competing message (the story of Davy Crockett) is presented from another loudspeaker 180° from the first one. To test a CROS fitting, the person is seated first at 90° and then 270° azimuth in relation to the loudspeaker from which the sentences are presented. The unaided scores for several message-to-competition ratios are compared with the same ones for the aided condition. Although the test-retest variability in scores (15.6% for 2 standard deviations; Madory 1978) is too great to distinguish between aids with similar electroacoustic characteristics, this test is useful to compare monaural versus CROS amplification. Furthermore, the aided test results can be compared with those from normal-hearing individuals to indicate realistic expectations the individual should have for understanding speech with the hearing aid.

[11]One study of test-retest reliability for the SRT test is by Chaiklin and Ventry (1964).

usually are aware of the internal noise of the hearing aid as well as amplified environmental noise.

The second procedure is an adaptive one in which the level of the test words is kept constant at 65 to 70 dB SPL and the level of the competing sound is changed every two to four words until the signal-to-competition ratio at which 50 percent of the words are correctly indentified is determined. The level of the speech minus the level of the competition is called the signal-to-competition ratio.[12] This test, which is similar to one of the tests in the original Carhart procedure, takes about three minutes for each aid.

The third procedure is to present a list of words or sentences (ten, twenty-five, fifty, or a hundred items long) at a conversational level (such as 50 to 55 dB HL) in quiet or in noise; the person responds by saying or writing what is heard. This is the traditional speech-discrimination test used by many clinicians. As described above, its test-retest reliability is not high enough to detect significant differences among aids that provide the pre-scribed frequency/gain characteristics. However, this procedure is valuable in comparing aided with unaided performance because of the relatively large changes in score associated with increased audibility provided by the hearing aid. For this comparison the speech is presented at the same level both aided and unaided. The person taking the test can often readily see how much easier it is to hear with the hearing aid than without it. It takes approximately five to ten minutes, depending on the length of the word list, to obtain unaided and aided scores using commercial recordings of mono-syllabic words for each condition.

Judgments of the nonacoustic characteristics of the aids.   No two hearing aids are exactly alike. They differ in size, physical fit, ease with which controls can be adjusted, potentiometers available for adjusting acoustic characteristics, presence of a telecoil, color, battery life, price, warranty period, and repair record. Some of these factors may mean as much as the acoustic dimensions of sound quality and speech intelligibility to the individ-ual who is getting a new hearing aid. These nonacoustic factors should be taken into account in choosing one among several aids.

Basis for choosing one aid.   All the information gathered from the judgments and tests described above should be considered in concert with the amount of reserve gain and the remaining electroacoustic flexibility of the SSPL90 and frequency-gain characteristics of the aids. Although the clinician is in the best position to evaluate the technical aspects of the choice, most hearing-impaired individuals appreciate contributing to the decision. When the individual contributes, s/he may make more of an effort to adapt to and use the aid effectively.

---

[12]This procedure is described by Tecca and Binnie (1982) using the California Conso-nant Test (Owens and Schubert 1977).

Determining the Acceptability of a Hearing Aid

Anecdotal observation by individual.   Most adults and older children can judge whether the sound amplified by a hearing aid is acceptable and whether it is comfortable to wear, is cosmetically acceptable, and has the kinds of adjustments desired. Since our clinical tests cannot simulate accurately the listening demands the person will encounter in everyday life, it is important (and legally required) to include the thirty-day trial period in the evaluation of the acceptability of the aid. The person should be guided by the clinician to take full advantage of this trial period by critically listening to sounds in a variety of environments before deciding whether a hearing aid is acceptable.

Observations of the person's response to the hearing aid.   It is important to observe the person's response to the aid. Does it fit comfortably, does loud sound cause discomfort, does the aid make it easier to communicate, and is the person more aware of environmental sounds? These observations give clues of how to evaluate the individual's comments and decide whether further adjustments are needed. For very young children and others who cannot say whether the aid is acceptable, these observations may be the major way to evaluate whether the prescribed characteristics are appropriate.

Readjustment of the Hearing Aid and/or Earmold

Some people are particularly sensitive to loud sound or to noise. They may need a lower setting of the SSPL90 control, use of an AGC circuit, and/or less low-frequency gain between 250 and 500 Hz than was originally prescribed. Others are irritated by amplified sound between 3000 and 6000 Hz, particularly those who have worn hearing aids for many years and have not heard these sounds before. For some of these people the gradual increase in the amount of gain in this region (for example, by using the various diameters of tubing inserts, as shown in figure 8.9) over a period of weeks may enable them to learn to use these high-frequency cues effectively. Others may continue to find them irritating, and they will need to have the hearing aid adjusted to eliminate them. If a closed earmold is used, some people will object to the booming quality of their own voices. For those with mild to moderate hearing losses, it may be feasible to use a 1- to 2-mm vent without acoustic feedback and too much loss of low-frequency gain. In other cases, a closed mold may be essential to give sufficient amplification without feedback, and these people may adapt to it over a period of weeks. If a person does not adapt, it may be better to give insufficient amplification with an aid that the person will wear than not to have her or him wear the aid at all. For some people a capillary vent that allows air pressure equalization will make the earmold and aid more comfortable to wear. A windscreen over the microphone of the hearing aid, if it is not already provided, may be helpful in reducing hissing, rumbling noise.

It is important that these changes in the prescribed frequency/gain characteristics and SSPL90 be made, so that the person will wear the hearing aid and gain experience with it. If these changes are not made, the person may choose, as so many others have, to put the aid in the dresser drawer. Once these changes are made, it is equally important to encourage the person to wear the aid so that s/he can adapt to hearing the amplified sound. There is evidence of this adaptation process from experienced hearing aid wearers who report that they become so accustomed to the sound through their aids that they need some time to readjust when their aids are repaired (and the characteristics are changed slightly).

The process of adjusting and readjusting the hearing aid and/or earmold to make them comfortable and acceptable to the individual in everyday life is as important as any other part of the hearing aid evaluation. It is essential for achieving the goal of a successful fit, and it gives information that validates the prescriptive procedure used or provides a basis for modifying it.

FINAL RECOMMENDATION

The final recommendation of a hearing aid and/or earmold should be made when the aid and earmold fit comfortably and acoustic output is adjusted so that it is acceptable and beneficial to the individual.

SUMMARY

The goal of a hearing aid evaluation is for the hearing aid and earmold to be comfortable, provide acceptable sound quality, and make understanding speech as easy as possible. An evaluation process for successfully fitting aid and earmold is described in this chapter and summarized in the chart in figure 9.1.

There are several key elements in this process. When the hearing aid or aids (and earmold) are preselected, their electroacoustic characteristics are set to provide what theoretically will (1) give the best speech intelligibility and (2) limit the maximum acoustic output so that it is not uncomfortable.

Since there are often large individual differences between the estimated and actual real-ear gain and SSPL90 of the hearing aid coupled to the ear, it is essential to obtain either functional-gain or insertion-gain measures with the hearing aid set so that (1) conversational speech is most intelligible and comfortable and (2) loud speech is not uncomfortably loud. If the actual frequency/gain and SSPL90 characteristics are not close to the prescribed characteristics, then adjustments are made before an aid is evaluated further. If several aids are compared, they are all adjusted in this manner. The aids then can be compared using judgments of speech intelligibility, ratings of sound quality, tests of speech recognition in quiet or noise, and judgments of nonacoustic characteristics of the aids. In many cases the tests or judgments used may not be reliable enough for differentiating between aids, but the experience the person gets critically listening with each aid is important for the total rehabilitative process. In addition, this listening gives him or her an opportunity to participate in the selection of an aid.

The process of evaluating whether the aid is acceptable to the individual (and adjusting the aid, if necessary) is as important as any other step in achieving a successful fit. In addition, this evaluation gives the clinician an opportunity to decide whether the prescriptive criteria chosen are valid indicators of success in everyday life or whether they need to be modified for future use.

Chapter Ten
COUNSELING AND HEARING AID ORIENTATION

THE HELPING RELATIONSHIP
Clinician-Counselor
Client and Family

EXCHANGE OF INFORMATION PRIOR TO HEARING AID EVALUATION
Confirmation of Hearing Impairment
Determination of Problems
Interview
Self-Assessment Scales
Recommendation of Hearing Aid Evaluation
Recommendation of Aural Rehabilitation

HEARING AID USE
Parts of an Aid
Operating a Hearing Aid
Hearing Aid
Batteries
Controls
Earmold and Tubing
Acoustic Feedback
Cord and External Receiver
Bone-Conduction Vibrator
Daily Listening Check
Troubleshooting
Repairs
Listening with a Hearing Aid
Using a Telecoil
Are Adjustments Needed?

WAYS TO IMPROVE COMMUNICATION
Environmental Factors
Factors That Facilitate Hearing
Factors That Facilitate Seeing

Cognitive Skills, Knowledge, and Experience
Attitudes for Enhancing Communication
Ways Family, Friends, and Co-workers Can Help
Problem Solving

SUMMARY

The focus of counseling before, during, and after a hearing aid evaluation is to determine the hearing and communication problems of the client and to create an environment in which the client seeks solutions to these problems with the guidance and support of the clinician-counselor. The wealth of information that clinicians have about using a hearing aid and ways to improve communication can be assimilated by a client only when s/he is emotionally ready. Consequently, the helping relationship described in the first section in this chapter is vital for providing the client with the best opportunity for learning to communicate more effectively.

Many times the client is an adult; when the client is an infant or child, the parents play the key role in helping their child. Much of the information in this chapter is written about counseling the adult client, but it can be adapted for parents of a hearing-impaired child. In addition, parents should receive guidance and support in choosing appropriate educational placement for their child. Criteria for making this choice and other specific issues in counseling parents of hearing-impaired children are beyond the scope of this chapter.

The families and caretakers of elderly people who have decreased hearing or cognitive and physical function can help bridge the sense of isolation and lack of communication that the elderly often endure. Although the basic information about hearing impairment, hearing aids, and improving communication is covered in this chapter, it may need to be adapted for particular situations in which these families and caretakers communicate with the elderly.

THE HELPING RELATIONSHIP

There are a number of different approaches to helping someone develop more satisfying, fruitful patterns of behavior. The human-potential approach[1] is one that clinicians have followed in guiding hearing-impaired individuals and their families to communicate more effectively. The basic assumption in this approach is that human beings have an innate capacity and drive to achieve their maximum potential. The role of the clinician is to facilitate growth by providing information and a supportive, accepting relationship in which the client makes decisions and takes courses of action that will lead toward achieving her or his potential.

[1]The human-potential approach to counseling is attributed to Carl Rogers, whose books *Client Centered Counseling* (1951) and *On Becoming a Person* (1961) are well known. Lawrence Brammer's book *The Helping Relationship* (1985) specifically addresses many facets of counseling that are applicable for aural rehabilitation from the perspective of the human-potential approach. Luterman (1976, 1979, 1984), Sanders (1975), Kaplan (1982), Wylde (1982), and McCarthy and Alpiner (1982) are audiologists who have espoused this approach to counseling people with hearing impairment.

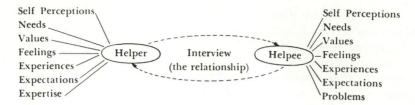

FIGURE 10.1.   Diagram of the helping relationship. From Lawrence M. Brammer. *The Helping Relationship: Process and Skills*, 3rd ed. Copyright 1985. Reprinted with permission of Prentice-Hall, Inc., Englewood Cliffs, N.J. and the author.

A diagram of the relationship between the clinician (helper) and the client (helpee) is shown in figure 10.1. The major difference between these two people is that the client has a problem and the clinician has expertise. Both people bring "needs, values, feelings, experiences, and expectations" to the relationship (Brammer 1985). As clinicians, we can be most effective if we understand what we bring and discover what the client brings to the relationship.

Clinician-Counselor

An understanding of our "needs, values, feelings, experiences, and expectations" evolves when we, as clinicians, are willing to directly assess them over a period of months and years. This self-assessment usually uncovers some attitudes and habits with which we are not satisfied, but it often takes times of personal crisis to enable us to see clearly that changes are necessary. These changes are often unsettling and sometimes painful, but if we decide to make them, they eventually enable us to experience new levels of understanding that bring satisfaction and joy. This process of change and growth makes us much more aware of our human fallibility and our need for love and unconditional acceptance. When we follow this path of personal growth, it is easier for us to provide the accepting and nuturing relationship within which those we counsel can explore ways to communicate more effectively.

In counseling we need to *listen openly and empathize* with our clients. Most of us do not have a hearing impairment and, therefore, have not experienced life the way hearing-impaired people do. Furthermore, we cannot assume that all people will experience the effects of their hearing impairment in the same way. There are some general, unifying concepts, but each person's perception is unique; it depends on the person's personality style, past experiences, patterns of behavior, and network of human relationships, especially with those closest to her or him. Therefore, we need to *listen* with complete attention to the information s/he conveys. This information is conveyed at a *content* and an *emotional* level at the same time, both of which need to be recognized and acknowledged. We can listen and empathize only if we consciously cease judging a person based on our own values and life experiences.

If we assess our own needs, it is clear that we make positive changes in our lives when our mentors *accept* us at the level at which we are functioning now and have confidence we will change when we comprehend the appropriate information and are emotionally ready. This acceptance, confidence, and information are exactly what those we counsel need from us. The acceptance and confidence provides the emotional context in which to consider the information about hearing aids, the effect of hearing impairment on communication, and skills needed to maximize communication. Within this context the individual and the family can weigh and balance the alternatives that are offered together with the internal factors that impinge on them, to choose the best course of action. In contrast, pressure or persuasion based on a preconceived notion that we, as clinicians, know what is best, usurps the responsibility of people to make this choice.

Since growth occurs through a process of trying new experiences and making mistakes, it is impossible to predict the time needed to understand and assimilate new patterns of behavior into our lives. For counseling to be most effective, we need to be sensitive to how much information should be presented, and at what level, for people to maintain their interest and attention. For some, it may be necessary to describe a concept in several different ways and to provide experiences, such as hearing through a hearing aid for the first time, for them to understand. Some people will fail to respond, will resist understanding, or will choose not to take advantage of the information we offer. Others will make some progress and then have periods of no growth. After experiencing satisfaction when someone we counsel grows and feels joyful about this growth, we may find it disappointing when a client chooses not to grow or seems blocked from within. It is important to recognize our disappointment, accept it, and stand back and be patient; this shifts the responsibility to client and family, which is where it should be.

When we have genuine concern and respect for the people we counsel and do all in our power to make the helping relationship a productive one, this creates an environment in which an individual can feel safe to reveal the communication problems s/he is having (that are directly related to the hearing impairment) and to learn ways to solve them. This growth in the ability to solve one's own problems involves learning to identify problems, analyze them, explore alternative ways to handle them, plan a course of action, and take the final step of changing behavior. The final goal is self-sufficiency.

Client and Family

In the helping relationship diagrammed in figure 10.1, the client with the hearing impairment is the "helpee." With an adult, the family may or may not be willing to participate in this relationship, whereas with children, the parents are key participants.

The reason the client and family enter into this relationship is that they are having problems directly related to the hearing impairment. These problems cover the whole spectrum from relatively simple ones, such as a hearing aid that needs repair or replacement, to much more complex ones, such as a six-month-old infant whose profound hearing impairment has just been confirmed and whose parents are finding it very difficult to cope with the news.

Some people grasp new information quickly, incorporate it in new patterns of behavior, and can deal effectively with the feelings they have during this process. Others have some difficulty finding satisfying ways to cope with their hearing impairment, and they need the guidance and support that a skillful clinician can give as they learn to become self-sufficient. Some will have emotional difficulties, beyond those directly related to the hearing impairment, that are severe enough to warrant referral for professional psychological guidance.

Hearing impairment is a loss of the physical integrity of the auditory system. This impairment often causes distortion that makes the signal reaching the brain incomplete and sometimes unrecognizable, and even with a hearing aid, very soft sounds may not be heard. Almost everyone whose hearing impairment occurs after early childhood experiences grief in response to this physical loss as do parents of hearing-impaired children. Grief usually evolves through five states of emotional response: denial, projection, anger, depression, and acceptance.

Denial occurs because facing the hearing impairment is too painful to accept. This is a time when one's emotions are regrouping to face this physical loss. The individual's perception of reality is that there is no problem. In the United States, where so much emphasis is placed on physical fitness and where relatively few young, healthy people have hearing impairment, there is a stigma attached to this physical problem. This stigma intensifies the difficulty one has in facing a hearing impairment.

Projection occurs when the individual recognizes that there is some breakdown in communication but states that the problem is caused by other people not speaking clearly or loudly enough. Although this may be true, the real problem is that caused by the hearing impairment.

Anger occurs in response to the hearing impairment and the problems caused by it. Examples of problems include the misunderstandings that result from not accurately hearing what people say or not hearing sounds that signal important events, convey a sense of safety, or give a feeling of aliveness to existence; feelings of isolation and inadequacy; and having to expend much more effort to communicate. Although this anger may be a generalized frustration with life, it is often focused on the person who is closest, such as a wife or husband. The anger compounds the difficulty the client is already experiencing because of the breakdown in communication due to the hearing impairment.

Depression can be defined as anger toward oneself for former behavior, for having a hearing impairment, and for feeling inadequate to cope with it. In this state one is miserable but may find it difficult to ask for help.

Acceptance occurs when the person knows (and accepts) that the problem is a hearing impairment and not related to his or her self-worth. Acceptance is necessary for facing change in old patterns of communication and learning to use a hearing aid effectively.

As human beings our emotional responses are much more complex than the descriptions of these states imply. Even when we achieve acceptance of a problem, we can be depressed or angry depending on the complex of circumstances at a particular time. Consequently, it is best for us, as clinicians, to focus on recognizing and accepting our client's emotional responses and realizing that s/he should not be categorized as being in one state or another. Furthermore, we need to realize that communication problems caused by hearing impairment are superimposed on (1) the long-standing communication patterns used by the client and her or his family, friends, and co-workers and (2) the client's own personality (for example, quiet or gregarious). Our counseling focuses only on those problems that are directly related to the hearing impairment and ways to compensate for it.

Clients who reach the stage of acceptance need to identify specific problems, get information on ways to solve these problems, choose ways that will be personally acceptable, and follow the needed course of action. Although the clinician-counselor is there to provide expertise and support, the responsibility for this change rests with the client or with the parents of a hearing-impaired child.

EXCHANGE OF INFORMATION PRIOR TO HEARING AID EVALUATION

Confirmation of Hearing Impairment

When the results of the hearing evaluation are explained, this may be the first time there has been a confirmation and documentation of the hearing impairment. Although the client may suspect a hearing impairment, this confirmation may provoke a number of questions and feelings. As clinicians, we need to explain the results in a clear, succinct manner and then ask the client or family to tell us what they understand. If they ask questions, these may be prompted by a desire for information, a desire for confirmation of their own beliefs, or a desire to convey feelings about the information. It may be important to explore their questions in greater depth before answering them with further information. In all cases, we should to be sensitive to both the content and the emotional aspects of this exchange of information.

Determination of Problems

Interview.   The interview may start with a discussion of the hearing-evaluation results, or it may occur at a subsequent time. The major goal of this interview is to help the client and/or family identify the problems that the hearing impairment is causing. The detail in which these problems are explored will depend on the resources you have to offer as a clinician in terms of time, expertise, and program and on the individual's need, commitment to work on the problems, and financial resources.

The focus of the interview should be on the individual—why did s/he come for help, what ways is the hearing impairment interfering with life and communication with other people, how does s/he feel about this, what information does s/he want, and does s/he want to use this information to make changes? These questions should be asked, not in the spirit of an inquisition, but rather in an open, unhurried context in which the individual feels as though we really want to understand and help clarify the issues before suggesting possible courses of action. It is our responsibility as clinicians to guide the interview so that discussion remains focused on the information needed for both us and the client to make decisions. This requires us to think clearly about what is happening and to be practical about time and attention constraints.

Self-assessment scales.   Self-assessment scales have been developed by a number of different groups (see table 10.1) to obtain information from adults (who developed language prior to acquiring a hearing impairment) about the

1. ability to understand speech and carry on a conversation in a variety of situtations,
2. ability to hear and recognize nonspeech sounds,
3. behavioral strategies used to communicate
    a.   are they maladaptive (for example, does the person hide the hearing loss, avoid situations where communication is required, pretend to understand, or ignore, interrupt, or dominate conversation?)
    b.   are they facilitory (for example, does the person watch a speaker's face, sit so the speaker's face is well lighted, choose a place to listen with less noise, ask for repetition only of words that were missed, use a hearing aid?)
4. personal adjustment to hearing impairment,
    a.   level of self-acceptance,
    b.   acceptance or denial of hearing impairment,
    c.   feelings of anger, guilt, anxiety, or stress; desire to withdraw,
5. communication environment of everyday life including
    a.   need for communication,
    b.   intensity levels at which people usually speak,

TABLE 10.1. Self-Assessment Scales for Adults with Hearing Impairment That Occurred After Language Development Was Complete.*

I. SCALES APPLICABLE TO GENERAL POPULATION

NAME	# ITEMS	# SCALES	SCALE	WAY GIVEN	CONTENT AREA	RELIABILITY	PURPOSE
Hearing Handicap Scale (High et al. 1964) (Forms A and B are equivalent)	20 for each form	1	5 points Almost always— almost never	Written	Ability to understand speech and carry on a conversation in a variety of situations. Ability to hear telephone and other sounds in everyday life.	Equivalence of two forms: correlation of means and SD is 0.96.	Screening for communication problems.
Hearing Measurement Scale (Noble and Atherley 1970)	48	7	5 points Always— never	Interview or written	Ability to hear and understand speech and carry on conversation in a variety of situations. Ability to hear nonspeech sounds. Ability to localize sound source. Emotional response to hearing loss. Response of others when have difficulty related to hearing loss. Attitude toward hearing loss. Tinnitus.	Test-retest reliability: correlation of means and SD on test and retest is 0.93	Screening for communication problems, emotional response, emotional response of others, attitude toward hearing loss.
Social Hearing Handicap Index (Ewertsen and Birk-Nielsen 1973)	21	3	Yes-No	Written	Ability to understand speech and carry on conversation in a variety of situations.	—	Screening for communication problems.
Denver Scale of Communication Function (Alpiner et al. 1978)	25	1 Items scored separately	7 points Agree-disagree plus comments	Written	Feelings about hearing loss and how they affect social interaction. Behavioral strategies used to communicate. Behavioral response of family. Ability to hear and understand speech and other sounds.	—	Questionnaire used at clinicial interview, emphasizing emotional response and response of family.

(continued)

313

TABLE 10.1. (Continued)

I. SCALES APPLICABLE TO GENERAL POPULATION

NAME	# ITEMS	# SCALES	SCALE	WAY GIVEN	CONTENT AREA	RELIABILITY	PURPOSE
Quantified Denver Scale (Alpiner 1982)	25	1	5 points (No comments)	Written	Same as above.	—	Same as above.
Profile Questionnaire for Rating Communicative Performance in a Home Environment Social Environment Occupational Environment School Environment (child observed by teacher) (Sanders 1975)	9 7 6 7	1 1 1 1	4 points (Little difference to great difference) plus 3 point (Happens often— happens seldom)	Written	Ability to understand speech and carry on a conversation in a variety of situations.	—	Short assessment of communication problems.
University of Northern Colorado Communication Appraisal and Priorities (Hull 1982)	15	1	3 points No problems— definitely problems (items ranked according to importance)	Written	Communication situations ranked according to importance to individual and difficulty they cause.	—	Short assessment of situations which cause difficulty.
Hearing Performance Inventory (HPI) (Giolas et al. 1979)	158	6	5 points Practically always— almost never	Written	Ability to understand speech and carry on conversation in a variety of situations including at work. Ability to detect and recognize speech and other sounds. Feelings about hearing loss and how they affect social interaction. Behavioral strategies used to communicate.	—	Detailed assessment of content areas. Can be used as basis for part of aural rehabilitation plan. Most sections can be used to assess change in patient scores pre- and post-treatment.

Instrument	No. of items	Scales	Scale points	Format	Content	Reliability	Purpose
Revised Hearing Performance Inventory (HPI, rev) (Lamb et al. 1983)	90	6	5 points Same as above	Written	Same as above.	Reliability coefficients for individual scales: 0.86–0.96 (Lamb et al. 1983); 0.86–0.99 (Demorest and Walden 1984) S_e:0.08–0.2 (Demorest and Walden 1984).	Same as above.
Hearing Performance Inventory for Profound and Severe Loss (PIPSL) (Owens Raggio 1987)	75	6 (15 items not in scale)	7 points	Written	Ability to understand speech and carry on conversation in variety of situations. Lipreading ability. Ability to detect and recognize environmental sounds. Behavioral strategies to communicate. Feelings about hearing loss. Response of people in family to hearing loss.	Reliability coefficients for individual scales: 0.86–0.90	Provide basis for planning aural rehabilitation program and assessing person's function pre- and post-treatment (e.g., hearing aid, vibrotactile device, or cochlear implant).
Hearing Problem Inventory (Hutton 1980)	51	1	4, 5, 6 points Words applicable to the question	Written	Ability to hear and understand speech. Ability to hear other sounds. Behavioral strategies to communicate. Feelings about hearing loss and problems it causes. Response of family and co-workers to person's hearing difficulties. Hearing aid and earmold benefit and usage.	—	Obtain information about hearing problems to guide person in solving them. Assess change in person's pre- and post-treatment function.

(continued)

TABLE 10.1. *(Continued)*

I. SCALES APPLICABLE TO GENERAL POPULATION

NAME	# ITEMS	# SCALES	SCALE	WAY GIVEN	CONTENT AREA	RELIABILITY	PURPOSE
McCarthy-Alpiner Scale of Hearing Handicap (1982, 1983) Form A (Hearing-Impaired Individual) Form B (Family Member)	34 each form	3	5 points Always—never	Written	Form A: Feelings person has about hearing loss and problems it causes. Behavioral strategies used to communicate. Emotional and behavioral response of others. Form B: Questions of Form A recast so that family member answers from observations of person with hearing impairment.	Reliability coefficient: 0.81 (within form reliability)	Identify problem areas for counseling person with hearing impairment and family members.
Communication Profile for the Hearing Impaired (CPHI) (Demorest and Erdman 1986a, 1986b, 1987)	145	25	5 points Frequency of occurrence (Rarely—almost always); Agreement (Strongly agree—strongly disagree); Importance for communicating effectively (Not important—essential)	Written	Ability to understand speech and carry on conversation in home, work, and social situations. Personal awareness of communication problems. Communication environment: need to communicate, physical characteristics, attitudes and behavior of others. Behavioral strategies to communicate. Emotional response to hearing loss (e.g., anger, denial, etc.).	Reliability coefficient of individual scales: 0.67–0.89; S_e:0.24–0.45	Detailed assessment of content areas to plan aural rehabilitation program. Testing pre- and post-treatment to evaluate change in person's function.

II. SCALES APPLICABLE TO A GERIATRIC POPULATION

NAME	# ITEMS	# SCALES	SCALE	WAY GIVEN	CONTENT AREA	RELIABILITY	PURPOSE
Denver Scale of Communication Function—Modified (Kaplan et al. 1978)	25	4	5 points Definitely agree— definitely disagree	Interview	Slight modification of wording of a few questions on original Denver Scale. Rearrangement of order. (Specifically adapted to geriatric population).	Test-retest reliability: correlation of item scores on test and retest for each individual 0.75–0.91	Questionnaire used as clinical interview with emphasis on emotional response to hearing loss, and response of family.
Hearing Handicap Inventory for the Elderly (HHIE) (Ventry and Weinstein 1982)	25	2	3 Yes, sometimes, no.	Interview (written)	Emotional response to hearing loss. Situations which cause difficulty.	Reliability coefficient: 0.88–0.95 Correlation of two subscales: 0.87	Assess self-perception of hearing handicap, identify communication problems, and evaluate function pre- and post-treatment.
Self-Assessment of Hearing (Manzella and Taigman 1980)	16	1	Yes-No	Interview or written	Questions about possible hearing problems in a variety of situations.	—	Screening test for possible hearing handicap.
Denver Scale of Communication Function for Senior Citizens Living in Retirement Centers (Zarnoch and Alpiner 1982)	7	1	Yes-No	Interview	Emotional response to hearing impairment. Behavioral strategies used to communicate. Response of family, friends, and staff to problems caused by hearing impairment.	—	Assess communication problems with family, friends and staff to plan ways that these might be resolved.

(continued)

TABLE 10.1. *(Continued)*

II. SCALES APPLICABLE TO A GERIATRIC POPULATION

NAME	# ITEMS	# SCALES	SCALE	WAY GIVEN	CONTENT AREA	RELIABILITY	PURPOSE
Communications Assessment Procedure for Seniors (CAPS) (Alpiner and Baker 1982)	35	6	3 points Always–never and not applicable	Interview or written	Situations in which person talks with others. Emotional response to hearing impairment; self-concept. Response of family, friends and staff to problems caused by hearing loss. Need and/or desire for aural rehabilitation.	—	Assess communication problems and plan ways that these might be resolved.
Nursing Home Hearing Handicap Index (Schow and Nerbonne, 1977) Resident's Form and Staff's Form	10 for each form	1	5 points Very often–almost never	Interview	Ability to understand speech in several situations. Emotional response to hearing problem. Response of other people to hearing problem.	—	Screening for hearing problems. Self-perception; staff perception; Use for planning ways to improve communication.

III. PREDICTING OR ASSESSING HEARING AID BENEFIT

NAME	# ITEMS	# SCALES	SCALE	WAY GIVEN	CONTENT AREA	RELIABILITY	PURPOSE
Feasibility Scale for Predicting Hearing Aid Use (FSPHAU) (Rupp et al. 1977)	12 (weighted according to importance)	1	6 points	Interview	Motivation. Emotional response to hearing impairment and life. Audiologic data. Acceptance of hearing aid. Age. Hand and finger dexterity. Visual ability. Financial resources. Significant other person. (Intended for geriatric population.)	—	Predict success with hearing aid.
Hearing Aid Performance Inventory (Walden et al. 1984)	64	1	5 points Very helpful–hinders performance	Written	Rating of benefit provided by hearing aid. Majority of items are situations in which individual is trying to understand someone talk.	Reliability coefficient: 0.96	Assess benefit of a hearing aid.

    c. level of background or competing sounds,
    d. reactions of family, friends, and coworkers,
        i. acceptance or denial of problems,
       ii. willingness and ability to facilitate communication, and
6. use of a hearing aid.

These are the major areas of concern in evaluating the handicapping effect of hearing impairment on an adult.

    The advantages of using a self-assessment scale are that more information can be obtained than in an interview, the client has an opportunity to focus attention on areas that may have been ignored in the past, a program of aural rehabilitation can be designed for the client's specific needs, the procedure is standardized, and the results can be quantified and analyzed statistically. Standardization and statistical analysis are important if the data are going to be used to measure the benefit of a hearing aid or the client's progress in aural rehabilitation (Demorest and Walden 1984). This measure of benefit or progress is one way to evaluate the quality of care and to modify the program if indicated.

    The choice of a self-assessment scale should be based on what aspects of function you want to assess, whom you are assessing, and for what purpose you want to use the results. The scales in table 10.1 are all designed for adults who understand and speak English fluently, and most are for those with mild to moderately severe hearing impairment. One is for people with profound impairment, and several are designed for elderly people. One or more of the existing scales may be appropriate; if not, a scale can be specifically designed for the population and issues you want to assess.

    Although a wealth of information can be obtained with a self-assessment scale, it should be used in conjunction with the interview. The relationship between the clinician-counselor and client is initiated in the interview, and much information is exchanged that is essential for interpreting the results of a self-assessment scale and making recommendations.

Recommendation of Hearing Aid Evaluation

    A number of factors should be considered before recommending a hearing aid evaluation. They include

1. degree of hearing impairment,
2. handicapping effects of hearing impairment,
3. acceptance of the hearing impairment,
4. willingness to try a hearing aid,
5. understanding of the benefits and limitations of an aid, and
6. financial resources to pay for the aid and other services.

The only time a hearing aid should not be considered is when the pure-tone thresholds between 250 and 2000 or 3000 Hz are all 15 to 20 dB HL or less.

If the thresholds are greater than this, then the handicapping effects of the hearing impairment should be considered. For mild hearing impairment, there may or may not be sufficient need for amplification, depending on the listening demands in the individual's life. With greater degrees of impairment, the handicapping effects are likely to be greater, and a hearing aid may be of significant benefit.

As listed above, other factors need to be considered before a recommendation is made. First, the client (or parents of a child) has to acknowledge that there is a hearing impairment and be willing to try the hearing aid before s/he will face the difficulties of learning to use it effectively. As mentioned in chapter 1, it is better to postpone the recommendation of a hearing aid evaluation if the client or parents are strongly resistant to the aid. Given information about an aural-rehabilitation or parent-infant program, they may be willing to take this step first.

Second, the benefits and limitations of a hearing aid have to be clearly understood. The benefits include

1. speech and other sounds can be heard louder and may be clearer than without an aid, and consequently,
2. recognition of what is said will be more accurate,
3. carrying on a conversation, particularly in a quiet place, will be easier and more satisfying, and
4. less attention will be needed to listen; this will mean less stress and fatigue.

The limitations include

1. it will take time to get used to the sound produced by the hearing aid and to the fit of the earmold in the ear,
2. the sound may never sound as natural as when hearing was normal,
3. noise or reverberant rooms will make it more difficult to understand speech (binaural hearing aids with directional microphones or assistive listening devices such as direct audio input, FM, or infrared systems may be of some help),
4. the hearing aid and earmold will need care to keep them functioning properly,
5. the aid may not provide enough information without speechreading and other cues to compensate fully for the hearing impairment.

Most people (including clients and their families) have false expectations—both positive and negative—about hearing aids. The formation of realistic expectations, based on information provided and subsequently the client's experience wearing an aid, is vital to its ultimate acceptance.

The cost of a hearing aid evaluation and a hearing aid varies substantially from center to center. In addition to the cost of the hearing aid, the total cost of the fitting will vary depending on the services and supplies offered (such as hearing aid evaluation, hearing aid checks within or beyond the thirty-day trial period, counseling, hearing aid orientation, batteries, battery testers, and Dri-Aid kits). It is important to counsel each client about specific services, supplies, and costs to consider. If these costs are too much, every effort should be made to find a way for the person to get a hearing aid.

After all this information has been considered within the context of the helping relationship, it is the clinician-counselor's decision whether to recommend a hearing aid evaluation. It is the client's decision whether to proceed with a hearing aid evaluation.

Recommendation of Aural Rehabilitation

Aural rehabilitation is a complex area of audiology in which hearing-impaired individuals are guided in learning to use their residual hearing to full advantage, to use other senses, primarily visual, to supplement hearing, and to develop communication strategies to compensate for their hearing impairment. The goal is to make communication more effective and, therefore, less stressful.

A recommendation of aural rehabilitation for adults will depend on a number of factors including

1. availability,
2. extent of aural rehabilitation included in the hearing aid evaluation process,
3. needs of the hearing-impaired person,
4. motivation of that person to participate,
5. cost.

A realistic appraisal of each of these factors should be made jointly by the client and the clinician-counselor. It is best to discuss the concept of aural rehabilitation from the beginning so that the client realizes that the hearing aid is an integral part of the aural-rehabilitation process and that there are a number of ways in which s/he can facilitate this process. One way is to read about the effects of hearing impairment and how to cope with them; selected references on this topic are listed in Appendix 10A. Samples of typical exercises that may be included in an aural-rehabilitation program are listed in Appendix 10B. Some people can read, practice new skills, and incorporate them into everyday life by themselves. Many others require the interpersonal experience of either individual or group therapy to understand, accept, and form new attitudes and strategies to improve communication. A number of these concepts are described in the section "Ways to Improve Communication."

Although many people with hearing impairment would benefit from an aural-rehabilitation program, it is the client's decision whether to spend time and money for a formal program of individual or group therapy.

All children who have a hearing impairment should receive aural habilitation so that language and speech development will progress at a pace that is optimum for the individual. Recommendations of programs that offer this training should be discussed with the parents. Support should be given until they are well settled in the program of their choice.

HEARING AID USE

After a hearing aid has been selected and adjusted and provides the needed characteristics (as described in chapter 9), it is essential to guide the client in how to use it. This is true even for people who have worn hearing aids for a number of years, because the new aid is usually different in some respects. The client (or parents of a young child) should actively participate in this process. The first step will include learning

1.   the parts of a hearing aid (see figure 10.2),
2.   correct insertion of the battery,
3.   manipulation of the switches,
4.   correct insertion of the earmold,
5.   to make sure the tubing is not twisted for behind-the-ear aids, and
6.   to adjust the volume wheel for comfortable listening in a variety of conditions.

Many of these tasks require eye-hand coordination and may seem awkward for a person doing them for the first time. Consequently, the client may require practice and patience until the tasks are mastered. This is a time when it is particularly important for the clinician to be quietly supportive. Since this mastery is essential for successful use of the hearing aid, enough time must be spent, even if it requires a second visit before the client takes the aid home.

A hearing aid provides the most benefit when the person who wears it knows about its function and operation, how to solve simple problems that arise, and how to listen to sound with it. This information is given in the sections that follow. Some of this information is presented in appropriate

FIGURE 10.2.   Parts of a hearing aid. Adapted from figure 11.1 in "Learning hearing aid use" by W. R. Hodgson. In *Hearing Aid Assessment and Use in Audiologic Habilitation*, 2nd ed. Ed. W. R. Hodgson and P. H. Skinner 1981a. Copyright 1981, Williams and Wilkins Co., Baltimore. Reproduced with permission of author and publisher.

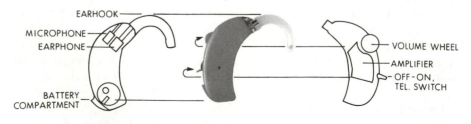

form for the client in booklets provided by some manufacturers of hearing aids. In addition, it may be helpful to develop you own materials based on information your clients can understand and use. Written materials should be taken home for future reference.

It takes time to learn about operating a hearing aid. Some will learn faster than others, and some will be able to solve problems as they arise more readily than others. It is essential to adjust the level and speed with which the material is presented to that which is best for the individual. The information in the sections that follow should be modified accordingly.

Parts of an Aid

The major parts of a hearing aid are microphone, amplifier, volume wheel, switches, receiver (or bone-conduction vibrator), tubing and earmold, and battery. These are shown for a behind-the-ear aid in figure 10.2. The following are short descriptions of these parts and their function.

1. Microphone: picks up sound and changes it into an electrical signal.
2. Amplifier: increases the electrical signal from the microphone.
3. Volume wheel: moving the wheel up or down makes the sound louder or softer; sometimes the lowest setting will turn off the sound.
4. On/off switch: turns the hearing aid on and off; often the telephone switch, if there is one, is on this switch.
5. Tone-control switch: controls the amount of low-pitched sound. Usually there are N(ormal) and H(igh) settings on this switch. The (H)igh position cuts out some of the low-pitched sound; this is particularly useful in noisy places.
6. Receiver: a miniature loudspeaker that transforms the amplified electrical signal to sound; it usually is inside the hearing aid case, but for body aids it is in a separate case. As in figure 10.2, the receiver may be called an earphone.
7. Bone-conduction vibrator: a device that transforms the amplified electrical signal to vibrations. The vibrator is held against the head with a head band so that the vibrations are transmitted to the skull and thereby to the inner ear.
8. Cord: used to attach a bone-conduction vibrator or an external receiver to a hearing aid.
9. Tubing and earmold: these direct the amplified sound from the receiver to the ear.
10. Battery: provides the power necessary to amplify the sound.

Operating a Hearing Aid

Hearing aid.   A hearing aid is a delicate instrument that may be damaged by:

1. being dropped on a hard surface,
2. being exposed to high temperatures (such as on a radiator, near a hair dryer, heater, or stove, or closed in a car on a hot day),

3. being immersed in water or exposed to excessive perspiration or moisture (placing the hearing aid in a plastic bag or jar with fresh silica gel each night will help prevent moisture damage),

4. being exposed to excessive dust or dirt,

5. using hair spray or perfume spray that can damage the microphone or volume wheel,

6. leaving a battery in it until it corrodes the terminals,

7. inserting a foreign object into it, or

8. attempting repairs beyond those recommended in the troubleshooting chart (see table 10.2).

When a hearing aid is not being used, it should be kept in the same safe place each day, out of the reach of children and pets.

Batteries. Batteries are made of several different materials. Some are made from mercury, and they last about half as long as zinc-air batteries but are about half as expensive. The zinc-air batteries are activated when the paper tab is removed to allow air to reach the zinc inside the battery; until this tab is removed, the batteries will remain fresh. Since the zinc-air batteries require air for activating them, they occasionally appear dead when used in tightly closed battery compartments. On the other hand, mercury batteries lose some of their power if they are not used within a period of months after they are manufactured. Mercury is poisonous, so it is important to dispose of used batteries so they do not cause pollution. Silver batteries provide 0.1 volt more power than mercury batteries, but they are more expensive than mercury or zinc-air batteries. Alkaline (size AA) batteries are used with body hearing aids; these are readily available because they are used for many other electronic devices such as calculators, portable radios, and children's toys.

Batteries come in a number of different sizes, and usually there is one correct size for a particular hearing aid. Behind-the-ear aids usually require a 675 battery, but small ones may require a 13 battery. In-the-ear aids usually require a 13 battery, but they may require a 312 battery. Canal aids usually require a 312 battery.

The following are suggestions for the use and care of batteries:

1. Buy mercury, silver-oxide, or alkaline batteries from a source that has a rapid turnover of stock; batteries will lose some of their strength if they are not used for a long time after they are manufactured.

2. Buy two to six batteries at a time. Store them in a cool, dry place (such as a refrigerator) and don't let them make contact with other metal objects.

3. Do not use a battery that appears to be leaking or corroded (it can damage the hearing aid); white power or brown fluid usually indicates leakage.

4. Keep the battery terminals clean (and noncorroded) by rubbing them gently using a pencil eraser or emery board. Remove any particles of corrosion, eraser, or emery board from the hearing aid.

TABLE 10.2. Troubleshooting Chart to Use When Hearing Aid Is Not Functioning Properly. (Asterisks denote the most common problems.)

SYMPTOMS	POSSIBLE CAUSE (SEE CHART NUMBER)
Hearing Aid:	
Produces no sound at all	1,2,3,4,5,6,8,9,11,14,15,16,17,18,19,22,23,24,25,32,35
Sounds weak:	
Microphone setting	1,2,3,5,6,12,20,22,23,24,25,32,35,38,39
Telephone setting	1,12,31
Sound is intermittent or fades	1,5,6,11,14,15,17,18,19,22,23,24,25,35
Whistles (sometimes or continuously)	13,20,21,26,27,28,29,30,34,37
Sounds noisy, raspy, or shrill	1,10,13,14,15,18,19,33,34
Sounds hollow, mushy, or muffled	1,10,22,23,24
Has poor sound quality	1,10,13,14,15,19,24
Batteries need to be replaced too often	7

LOCATION	POSSIBLE CAUSE	TEST	REMEDY
Battery (all aids)	**1. Weak or dead	Use battery tester to check charge.	Replace battery.
	2. Wrong size	Check if battery is correct size.	Replace with fully charged battery of correct size.
	3. Dirty	Remove battery from hearing aid, and check for dirt on flat sides.	Rub flat sides of battery with pencil eraser.
	**4. Upside down in holder	Check to see that + side of battery matches + on battery case.	Insert battery in correct position.
	5. Leaking	Check for white powder or brown fluid on battery.	Discard battery, clean battery contacts, and insert new battery.
	6. Dirty or corroded battery contacts	Check for dirt or corrosion on battery contacts.	Use pencil eraser or emery board to clean contacts; remove all particles of dirt, eraser or emery board after cleaning.

(continued)

TABLE 10.2. *(Continued)*

LOCATION	POSSIBLE CAUSE	TEST	REMEDY
	7. Using higher gain or more complicated circuit than previous aid and/or hearing aid circuit is defective.	Note use/gain setting and # hours for each battery and compare with manufacturer's estimated battery life at use-gain setting.	Buy batteries at economical prices, if getting manufacturer's estimated battery life. If not getting estimated battery life, send hearing aid for repair.
Switches *(all aids)*	Wrong position of:		
	**8. Microphone/telephone switch	Check position of switch.	Place switch in correct position.
	**9. On/off switch	Check position of switch.	Place switch in correct position.
	10. Tone control switch	Check position of switch.	Place switch in correct position.
	11. Switch contacts are dirty	Turn switches back and forth several times; listen to sound. If no sound, test for other possible causes (1, 5, 6 . . . 39)	If test remedies problem, continue to monitor sound. If not, and another cause is not identified, take aid to dispenser.
Volume wheel *(all aids)*	12. Set too low	Turn up volume wheel; listen to sound.	Continue to monitor sound if test remedies the problem.
	13. Set too high	Reduce volume-wheel setting until speech sounds clearer.	Continue to monitor volume-wheel position if test remedies problem. Return to dispenser if volume not sufficiently loud.
	14. Contacts dirty	Rotate volume wheel back and forth several times; listen to sound.	If test remedies problem, continue to monitor sound. If problem persists, volume wheel will need to be cleaned or replaced.
	15. Volume wheel defective	Rotate volume wheel slowly and listen to sound; if sound comes on suddenly at loud level or there are dead spots, volume wheel is defective.	Have volume wheel replaced.

Cord (body or some behind-the-ear aids)	**16. Not completely plugged in	Check plugs; push in securely and check sound.	Push in securely; make sure it will stay in.
	17. Plug or plug sockets dirty	Push plugs in and out several times and check sound.	If test remedies problem, may need to repeat if problem occurs again.
	**18. Wires broken	With cord securely plugged into the hearing aid and receiver, volume wheel turned up, and a fully charged battery in the aid, listen to output of aid with stethoscope as gently roll cord back and forth between fingertips along full length of cord. If no sound is heard, or sound is intermittent, try same thing with new cord.	Replace cord if broken.
Receiver or bone-conduction oscillator (body, behind-the-ear, or eyeglass aids)	19. Broken	Try new receiver.	Replace receiver.
Earmold (all air-conduction aids)	**20. Not properly positioned in ear	Look in two mirrors to see if earmold is all the way in. Use fingertips to twist earmold to correct, fully inserted position and listen to sound.	Make sure earmold is positioned correctly.
	21. Does not fit snugly in earcanal; vent too large	Make sure earmold is properly positioned in ear. If it whistles when the volume wheel is turned up to a comfortable level, then coat tip with vaseline and/or plug vent.	Vaseline coating or plugging vent may be enough; if not, then a new, more tightly fitting earmold should be ordered, or if it is a Lucite earmold, try putting dental liner material around canal part.

(continued)

TABLE 10.2. (Continued)

LOCATION	POSSIBLE CAUSE	TEST	REMEDY
	**22. Clogged with ear wax	Remove earmold from hearing aid and examine visually. Blow through to see if passage is open.	Never put hearing aid in water. Remove wax with toothpick, wire or pipe cleaner. Clean earmold with warm (*not* hot) water. Remove excess water with earmold blower (See figure 10.4). Listen to sound.
	23. Clogged with moisture	Remove earmold from hearing aid and examine visually.	Remove moisture with earmold blower.
Tubing/earhook (behind-the-ear or eyeglass aids)	**24. Tubing twisted or sharply bent	Look in two mirrors to see if tubing is twisted or sharply bent.	Reposition aid so tubing is not bent. If necessary, shorten or replace tubing.
	25. Tubing clogged with earwax or moisture	Visually inspect tubing.	Remove tubing from hearing aid. Clean out wax with toothpick, wire or pipe cleaner. Wash with warm (*not* hot) soapy water. Use earmold blower to remove moisture.
	26. Tubing fits loosely around earhook	Visually inspect to see if tubing fits loosely around earhook.	Have dispenser replace tubing if it is loose.
	27. Tubing not glued into earmold	Visually inspect to see if tubing is unglued.	Have dispenser glue tubing into earmold.
	28. Earhook does not screw tightly onto hearing aid	Remove earmold and tubing from hearing aid. Screw earhook snugly against hearing aid. Turn up volume wheel to highest setting, and put finger over tip of earhook; if there is still whistling sound, earhook does not fit tightly enough.	Have dispenser replace earhook.

29. Crack or hole in earhook tubing	Visually inspect both tubing and earhook.	Have dispenser replace earhook and/or tubing.
30. Tubing wall not thick enough *or* Sta-Dri tubing used for high-gain aid	If tubing walls are thin, you are using a high-gain aid, and there is a whistling sound when you turn the volume wheel to a comfortable level, remove the aid and put your finger over the openings in the earmold. If there is whistling, and all the possible causes for whistling mentioned above have been eliminated, then the tubing wall is too thin (or the pores of the Sta-Dri tubing allow the sound to escape).	Have the dispenser replace the tubing with thick-walled tubing.
Telephone amplifier (aids with telephone switch)		
31. Amplifier too weak	Switch to telephone setting, put telephone receiver to hearing aid and turn volume wheel all the way up while talking with someone on the phone. Move the telephone receiver around the hearing aid to get the best reception. If sound is too soft, then the amplifier is too weak.	Have dispenser get telephone amplifier replaced with a stronger one and/or use an amplifier on the telephone.
Cold temperature (all aids)		
32. Hearing aid and/or battery are too cold to function normally	Warm aid and battery up to room temperature. Listen to sound through the aid at normal use-gain setting.	Warm up the aid.

(continued)

TABLE 10.2. (*Continued*)

LOCATION	POSSIBLE CAUSE	TEST	REMEDY
Hearing aid dysfunction	33. Internal noise	Put on aid and listen to someone talking with volume wheel set so the words are comfortably loud. Then go into a very quiet room and listen for the noise. If there is no noise, then the noise heard before was noise "in the world" amplified by the hearing aid. If there is still noise, this is internal noise from the hearing aid. This noise should not interfere with sounds you want to hear.	If internal noise is annoyingly loud, return aid for repair.
	34. Internal whistling (feedback)	If you have a behind-the-ear or eyeglass aid, take off the earhook and tubing, put your finger over the receiver hole and turn the volume wheel all the way up after being sure the battery is working. If the hearing aid whistles, this indicates it is coming from inside the hearing aid. The same test can be made with (1) a body aid by removing the earmold and putting your finger over the receiver hole, or (2) an in-the-ear aid by putting your finger over the receiver hole.	Return the aid for repair.

35. Hearing aid case cracked, or circuit loose inside hearing aid case	Visually inspect the hearing aid for cracks. Tap the hearing aid gently while listening to the amplified sound. If the sound is intermittent, or there is no sound, it needs repair.	Return the aid for repair.
36. Microphone port clogged with dirt	Visually inspect microphone hole for dirt. Use well-charged battery, insert it properly, turn the volume wheel up, and listen for it to whistle. If there is none, the microphone hole may be clogged.	Return the aid for repair.
Microphone too close to reflecting surface		
37. Microphone too close to wall, hand or another reflecting surface	Wear aid as you normally would; then move close to a wall, put hand up near the aid or cover with a hat or scarf. Listen for the whistling.	Move hand away from aid, move away from the wall, or remove the hat or scarf.
Blockage in ear		
38. Ear wax blocking earcanal	Have doctor examine earcanals.	Doctor will remove ear wax.
39. Blockage in middle ear	Have doctor examine ears.	Doctor will treat ears as needed.

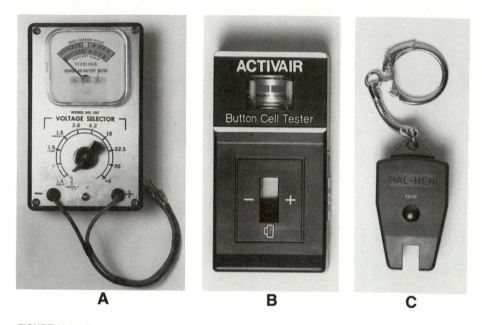

FIGURE 10.3. Battery testers. **(A)** Desk type battery tester appropriate to use in a clinic. **(B)** Battery tester for zinc-air batteries. **(C)** Minilite battery tester. **(B)** and **(C)** are inexpensive and often used by clients.

5. Use the right size battery.
6. When you insert the battery, be sure
    a. it is at room temperature,
    b. it is dry, and
    c. the + mark on the battery is placed so it matches the + sign on the battery case. (If the battery is forced in incorrectly, it may cause the battery case to break.)
7. Remove the battery from the hearing aid when it is not in use; even if the hearing aid is turned off, the battery may continue to drain as long as it is in the aid.
8. After extended use of a battery, the sound from the hearing aid will become weaker and sometimes noisy. The old battery should be removed and discarded and a new battery inserted. (Old batteries should not be left in the hearing aid because they tend to leak and corrode the battery terminals.)
9. Dead batteries can be sent to a collection agency that will pay for them. *Hearing Instruments* carries advertisements from these agencies.
10. Keep track of how many hours a battery lasts; if there is a sudden decrease in battery life, the aid may be defective. (Batteries last from approximately one day to three weeks depending on the type and degree of hearing loss, type of battery, circuit of the hearing aid, number of hours of use, and volume-wheel setting.)
11. Use a battery tester to check the battery when you are uncertain whether it is functioning well; the battery tester drains the battery so use it sparingly (see figure 10.3).
12. Do not use a battery recharger unless you have rechargable batteries.

Controls.

A. Volume wheel
   1. Purpose: Adjust the overall intensity of the amplified sound.
   2. The intensity does not always change the same amount for equal changes in the rotation of the wheel.
   3. Explore the effect of various volume-wheel settings on the comfort of amplified sounds in your everyday life.

B. On-off switch
   1. Turn the hearing aid on after earmold and aid are in place.
   2. Turn the hearing aid off before taking earmold and aid off. (Remove the battery if you are going to leave the aid off.)

C. Tone control switch
   1. When there is an external, normal/low-frequency switch, use the normal or low-frequency setting in quiet situations, and the low-frequency setting in very noisy situations.
   2. Internal tone-control switches should be adjusted by the dispenser. Occasionally, the person wearing the aid will want the flexibility provided by these controls; s/he may be instructed in their use.

D. Microphone/telephone switch
   1. When the switch is in the microphone position, sound from sources that are close enough will be amplified.
   2. When the switch is in the telephone position, only electromagnetic energy will be sensed and amplified by the hearing aid. If the switch is in the telephone position by mistake, the battery and/or hearing aid will appear to be *dead*.

Earmold and Tubing.

A. The earmold should fit comfortably in the pinna and earcanal; if it irritates the skin, the earmold should be modified or remade with non-allergenic material.

B. Keep the earmold clean and unclogged by wax or moisture.
   1. *Detachable earmold*: Gently detach the earmold, clean the ear wax out with a toothpick or pipe cleaner, clean with warm (*not hot*) soapy water, rinse, and dry completely. Blow moisture out of tubing and vent with an earmold blower (see figure 10.4); a drop of moisture can prevent sound from passing through the tubing, and moisture can damage the hearing aid. Do *not* use alcohol or carbon tetrachloride to clean the earmold. Reattach the earmold tubing to the earhook.
   2. *All-in-the-ear aids*: Gently use the wire loop provided by the manufacturer to get behind and pull out the ear wax. (Do not push the wax inward so that it blocks the sound from the receiver.) Wipe the outside of the earmold with a damp cloth; dry immediately.

C. Inspect the tubing to make sure it
   1. fits snugly around the earhook,

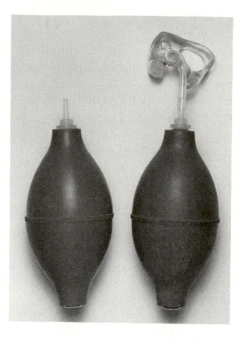

FIGURE 10.4.
Earmold blower. After A. M. Loavenbruck and J. R. Madell 1981. *Hearing Aid Dispensing for Audiologists.* Reproduced with permission of Grune & Stratton, Inc. and the authors.

2.   is glued securely in the earmold, and
3.   has no cracks that will allow the amplified sound to cause feedback.
If the tubing is loose, hard, stiff, or cracked, it should be replaced.

Acoustic Feedback.   Acoustic feedback is the familiar squeal that occurs when amplified sound gets back to the hearing aid microphone at a high enough intensity and is amplified again. This can occur when the hearing aid is turned on and

1.   the earmold is not placed properly in the ear,
2.   the earmold does not fit tightly enough in the ear,
3.   there is a vent in the earmold,
4.   the tubing walls are not thick enough,
5.   there is a crack in the tubing, earmold, or earhook,
6.   a reflective surface such as a wall, pillow, or your hand is too close to the microphone and receiver, or
7.   the hearing aid is defective.

Cord and external receiver.   In a body hearing aid (and occasionally in a behind-the-ear or eyeglass aid) the external receiver is connected to the hearing aid by a replaceable cord. Since the receiver and cord are fragile, they should be handled with care.

A.   Cord wires
   1.   will break eventually through extended use and bending,
   2.   will break if they are allowed to knot or twist,

3. will cause either intermittent or no sound if they are broken,
4. will need to be replaced with a new cord if they are broken (keep a spare one for this purpose).

B. Receiver
   1. is often attached to the earmold with a plastic washer to prevent feedback,
   2. should not be dropped or hit,
   3. should not be immersed in water or other liquid,
   4. will distort and/or greatly reduce the amplified sound when it is broken or defective,
   5. needs to be replaced when it is broken (keep a spare one for this purpose).

Bone-conduction vibrator.   A bone-conduction vibrator is delicate and should not be dropped or immersed in water. It is usually coupled to the head with a headband, which must be adjusted to give sufficient pressure to make good contact but not so much pressure that it slips or is uncomfortable.

Daily listening check.
A. Check the battery.
   1. Are the battery terminals clean?
   2. Is the battery leaking?
   3. Is the battery weak? (Use a battery tester.)
B. Check the switch positions.
   1. On/Off (set "on").
   2. Microphone/telephone (set on microphone).
   3. Tone control (set on most frequently used position).
   4. Volume wheel (lowest setting).
C. Check tubing and earhook for stiffness, holes, or cracks. (If body aid, check the cord.)
D. Check the earmold. Clean it if necessary and blow out any moisture with an earmold blower, after it has been removed from the hearing aid.
E. Listen to the sound with the volume wheel set at a comfortable listening level. If there is excessive noise, abnormal sound quality, whistling, then consult the troubleshooting chart, table 10.2.

Troubleshooting

It is much easier to wear a hearing aid when one knows how to solve simple problems that inevitably occur. The most common problem is that the aid produces no sound at all. Often a switch is turned to telephone or off instead of to microphone, a battery is dead, the battery is inserted upside-down, the earmold is plugged with wax, the tubing is sharply twisted or blocked by moisture, or the cord is broken. Another common problem for someone using an aid for the first time is the sound being too weak or a whistling sound caused by inserting the earmold so that it is not properly positioned. These common causes, which are indicated with asterisks on the troubleshooting chart, table 10.2, are the first things to investigate.

Once solutions to these common problems become second nature, one can turn to learning the possible causes, tests, and remedies for other symptoms of hearing aid dysfunction. Many of these are listed in the troubleshooting chart. Mastery of this information usually occurs when the hearing aid does not work properly, and the person who wears it learns to solve the problem by tracking down the cause and remedying it or realizing that the dispenser or manufacturer needs to repair it. One way to facilitate the mastery of this information is to offer a session in which a number of aids are set to malfunction and the participants are guided in learning to remedy the causes.

Some of the causes of problems listed in the troubleshooting chart, such as dirty switch contacts or earhooks that do not screw on tightly, will require greater understanding to resolve than hearing aid users have. These can be resolved by the clinician who dispensed the aid.

Repairs

Occasional servicing and repair are needed for all hearing aids. Tubing and earhooks become worn and need replacement, and the hearing aid switches or circuits may need repair or replacement.

Manufacturers of hearing aids always give a one-year warranty with new hearing aids, and some give two- or three-year warranties. For an additional cost, the original warranty can be extended. These warranties cover the cost of repair by the manufacturer, provided that repair has not been attempted by someone else. For aids that are not under warranty at the time of repair, a three-, six-, or twelve-month guarantee should be given at the time of the repair. The length of this guarantee usually affects the cost of the repair to a small extent. Repairs of out-of-warranty aids may be provided by the manufacturer, a company that specializes in repairs, or if a dispenser's operation is large enough, s/he may have a technician to repair hearing aids.

Listening with a Hearing Aid

Listening to sound through a hearing aid for the first time can bring joy and at the same time be unsettling. There will be many sounds that the person has not heard, particularly high-frequency sounds, such as a telephone ringing or birds singing, and soft sounds, such as someone talking in the next room. Noises such as a refrigerator running, dishes and silverware clinking together, or many people talking, will seem loud and perhaps annoying. All sound, not just the sounds the person wants to hear, will be amplified. It may be very difficult to pay attention to the significant sounds and ignore the background sounds. One's own voice will sound loud and unnatural. If the client knows that these experiences are normal, it should be easier to deal with them. Table 10.3 lists some common complaints and an explanation for them.

TABLE 10.3.   Hearing Aid User Complaints. From *Coping with Hearing Loss*. Copyright 1985, Susan V. Rezen and Carl Hausman. Reprinted with permission of Dembner Books, New York, N.Y.

PROBLEM	EXPLANATION
When I work in the kitchen, the sound of dishes clinking together drives me crazy.	You are bothered by sudden high-frequency sounds, such as dishes clinking. It is probably quite annoying because you haven't heard these sounds in a while, or you have only heard the low frequencies in these sounds. In some cases, a condition called *recruitment* (an abnormal sensitivity to loudness) will cause sudden, high frequency sounds to be uncomfortable. You may soon adjust to the new sounds coming through the hearing aid, though. If you can't get used to them, the hearing aid dispenser may adjust the aid.
I hate the unnatural sound of the hearing aid.	Since you have a hearing loss, "natural" for you means not hearing well. As mentioned earlier in the chapter, the hearing aid must change the nature of sound; the change, while less natural-sounding, will allow better hearing. Most hearing aid users become accustomed to this different type of sound.
I get so much wax in my ears, now that I wear a hearing aid.	The presence of the earmold may stimulate wax production. People who don't wear hearing aids get wax in their ears, too, but it gradually falls out of the earcanal. With an earmold in place, much of the wax is retained. You may have to visit a physician from time to time and have the wax removed; this is a simple and painless procedure.
The earmold hurts.	In the beginning, the earmold will be slightly uncomfortable. It's much like wearing a new pair of shoes, and you will probably soon become used to it. However, if the earmold still is uncomfortable after a few days, or if you notice irritated spots in your ear, go back to the dispenser and have the earmold altered.
Everything is so loud! I can't stand it.	When you're coming out of a movie theater into bright sunshine, the light hurts your eyes. Much the same situation occurs when you have become used to a hearing loss and suddenly put on an aid. It may take days or weeks for you to adjust to your newfound hearing when you first get an aid. If you still are bothered after three or four weeks, or if it is actually painful to wear the aid at any time, return to the dispenser. Having the characteristics of the aid readjusted may allow a compromise between good hearing and tolerance of the sound.
I wore my new hearing aid to a meeting yesterday and it was unbearable.	A hearing aid takes getting used to, and a room full of people is not the place to start. Begin by wearing the aid alone in a quiet room, and read aloud. After you've become used to the sound of your own voice, invite another person in to speak with you. Gradually increase the number of people in the communication situation; you may also want to experiment with various levels of background noise to simulate real-world conditions. Putting on the aid and immediately venturing into a difficult communication situation can quickly alienate a new wearer; this is one reason why so many aids wind up in the drawer after only one use. You will probably want to allow three or four weeks before you are

(continued)

TABLE 10.3. *(Continued)*

PROBLEM	EXPLANATION
My own voice sounds strange.	wearing the aid full time in all types of situations. This is normal because you are not used to hearing yourself as others hear you. Remember the first time you heard yourself on a tape recorder? You will adjust to the "new voice" within a few days. But if your voice continues to sound hollow or it echoes (or you have a "full" feeling in your ear) report this problem to your hearing aid dispenser, who can adjust the aid and/or your earmold.

Some clinicians recommend wearing a new aid a few hours each day initially and increasing this time until it is worn all day. Others recommend wearing it all day immediately. The length of time a new aid is worn should depend on the environment and the individual's response to hearing the amplified sound. For adults, it is best to start with quiet environments listening to (1) sounds that were not audible before (such as the newspaper rattling), (2) sounds that are louder and have a different quality now (such as footsteps, keys jingling), (3) one's own voice, and (4) one other person talking. The individual needs to experiment with various volume-wheel settings to discover which will make the sounds loud enough to be easily recognized and also comfortable; just barely turning it on is usually not high enough. With practice it should become automatic to set (and reset) the volume wheel depending on the listening conditions. When it is relatively comfortable to listen in quiet environments, then more difficult listening situations can be tried; a suggested hierarchy is given in table 10.4. With practice the hearing aid will be helpful in some situations, such as talking with one person in a quiet place, marginally helpful in some, such as listening in the midst of background noise, or hazardous in some, such as listening to industrial noise at high intensity levels (the hearing aid should not be used in these situations). It is important for the client to adjust expectations according to the degree of hearing impairment and listening environment. Wherever possible s/he should modify the environment for better sound reception (suggestions are given later in this chapter).

With infants and small children, parents, teachers, and audiologists make decisions about where to set the volume wheel and how long to leave the aid on. The audiologist should recommend a volume-wheel setting based on the test results, but the parents and/or teacher need to observe the child's reaction to the sound. Initially, it may be necessary to insist firmly that the child keep the aid on. The next step is to determine whether the child seems to be getting the appropriate sound level (is it too high or too low?) and then set the volume wheel accordingly. The level should be high enough for the child to show an awareness of sound in the environment (as demonstrated by a "listening" quietness or vocalization). The level should not be so high that the child winces or starts to cry when a loud sound occurs (in some

TABLE 10.4.   A Hierarchy of Listening Experiences Ranked from Simple to Complex; the Listening Difficulty Increases as the Experiences Become More Complex. Adapted from W.R. Hodgson, "Learning Hearing Aid Use." In *Hearing Aid Assessment and Use in Audiologic Habilitation*, 2nd ed. Ed. W.R. Hodgson and P.H. Skinner. Copyright 1981, Williams and Wilkins Co., Baltimore. Reprinted with Permission of the Author and Publisher.

1. Listen to background sounds like water running, your footsteps as you walk, the doorbell, and kitchen appliances.
2. Listen to a simple conversation with one person talking to you in a quiet room with many sound-absorbing surfaces. Practice with the speaker at different positions and distances.
3. Listen to one person talking with some background noise, such as water running at different levels in the kitchen sink. Make sure the noise is relatively quiet so it does not completely mask what the person is saying.
4. Listen to TV programs in which the individuals speak clearly about topics you know (such as a news broadcast). The room should be quiet except for the TV.
5. Listen to one person talk at a quiet dinner table.
6. Listen to conversation with two, then three or four other people.
7. Listen outside in quiet, such as in the backyard, where there will be some wind noise.
8. Listen over the telephone; try the telecoil.
9. Wear the aid at church, a lecture, or a play.
10. Take a quiet drive in the country with the car windows up.
11. Walk along the street in a quiet neighborhood.
12. Take a drive with the car windows open.
13. Go shopping.
14. Try wearing the aid at a restaurant, at a party, or in a room where a large number of people are talking.

cases the level *may* be all right but the SSPL90 may need to be lowered). It may take a period of weeks and months of evaluation to determine the best setting of the hearing aid.

For the first few days the aid should be put on for short periods of time (thirty to sixty minutes), several times a day, when the child is rested and the room is quiet. Then it should be put on for successively longer periods, until it is worn all day.

Once people are used to wearing an aid, adults with mild hearing losses may wear it only for specific listening situations, whereas those with moderate, severe, or profound hearing losses usually wear it all day. Since the perception of one's own voice and sounds in everyday life is different with a hearing aid than without it, wearing the aid all the time should be less confusing and more helpful than wearing it only occasionally. For hearing aids that have a maximum acoustic output greater than 132 dB SPL, it is wise to turn it off several times a day (preferably once an hour) to give the ear a chance to rest.[2]

[2]Although there are no formal studies of the effect of rest periods on the auditory fatigue experienced by people who wear hearing aids with SSPL90s greater than 132 dB SPL, the results of research with animals and humans support the use of rest periods (Bohne, Zahn, and Bozzay 1985; Ward 1976).

It takes considerable time to become thoroughly familiar with sound amplified through a hearing aid. Those who use aids most effectively report that it takes as long as a year to recognize the minimally audible or discriminable cues of speech and other sounds. When their aids are repaired or they change to another aid, it often takes some time to adjust to the change in sound.

Some people are able to learn to listen by themselves; others are more successful if they have some guidance (see Appendix 10B for examples of listening exercises). This is particularly true for infants and young children, who are in the process of learning language. For infants and children, it is best if the parents and child are guided by a teacher of the hearing impaired and routinely evaluated audiologically. If this is impossible, a correspondence course, such as that provided by the John Tracy Clinic,[3] should be followed. For adults, reading materials may provide sufficient information (see the reading list in Appendix 10A). Some people may prefer individual or group aural rehabilitation to learn effective ways to listen with their aids.

Using a Telecoil

If the aid is equipped with a telecoil, the client should be guided in how to use it. The first step is to discover how to place the telephone receiver over the hearing aid case to get the best sound level (with the volume wheel adjusted appropriately). This can be done while listening to recorded public-service messages that are available from the local telephone company. Most hearing aids do not have telecoil amplifiers that are as strong as the microphone amplifiers. Therefore, in some cases a booster amplifier will be needed for the telephone. This is particularly true for people with severe or profound hearing losses. As mentioned in chapter 8, some telephone receivers do not radiate enough electromagnetic energy to drive the telecoil, and a special adapter is needed. In addition, the signal from some telephone companies is not clear enough for people with severe or profound hearing losses to understand the message. Despite all these possible problems, many people use the telecoil of their hearing aids to hear well over the telephone.

It takes practice to change the switch position, adjust the volume wheel (if necessary), and answer the phone. In the beginning people are often anxious when the telephone rings. Until answering becomes an automatic response, it is helpful for the client to ask the person calling to wait until s/he has adjusted the aid.

Are Adjustments Needed?

After wearing a hearing aid for several weeks, listening to many kinds of sounds in a variety of situations, and learning to adjust the volume wheel to the best listening level, the client may find further adjustments needed. If

[3]This correspondence course is available from the John Tracy Clinic, 806 West Adams Boulevard, Los Angeles, Calif. 90007.

sounds are intolerably loud, the SSPL90 or compression settings may need to be reduced or an acoustic damper placed in the earhook or tubing. If the sound is too shrill or high-pitched sounds are irritating, the gain in the high frequencies may need to be reduced, either by internal adjustments or by modifying the earmold. If the sound is hollow, particularly one's own voice, a vent may resolve this problem. If low-pitched sound seems to drown out higher-pitched sounds, then the low-frequency gain may need to be reduced internally. Resolving problems such as these may make the difference between the client's wearing the aid successfully or putting it in the dresser drawer. Even if less of the speech spectrum is audible as a result of these adjustments, it may be possible to give more gain in specific frequency regions at a later date.

WAYS TO IMPROVE COMMUNICATION

The major impact of hearing impairment is on communication with other people. Although a hearing aid can make sound comfortably loud for most people, it cannot restore normal hearing function. Consequently, a hearing-impaired person should develp a number of strategies that will help compensate for the remaining deficits. These strategies include learning what

1. environmental factors make it easiest to hear and see what someone is trying to communicate,
2. cognitive skills, knowledge, and experience are helpful in figuring out what was said,
3. attitudes are important for enhancing communication,
4. ways family, friends, and associates can help, and
5. ways to identify and solve particular difficulties.

Environmental Factors

Factors that facilitate hearing.   Speech can be understood most easily when what is said is clear, comfortably loud, and not masked by noise. The client can maximize his or her reception of speech by understanding

1. what the person talking needs to do to speak clearly,
2. what to do about minimizing the effects of noise,
3. what room reverberation does to reception of speech, and
4. how to position oneself in relation to the person talking.

The person talking can make it much easier for the individual with the hearing impairment to understand by doing the following:

1. articulate the words clearly, being careful not to overarticulate or cut off the ends of words,

2. speak at a normal loudness level, trying not to drop the level much at the end of a sentence,

3. speak at a rate that the person with the hearing impairment can easily follow (the greater the hearing impairment, the more the rate may need to be slowed; elderly people may also need the rate slowed),

4. do not speak while eating, chewing gum, or smoking,

5. speak at approximately 5 ft. from and directly facing the person with the hearing impairment (this distance is a compromise between the best distance for hearing, which is 1.5 to 3 ft., and the best distance for speechreading, which is 6 to 9 ft; at 3 ft. speech is at a reasonable level [for each doubling of the distance between the sound source and listener in a free field, there is a 6-dB drop in level], and it will reach the person before it reverberates within the room; at 6 to 9 ft., s/he can see all the lip, face, and body movements for speechreading.),

6. answer questions with a sentence because it is often easier to guess when there are contextual cues,

7. stress keys words by making them a little louder and longer than other words in the sentence,

8. use a definite rising inflection when asking a question,

9. shout only when there is an emergency, and

10. use gestures and facial expressions to get the message across.

If the person with the hearing impairment knows about these techniques, s/he will be better prepared to guide family, friends, and co-workers in communicating effectively.

Background noise can cause difficulty, depending on how loud it is (particularly in relation to how loud the speech is), the content of the noise, and how much effect the hearing impairment has on the person's ability to hear speech in the midst of noise. The best strategy is to eliminate the noise source or lower its level, if this is possible. Certain noise sources, such as the TV, radio, tape recorder, dishwasher, fan, or running water, can be eliminated by turning them off. The noise level can often be lowered by moving away from the noise source (for example, select a seat in a restaurant as far from the kitchen as possible) or closing a door or window (and closing the car window in busy traffic). If the noise cannot be avoided in certain situations, such as at a large gathering, focusing only on what one person is saying may help.

The reverberation in a room, auditorium, theater, or church can adversely affect the intelligibility of speech if

1. it takes a long time for the reverberant sound to cease (a long reverberation time),

2. the person listening is a considerable distance from the speaker (or a loudspeaker) so that the reverberations combine with the direct sound, and

3. the person is sitting close to a hard wall where the reverberant sound level is relatively high.

One can reduce the reverberation time at home by using sound-absorbing materials, such as carpets, draperies, acoustic tile on the ceiling, and upholstered furniture. If reverberation causes difficulty, the client should find out which theaters and meeting places have good amplification systems, relatively short reverberation times, or assistive listening devices such as direct audio input, FM, or infrared communication systems.

Since speech is most understandable when the person listening is approximately 5 ft. from the speaker (or loudspeaker) and the noise level is as low as possible, it is important for the person with a hearing impairment to consciously choose the best place to sit or stand depending on the situation. The following are examples:

1. *small group of people in a living room*: sit in a chair facing the other people instead of side by side on a sofa; position the chair chose enough to the other people that their voices are comfortably loud when the gain of the hearing aid is adjusted appropriately;

2. *meeting in an auditorium*: sit as close to the speaker or loudspeaker and away from the walls (come early to get an appropriate seat);

3. *talking in a car*: sit so that the aided ear is toward the person with whom you are talking (sometimes with binaural aids it is helpful to turn off the aid nearer the window) or use a direct audio input system with the microphone placed near the other person's mouth;

4. *eating in a restaurant*: choose a table as far from the major noise sources as possible; either face or have the aided ear nearest the people who are most important to hear;

5. *at home*: if someone speaks from across the room or from another room, move close enough the hear easily; if the person speaking is near an interfering noise source, either turn it off, or both move to a quieter place.

Factors that facilitate seeing. A number of visual cues can provide important information about what someone is saying. These include

1. lip, tongue, mouth, and facial movements,
2. bodily gestures, and
3. contextual cues.

Close observation of the movements of the lips, tongue, and mouth to try to understand what is being said is called *lipreading*. Without sound it is impossible to understand everything by lipreading. A number of the speech sounds, (such as *k* and *g*), cannot be seen because they are formed in the back of the mouth. Some speech sounds (such as *p*, *b*, and *m*), look the same on the lips; these are called a *homophonous* group. In addition, we cannot follow all the lip movements of natural speech with our eyes as quickly as they are made. Nevertheless, the cues that are present on the lips, when combined with sufficient auditory cues, can enable many hearing-impaired people to understand much or all of what is being said. For this reason, it is important for people with hearing impairment to learn the basic principles of lipreading (see, for example, the exercises for adults in Appendix 10B) to enhance the natural tendency we all have to look for visual cues.

The cues of lipreading are best seen when

1. the face of the person speaking is well lighted, preferably with diffuse light so there are no shadows,
2. the face of the person speaking is at a comfortable distance for the person with the hearing impairment to focus clearly on the face movements (approximately 4 to 6 ft.),
3. the person speaking uses clearly visible movements that are not obscured by a beard or moustache, holding one's hand or a paper in front of the mouth, or chewing,
4. the person with the hearing impairment does not have light shining directly into his or her eyes,
5. the person with the hearing impairment faces the people whom s/he is lipreading,
6. their faces are at the same level.

With these facts in mind, the person with a hearing impairment can unobtrusively arrange the seating and lighting accordingly, whenever possible.

Facial and bodily gestures such as raising the eyebrows, a nod of the head, or a shrug of the shoulders, often convey attitudes or emotional information about what is being said. Many times these cues are consistent with what is being spoken; however, sometimes they convey a different message, one that the person may not be aware of but that is nevertheless important.

It is also important to see what is happening at the time the person is speaking. This often gives clues to what is being said. The observation of this contextual information, facial and bodily gestures as well as lipreading, and integrating all this information to guess what is being said, is called *speech-reading*. Observing facial and bodily gestures is best done at 7 to 9 ft.

Cognitive Skills, Knowledge, and Experience

People with hearing impairment need to use all their cognitive skills, knowledge, and experience to compensate for insufficient auditory cues. Examples of important cognitive skills are

1. the ability to learn the visual cues of lipreading,
2. the ability to use distorted or minimally audible cues to recognize speech sounds,
3. the ability to integrate the visual and auditory cues of speech,
4. the ability to use one's knowledge of the language, the situational and contextual clues, and an understanding of the logical sequence of events to deduce the meaning of what was said without having to hear and see every word or speech sound accurately, and
5. the ability to focus on main ideas and concepts rather than on isolated words.

People with hearing impairment can actively expand their knowledge of

1. local, national, and international affairs,
2. the topics to be covered in meetings,
3. the script of a play,
4. the particular interests of family and friends, and
5. the vocabulary, sentence structure, accent, and facial expressions that family and close friends use when they talk . . .

so they can draw on this information when they try to understand what is said. Personal experiences of all kinds are also valuable sources of information.

Attitudes for Enhancing Communication

The most important attitude is the desire and motivation to communicate that is strong enough to surmount the difficulties that inevitably arise. This attitude is natural for babies and young children, but it needs to be nurtured by parents and teachers. For adults, this attitude is necessary to change old attitudes and patterns of communicating to ones that will help compensate for the hearing impairment. Some of these attitudes are

1. be committed to using a hearing aid or aids that are well fitted and adjusted so the sound is comfortably loud,
2. be committed to learning speechreading and about environmental factors that affect speech reception,
3. be committed to arranging the situation to hear and see best, if it is feasible, such as
   a. turn off a noisy TV, dishwasher, etc.,
   b. move closer if someone speaks at too great a distance,
   c. choose an appropriate seating arrangement (the criteria for making this choice are described in the Environmental Factors beginning on p. 341),
   d. choose to attend plays and movies in theaters that have good room acoustics, amplification systems, and other assistive devices, such as infrared devices,
   e. arrive early for meetings, movies, etc., to get an appropriate seat.
4. be willing to tell people that you have a hearing problem,
5. be willing to ask people for help, such as
   a. moving with you to a location where you can see and hear better,
   b. getting your attention (for example, by calling your name or gently touching your arm or shoulder) before they talk to you,
   c. telling you the topic of the conversation
      i. before they start,
      ii. when you get lost in the middle, or
      iii. when you enter an ongoing conversation,
   d. repeating the part of a sentence that you did not understand, after you repeat the part you did understand (this indicates that you were listening and want to understand),
   e. rephrasing or simplifying a complex sentence,
   f. speaking louder, more softly, or more slowly,

    g. not covering their faces, and
    h. writing down crucial information.

6. understand that the attitude you have in asking will often affect the response you get; if you ask openly, expecting a positive response, you often will get one; if you ask with clenched teeth and expect a negative response, you often will get one!

7. understand that some people are not willing or are unable to expend the extra effort to help you; realize that that is their choice and you can manage if they refuse,

8. encourage conversation rather than monopolizing the conversation,

9. set realistic expectations on listening abilities
    a. know the limits of what you can hear, given your hearing impairment and the situations you normally encounter in everyday life,
    b. when you are tired or ill, you do not have the energy to hear and compensate for your hearing impairment as well as when you are well rested,

10. be patient about how long it takes to learn new skills and habits,

11. relax; you can understand more when you are not tense,

12. be willing to take the risk of being wrong; everyone is sometimes!

13. have a sense of humor—be able to laugh with others about your mistakes.

Although some clients can adopt these attitudes and behavioral strategies after reading about them, many learn more quickly when they participate in an aural-rehabilitation program where they can role play typical situations and get to know other people who have similar problems and make similar mistakes.

Ways Family, Friends, and Co-workers Can Help

Family, friends, and co-workers of a person with a hearing impairment can help communication in a number of ways. Many of these ways are described in the sections above; they include speaking clearly, choosing a well-lighted, quiet place to talk, and helping the person when s/he asks. In addition, it is important to understand that noise, which normal-hearing people have learned to ignore, may cause significant difficulty for the person with a hearing impairment. It helps to become particularly aware of the background noise and eliminate it where possible or move to a quieter place to talk.

Successful communication is vital to maintaining and developing a relationship. Family, friends, and co-workers can show their commitment to successful communication by

1. speaking directly to the person with the hearing impairment,
2. being sensitive to whether s/he understands what is being said from facial expressions and responses,
3. finding ways to convey meaning accurately, and
4. being patient.

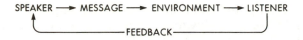

This process takes more effort than talking with a normal-hearing adult, but it is essential for maintaining communication. When these people experience how much effort it takes, it will be easier to understand how much energy it takes their hearing-impaired friend to communicate. In addition, they need to understand that it is not an intellectual impairment but a hearing impairment that makes it difficult for the person to understand what is being said.

Family, friends, and co-workers who understand the difficulty a hearing impairment can cause, and who take the initiative to learn ways to facilitate communication, will make it much easier for the person with a hearing impairment to develop new skills and habits than if s/he does not get this support.

Problem Solving

When a person with a hearing impairment has difficulty communicating, it is very helpful to analyze what is causing the problem. The diagram in figure 10.5 is a model of communication that can be used to determine where the breakdown is occurring. For example, it may be that the speaker is not talking clearly enough, that the message is either unfamiliar or uninteresting, that there is too much noise to hear what is being said, that the hearing aid is not adjusted properly, or that the listener is too tired. It is essential to assess logically where the problem lies, before it is possible to remedy it. There may be one source of difficulty or several. After determining problems, it is satisfying to solve them. However, in some cases there may be no feasible solution, and knowing this often makes it easier to accept the status quo.

SUMMARY

As clinicians, we can use our technical expertise to select and adjust a hearing aid for an individual so that speech and other important sounds are comfortably loud, speech is as understandable as possible, amplified loud sounds do not become uncomfortably loud, sound quality is acceptable, and the earmold is comfortable. We can also provide a wealth of information about how to operate the hearing aid, about how to solve simple problems when it is not functioning correctly, and about ways a client can improve communication by optimizing her or his ability to see and hear and by developing positive attitudes and strategies for understanding what people are saying.

However, this information can be assimilated by the hearing-impaired individual only when s/he is emotionally ready. We, as clinicians, can be most helpful if we understand our own need for personal growth and show genuine concern, respect, and acceptance for the client and his or her family. Within this emotional context we can encourage her or him to identify the communication problems s/he is having and provide the support and guidance for him or her to discover ways to solve, alleviate, or accept these problems. Although we can provide the supportive environment for this discovery, it is the responsibility of the client to make the changes necessary for learning to use the hearing aid effectively and compensating for the effect hearing impairment has on communication with other people.

If we, as clinicians, will continually seek out information on how we can best select and adjust hearing aids and earmolds as well as techniques for improving speechreading and listening skills, evaluate this new information through personal experience, and be committed to our own personal growth, our clients will have the best opportunity to benefit from their aids.

APPENDIX 10A

The following books or journals give information about hearing impairment and how a number of people have coped with it. Reading these has been helpful to provide both factual information and emotional release. (Some of these references are from Wylde 1982.)

FOR ADULTS

CALKINS, E. E. 1969. *And hearing not*. New York: Doubleday.
HEINER, M. H. 1949. *Hearing is believing*. New York: World Publishing.
HELLENBERG, M. M. 1979. *Your hearing loss: How to break the sound barrier*. Chicago: Nelson-Hall.
REZEN, S. V., and C. HAUSMAN. 1985. *Coping with hearing loss: A guide for adults and their families*. New York: Red Dembner Enterprises.
SHHH Journal. Published by Self Help for Hard of Hearing People, 4848 Battery Lane, Suite 100, Bethesda, MD 20814 (301-657-2248; TTY 301-657-2249). (Six issues of the journal are published each year and sent to members; membership fee is $10 annually.)
WARFIELD, F. 1957. *Cotton in my ears*. New York: Viking.
WARFIELD, F. 1957. *Keep listening*. New York: Viking.

FOR PARENTS OF HEARING-IMPAIRED CHILDREN

A. G. Bell Association. *Parent kit*. Available from the A. G. Bell Association, 3417 Volta Pl., N.W., Washington, DC 20007.
BIKLEN, D. 1974. *Let our children go*. Syracuse, N.Y.: Human Policy Press.
BITTER, G. B. 1978. *Parents in action*. Washington, DC: A. G. Bell.
DAVIS, J. M. and E. J. HARDICK. 1981. *Rehabilitative audiology for children and adults*. New York: Wiley (Especially chapter 10, Educational management, and chapter 11, Assessment and treatment of psychosocial problems.)
FEATHERSTONE, H. 1978. *A difference in the family*. New York: Basic Books.
FERRIS, C. 1980. *A hug just isn't enough*. Washington, DC: Gallaudet.
FREEMAN, R. D. 1981. *Can't your child hear*? Baltimore: University Park Press.
Gallaudet College Public Service Programs. *Parent Packet*. Available from Gallaudet College, 7th and Florida Ave., N.E., Washington, DC 20002.
GLICK, F. P. 1982. *Breaking silence*. Scottsdale, Pa.: Herald Press.
GREGORY, S. 1976. *The deaf child and his family*. New York: Wiley.
GRIFFIN, B. F. 1980. *Family to family*. Washington, DC: A. G. Bell.
HARRIS, G. A. 1983. *Broken ears, Wounded hearts*. Washington, D.C.: Gallaudet.
Illinois Annual School for Mothers of Deaf Children. 1965. *If you have a deaf child*. Champaign, IL: University of Illinois.
LERMAN, S.R.F. 1980. *Parent awareness training: Positive parenting for the 80's*. NY: A & W Publishers.
McARTHUR, S. H. 1982. *Raising your hearing-impaired child: A guideline for parents*. Washington, DC: A. G. Bell.
MEADOW, K. P. 1980. *Deafness and child development*. Berkeley: University of California Press.
MURPHY, A. T. 1979. *The families of hearing-impaired children*. Washington, DC: Gallaudet.
OGDEN, P.W., and S. LIPSETT. 1982. *The silent garden*. New York: St. Martin's.
SPRADLEY, T. S. and J. P. SPRADLEY. 1985. *Deaf like me*. Washington, DC: Gallaudet.

FOR CHILDREN

LaMore, G.S. 1985. *Now I understand.* Washington, DC: Gallaudet. (Grade-school children.)

Litchfield, A. 1976. *A button in her ear.* Chicago: Albert Whitman. (Preschool and grade-school children.)

Peterson, J. W. 1977. *I have a sister, my sister is deaf.* New York: Harper & Row. (Preschool and grade-school children).

Scott, V.M. 1985. *Belonging.* Washington, DC: Gallaudet. (Adolescents.)

APPENDIX 10B

These exercises by Rezen and Hausman, written for hearing-impaired adults to try at home, are representative of speechreading and listening activities that are often included in aural-rehabilitation programs for adults. (From *Coping with Hearing Loss*, 1985 by Susan V. Rezen and Carl Hausman. Reprinted with permission of Dembner Books, New York, NY).

Exercises like this are extremely valuable in enhancing speechreading skills. Here are some exercises that are commonly used in hearing therapy groups. Try and make up some of your own after you finish these.

Exercise 1: Being aware of facial expressions and gestures. Try these activities to practice getting as much information as possible from facial expressions and gestures:

- Look at photographs in magazines and newspapers and guess at what might have been said by the subject of the photo. Does the subject look angry, questioning, sad? Does the subject appear to be talking or listening?
- Watch television with the sound off. Try to imagine—from the gestures and expressions you see—what is going on and what is being said.

Exercise 2: Picking up cues from various situations. Since speechreading is really a series of educated guesses, the more possibilities you can anticipate (things likely to be said) the better. To develop the habit of giving yourself more cues to the content of the message, stop and think for a moment before you go into a familiar situation. Try to predict the things that may be said to you. You'll have a better chance of understanding conversation when you know what to expect. Using your past experience, predict what is likely to be said in the following examples (we've given a few samples; try to make up some more of your own):

Situation	What might be said
Out to dinner	How many in the party?
	Something from the bar?
	Are you ready to order?
	We have beans, carrots, and corn.
	Please pass the salt and pepper.
	I'll get the check.

Situation	What might be said
At the gas station	Fillerup?
	Back up, please.
	No-lead or super no-lead?
	Should I check under the hood?
	Your right front tire looks low.
	Sorry, we don't take credit cards.
Registering at the hotel	Do you have a reservation?
	Double or twin beds?
	Sign here, please.
	The bellman will take your bags.
	Please pay the cashier when you leave.
At the bank	Can I help you?
	Is this for savings or checking?
	Do you want tens or twenties?
	Would you sign the back of the check?
	Could I see some identification?
At the doctor's	Have you been here before?
	Which doctor is your appointment with?
	Fill these out and bring them back.
	Have you been staying on your diet?
	Describe the pain for me.
	Your insurance will not pay for this.

Exercise 3: Recognizing the homophonous groups.   Go back and review what the groups of sounds look like on the lips. Following are lists of identical-looking words within each group. Have a helper say one of the words to you silently. Be sure your partner uses normal lip movements; exaggerated lip movements will only prove distracting. You should try to determine what *group* the beginning or final sound of the word is in—the *p, b,* and *m* group; the *f* and *v* group; the *th* group; the *w* and *r* group; or the *ch* and *sh* group. *Don't try to guess the word—that's impossible, and you'll only get frustrated.* Guess the *group.* For example, if your partner silently says "boot" in an exercise dealing with the beginning sound, your response should be "the p, b, and m group." If your partner silently says "bath" in an exercise dealing with the end of words, your response should be "the th group."

The only reason we are using words is that having your partner say individual sounds would be worthless, since the lip movements would be distorted. By the way, your partner should skip around among these lists; it will be a bit obvious if all the words from the *p, b,* and *m* group are said one after the other. Your partner should tell you whether the group sound you are guessing occurs at the beginning or end of the word.

Words beginning with sounds from the *p*, *b*, and *m* group:

BOOT	MAT	POLE	MOLE	BONE	BORE
MADE	MAKE	BAT	BEAT	MIKE	PIKE
PAT	BAKE	MORE	MUD	BUD	MEAT
PAID	POUR	BIKE	POOL	PEST	BACK

Words ending with sounds from the *p*, *b*, and *m* group:

LAMB	SLAB	TOM	TOP	LAP	LAB
SLIM	COP	SLAP	CALM	SLIP	SLAM

Words beginning with sounds from the *f* and *v* group:

FAN	FEND	VAULT	FAT	VENT	VAN
VEST	VINE	VAT	FINE	FAULT	FILL

Words ending with sounds from the *f* and *v* group:

LEAF	STRIFE	STRIVE	LIVE
LEAVE	SAFE	LIFE	SAVE

Words beginning with sounds from the *th* group:

THIS	THAT	THROW	THINK

Words beginning with sounds from the *w* and *r* group:

WING	WOUND	WAIT	WEAK	WAIL	RAIL
RATE	RUN	RING	ROUND	RAKE	WON

Words beginning with sounds from the *sh* and *ch* group:

SHOW	SHOES	SHIP	SHIN
CHIP	CHIN	CHEW	CHOOSE

Words ending with sounds from the *sh* and *ch* group:

LEASH	WISH	WHICH	MUSH
WASH	WATCH	LEACH	MUCH

Exercise 4: Guessing words. Now's your chance to guess the whole word. Below are sets of three words (note that the words are not from the same homophonous group). You choose a set of three words. Your partner will mouth one of the three words; you must select the word based on the lip movements you see.

PAY, WAY, THEY
BAT, THAT, CHAT
LIME, LIVE, LIAR
RAIL, BAIL, FAIL
BOAT, VOTE, WROTE
POUND, ROUND, FOUND
MEAT, WHEAT, CHEAT

FINE, WINE, MINE
BOO, FEW, SHOE
FAULT, VAULT, MALT
THINK, WINK, MINK
CHIN, THIN, FIN

Exercise 5: Guessing groups in a sentence.   Have your partner read each of these sentences silently, mouthing the words. You are to guess which *group of sounds* appears most frequently. Do not try to guess the sentence itself.

BOB BROKE THE BOY'S BIKE.
SHE CHOSE TO SHOW HER SHOES.
THEY RODE ROUND IN THE RED ROADSTER.
PUT THE PURPLE POLE ON THE PORCH.
THE VIEW FROM THE VILLAGE IS VIVID.
WILLIAM WENT TO WATERTOWN TO WEIGH HIS WAGON.
THE FLAT TIRE WAS FINALLY FIXED ON FRIDAY.
THERE ARE THREE THOUSAND THESPIANS IN THE THEATER.

Exercise 6: Practicing grammatical closure.   Your brain fills in information without any conscious effort on your part. Once you've learned a language, you apply the rules of grammar even when the message is heard incorrectly. Have your partner read the following sentences aloud—without saying the parts in parentheses. The sentences have intentional errors. The errors duplicate what people with a hearing loss might *think* they hear. Note how your knowledge of grammar enables you to correct the error without even thinking about it.

THE BOY(S) ARE GOING TO THE STORE.
THE MAN BOUGHT (A) CAR.
THAT IS SALLY('S) DRESS.

WHO (IS) COMING HOME?
HE IS GO(ING) TO THE BANK.
GIVE THE BALL (TO) JACK.
I LEFT MY KEYS (IN) MY CAR.
HE GO(ES) BACK HOME EVERY DAY.

Exercise 7: Practicing conceptual closure and flexibility.   Your past experience with language and with life helps you to figure out what was said by:

1. helping you judge what might have been said, even if you didn't hear the whole message correctly
2. enabling you to eliminate choices that just don't make sense.

However, in order to figure out what might have been said, you must remain open to many different kinds of possibilities—as long as they make sense. In the sentences below, fill in the blank in at least four different ways. Be flexible, and consider *all* the different possibilities; remember that there are many different shades of meaning in the English language. Some possible ways the sentence can be completed are given at the end of the exercise. See if you can come up with an equally wide range of possibilities.

1. I HAVE A BLUE _____.
2. I WENT TO _____ ON MY VACATION.
3. I DRIVE A _____.
4. I LIKE _____ SANDWICHES.
5. GET SOME _____ AT THE GROCERY STORE.
6. I FEEL _____.
7. WHERE ARE YOU _____?
8. THE BIRDS WERE _____.

Possible ways to complete the sentences:

1. sweater, car, rug, book
2. Europe, Chicago, bed, camp
3. car, motorcycle, Ford, hard bargain
4. ham, huge, fresh, club
5. milk, meat, lettuce, change
6. sad, lonely, soft, carefully
7. going, driving, at, looking
8. flying, eating, beautiful, singing

Exercise 8: Practicing flexibility and homophonous groups.   Now, here's a chance to combine some skills. Following are some sentences that don't make sense—but let's pretend this is the way you heard them. For each one, first decide why it doesn't make sense. Then replace one of the words in the sentence with one that would look like it on the lips (same homophonous group) but will be more sensibile. The correct replacement words are shown at the end of the exercise.

1. DID YOU TAKE A MATH?
2. THAT MAN IS VAT.
3. I LOST MY CHEW.
4. I DON'T LIKE TO RATE.
5. SHOP THE ONIONS INTO PIECES.
6. THE TRAIN CAME OFF THE WAIL.
7. SOMEONE CALLED A COB.
8. SIT ON HIS LAB.
9. WE HAD A VINE TIME.
10. THAT WAS VERY LEAN BEAT.
11. I'VE HAD TOO MUSH OF IT.
12. SHE IS REALLY GETTING SLIP.
13. THE BIRD HURT HIS RING.
14. THE DOG SHOULD BE ON A LEECH.
15. PUT THE SOUP IN THE POLE.

Replacement words:

1. bath
2. fat
3. shoe
4. wait
5. chop
6. rail
7. cop
8. lap
9. fine
10. meat
11. much
12. slim
13. wing
14. leash
15. bowl

Exercise 9: Practicing association. Fortunately, most people carry on a conversation so that the same topic is maintained for a period of time. Once you know the topic, using your past experiences you can predict what ideas and words might appear later in the conversation. Again, once you expect something, it is easier to figure out. A change in topic, of course, may throw you. Possibly you can prearrange a signal with a close companion. If the companion is talking he or she can verbally alert you to a topic change, such as "On another topic . . . " If a third person is talking, the companion can use a signal such as touching you in a certain way to indicate a topic change.

Given the following topics, think of at least ten words or ideas that might also be heard in the conversation. Don't be rigid—think of varied possibilities as shown in the lists at the end of the exercise.

1. BASEBALL
2. FOOD
3. GARDEN
4. INFLATION
5. ILLNESS

Words that might be heard:

1. bat, score, little league, stadium, run, hot dogs, beer, Yankees, strike, TV
2. dessert, diet, store, refrigerator, recipe, roast beef, cost, cook, splurge, cookbook
3. plant, rain, weeds, rototiller, flowers, fertilizer, seeds, rake, vegetables, bees
4. interest, banks, bills, Congress, prices, social security, economy, stock market
5. arthritis, medicine, hospital bed, bills, doctors, pain, aspirin, fever, heart

Exercise 10: Understanding key words.   Remember that because of your hearing loss and the limitations of lipreading, it is impossible to perceive every single sound or word in a conversation. But also remember that it isn't necessary to get everything to figure out the meaning of the message.

You are looking for ideas, not words. If you try to see/hear every word you will be hopelessly lost, because while you are trying to figure out some words the speaker will get ahead of you. You are not required in conversation to repeat exactly what is said; you only need to react to ideas. So concentrate on following ideas, not words. Once you have gotten a few key words, you can figure out the rest. Pick out the three or four key words in each of the following sentences. The answers are given at the end of the exercise.

1. JOHN CAUGHT THE THIEF YESTERDAY.
2. THE LITTLE BOY CRIED BECAUSE HE LOST HIS CAT.
3. THE FAST CAR HIT THE TRUCK.
4. HER CAT CHASED THE GREY SQUIRREL.
5. THE GIRL OPENED THE DOOR SLOWLY.

Key Words:

1. John, caught, thief
2. boy, cried, lost, cat

3. car, hit, truck
4. cat, chased, squirrel
5. girl, opened, door

Exercise 11: Using key words. Now, you can practice what you must do with the key words. Let's pretend that you only heard the following key words. For each item, give at least one—or maybe two—possible sentences that could include the key words. In conversation you would know which sentence is correct based on the context. Some possible sentences are given at the end of the exercise.

1.	ANN	BAKED	APPLE	PIE
2.	JOHN	STORE	YESTERDAY	
3.	BOOK	ON	FLOOR	
4.	PUT	FLOWERS	VASE	
5.	BOOKSHELF	OVER		
6.	YOU	READ	PAPER	
7.	WHAT	ON	TV	
8.	TURN	LIGHT	OFF	
9.	ANOTHER	LOG	FIRE	
10.	SALLY	SWAM	LAKE	

Possible sentences:

1. Ann baked an applie pie.
2. John went to the store yesterday.
   John bought a coat at the store yesterday.
3. The book fell on the floor.
   The book is on the floor.
4. Put the flowers in the vase.
   Put some flowers in that vase.
5. The bookshelf fell over.
   The bookshelf is over there.
6. Did you read the paper?
   You read the paper every day.
7. What's on TV tonight?
   What did you put on the TV?
8. Please turn the light off.
   Did you turn the light off?
9. Put another log on the fire.
   Another log fell off the fire.
10. Sally swam across the lake.
    Sally swam in the lake.

Exercise 12: Completing related sentences. Here is a chance to practice associating words and topics. Following are pairs of sentences that might follow each other in a conversation. Complete the second sentence using the topic of the first, word association, and your past experiences. For the first item one way of completing the sentence is given as an example.

1. I WENT TO THE STORE TO GET OLIVES.
   THEY DIDN'T <u>have any green ones</u>.
2. WE SAW THAT MOVIE LAST WEEK.
   I THOUGHT IT _____.
3. WHO DID YOU VOTE FOR?
   I DECIDED NOT _____.
4. THE RECIPE CALLS FOR TWO TABLESPOONS OF CORNSTARCH.
   I HAD TO USE _____.
5. THE FLOWERS WERE WILTED.
   THE WEATHER _____.

Exercise 13: Forming related sentences.   This time give an entire sentence that might follow the first one in conversation based on the first sentence's topic. The first item is completed as an example.

1. DID YOU READ THE PAPER THIS MORNING?
   (The president's speech was in it.)
2. TV SHOWS ARE GETTING POORER EVERY YEAR.
3. THE CAR SQUEALED ITS TIRES ON THE CORNER.
4. I LEFT THOSE COOKIES ON THE TABLE.
5. THE LIBRARY BOOKS ARE THREE DAYS OVERDUE.

Exercise 14: Speechreading related sentences.   Find your partner again and practice a lot of these skills together. Following are more related sentences. Your partner should read the first one aloud and then only mouth silently the second one. Using your skills of association, watching the lips and filling in (closure), try to get the general meaning of the second sentence.

1. THE PAPER BOY IS HERE.
   DO YOU HAVE ANY MONEY?
2. IT'S COLD IN HERE.
   PLEASE SHUT THE WINDOW.
3. WE'RE HAVING POTATOES FOR DINNER.
   DO YOU WANT THEM MASHED OR BOILED?
4. IT'S A BEAUTIFUL DAY TODAY.
   I MADE A PICNIC LUNCH.
5. MY CAR WOULDN'T START TODAY.
   THE BATTERY MUST BE WEAK.
6. MY SOCIAL SECURITY CHECK CAME.
   I'M GOING TO THE BANK.
7. IS THERE ANYTHING GOOD ON TV?
   I LIKE SOAP OPERAS.

8. WOULD YOU LIKE A SNACK?
   I HAVE SOME POPCORN.
9. I'M HAVING TUNA FISH FOR LUNCH.
   I ALWAYS EAT FISH ON FRIDAYS.
10. I'M WORKING IN THE GARDEN.
    I LOVE TO PLANT FLOWERS.

Exercise 15: Listening practice.   You need to practice listening with your new hearing aid(s). There are some sounds that will probably be very difficult for you. Following are some pairs of words that sound similar. Sit next to your partner and hold the book in front of you so you can see the words but so that you can't see your partner's face. Listen as one of each pair of words is read aloud to you. Try to determine which one was said. Practice a lot.

FEW, CHEW	SHOW, FOE
FIN, CHIN	SHORE, FOUR
FILED, CHILD	SHADE, FADE
FOUR, CHORE	LEASH, LEAF
FIT, KIT	ICE, EYES
FOUR, CORE	BUS, BUZZ
FIND, KIND	LICE, LIES
LAUGH, LACK	SEAL, ZEAL
LEASE, LEASH	FIVE, FIFE
SEW, SHOW	VASE, FACE
SIGH, SHY	LEAVE, LEAF
SAVE, SHAVE	VIEW, FEW
TAIL, PAIL	FINE, SIGN
CAT, CAP	FLAT, SLAT
CUT, CUP	CUFF, CUSS
TOLL, POLE	NICE, KNIFE
THIN, FIN	TIE, THIGH
THIRST, FIRST	TIN, THIN
THREE, FREE	MIT, MYTH
THOUGHT, FOUGHT	PAT, PATH
KICK, TICK	PIKE, PIPE
KITE, TIGHT	CAT, PAT
CODE, TOAD	CRY, PRY
PARK, PART	COAL, POLE
THUMB, SUM	THAN, VAN
PATH, PASS	THAT, VAT
THING, SING	THINE, VINE

BIBLIOGRAPHY

ALPINER, J. G. 1982. *Handbook of Adult Rehabilitative Audiology*, 2nd ed. Baltimore: Williams and Wilkins.

ALPINER, J. G., and B. R. BAKER. 1982. "Communications assessment procedure for seniors (CAPS)." In *Handbook of Adult Rehabilitative Audiology*, 2nd ed. Ed. J. G. Alpiner. Baltimore: Williams and Wilkins.

ALPINER, J. G., W. CHEVRETTE, G. GLASCOE, M. METZ, and B. OLSEN. 1978. 1971 Unpublished materials. In *Handbook of Adult Rehabilitative Audiology*. Ed. J. G. Alpiner. Baltimore: Williams and Wilkins.

Altec-Lansing Corporation. 1985. Brochure describing Altec-Lansing loudspeakers. Available from P.O. Box 26105, Oklahoma City, OK 73124

American National Standards Institute. American National Standard Specifications for Audiometers, ANSI S3.6-1969. New York: ANSI.

American National Standards Institute. Methods for the Calculation of the Articulation Index, ANSI S3.5-1969. New York: ANSI.

American National Standards Institute. American National Standard Specifications for Sound Level Meters, ANSI S1.4-1971. New York: ANSI.

American National Standards Institute/Acoustical Society of America. American National Standard Specification of Hearing Aid Characteristics, ANSI S3.22-1982. New York: ANSI.

American National Standards Institute/Acoustical Society of America. American National Standard Criteria for Permissible Ambient Noise during Audiometric Testing. ANSI S3.1-1977. New York: ANSI.

American National Standards Institute/Acoustical Society of America. American National Standard for an Occluded Ear Simulator, ANSI S3.25-1979. New York: ANSI.

American National Standards Institute/Acoustical Society of America. Specifications for Hearing Aid Characteristics, ANSI S3.22-1982. New York: ANSI.

ANIANSSON, G. 1974. "Methods for assessing high frequency hearing loss in every-day listening situations." *Acta Otolaryngologica* (Stockholm), Supp. 320, 1−50.

ANSI. *See* American National Standards Institute.

BALBI, C. M. R. 1935. United States Patent 2,003,875.

BARFOD, J. 1972. "Investigations on the optimum corrective frequency response for high-tone hearing loss." Technical University of Denmark, Acoustics Laboratory, Report no. 4. Copenhagen.

BEATTIE, R. C., and B. J. EDGERTON. 1976. "Reliability of monosyllabic discrimination tests in white noise for differentiating among hearing aids." *Journal of Speech and Hearing Disorders* 41:464−76.

BEATTIE, R. C., B. J. EDGERTON, and D. W. GAGER. 1979. "Effects of speech materials on the loudness discomfort level." *Journal of Speech and Hearing Disorders* 44:435−58.

BECK, L. B. 1983. "Assessment of directional hearing-aid characteristics." *Audiological Acoustics* 22:178−191.

BECK, L. B., R. W. LEATHERWOOD, and J. L. PUNCH. 1980. "Aided low-frequency response: Speech quality and speech intelligibility." Paper presented at the Annual Convention of the American Speech-Language-Hearing Association. Detroit.

A. G. Bell Association, Parent Kit. Washington: A. G. Bell Association.

BERGER, K. W., E. N. HAGBERG, and R. L. RANE. 1984. *Prescription of Hearing Aids: Rationale, Procedures, and Results*. 4th ed. Kent, Ohio: Herald.

BERGER, K. W., L. D. HARRISON, N. MONACK, and G. E. FERREN 1980. "Comfortable loudness judgments for discrete frequency signals." *Journal of Auditory Research* 20:119−27.

BERGER, K. W., and L. L. SOLTISZ. 1981. "Variability of thresholds and MCLs with speech babble." *Australian Journal of Audiology* 3:1−3.

Bernafon, Inc. 1984. Hearing aid specification sheet. Availabile from 1125 Globe Avenue, Mountainside, NJ 07092.

BIKLEN, D. 1974. *Let Our Children Go*. Syracuse, N.Y.: Human Policy Press.

BILGER, R. C., J. M. NUETZEL, W. M. RABINOWITZ, and C. RZECZKOWSKI. 1984. "Standardization of a test of speech perception in noise." *Journal of Speech and Hearing Research* 27:32−48.

BINNIE, C. A. 1985. "Effects of amplification on the residual hearing of children." *Seminars in Hearing* 6(3):299–307.

BIRK-NIELSEN, H. 1985. "Hearing aid fitting based on insertion gain measurements." *Audecibel* 34(1):16–19.

BITTER, G. B. 1978. *Parents in Action.* Washington: A. G. Bell.

BOHNE, B. A., and W. W. CLARK. 1976. "Growth of hearing loss and cochlear lesion with increasing duration of noise exposure." In *Effects of Noise on Hearing*, Ed. D. Henderson, R. P. Hamernik, D. S. Dosanjh, J. H. Mills. New York: Raven Press, 283–302.

BOHNE, B. A., S. J. ZAHN, and D. G. BOZZAY. 1985. "Damage to the cochlea following interrupted exposure to low frequency noise." *Annals of Otology, Rhinology and Laryngology* 94:122–128.

BRAMMER, L. 1979. *The Helping Relationship: Process and Skills.* 1985. 3rd. ed. Englewood Cliffs, N.J.: Prentice-Hall.

BREDBERG, G. 1968. "Cellular pattern and nerve supply of the human organ of Corti." *Acta Otolaryngologica* (Stockholm) Supplement 236:1–135.

BROOKS, D. 1973. "Gain requirements of hearing aid users." *Scandinavian Audiology* 2:199–205.

BYRNE, D. 1977. "The speech spectrum: Some aspects of its significance for hearing aid selection and evaluation." *British Journal of Audiology* 11:40–46.

———. 1978. "Selection of hearing aids for severely deaf children." *British Journal of Audiology* 12:9–22.

———. 1980. "Binaural hearing aid fitting: Research findings and clinical application." in *Binaural Hearing and Amplification*, vol. 2. Ed. E. R. Libby. Chicago: Zenetron.

———. 1981. "Clinical issues and options in binaural hearing aid fitting." *Ear and Hearing* 2:187–93.

———. 1983. "Theoretical prescriptive approaches to selecting the gain and frequency response of a hearing aid." *Monographs in Contemporary Audiology* 4(1):1–40.

———. 1984. *Evaluation of the National Acoustic Laboratories' Procedure for Selecting the Gain and Frequency Response of a Hearing Aid.* Unpublished Ph.D. thesis, Macquarie University, Sydney, Australia.

———. 1986a. "Effects of bandwidth and stimulus type on most comfortable loudness levels of hearing-impaired listeners." *Journal of the Acoustical Society of America* 80:484–93.

———. 1986b. "Effects of frequency response characteristics on speech discrimination and perceived intelligibility and pleasantness of speech for hearing-impaired listeners." *Journal of the Acoustical Society of America* 80:494–504.

———. 1987. "Hearing aid selection formulae: same or different?" *Hearing Instruments* 38 (1):5–6, 8, 11.

BYRNE, D., and H. DILLON. 1981. "Comparative reliability of warble tone thresholds under earphones and in sound field." *Australian Journal of Audiology* 3:12–14.

———. 1986. "The National Acoustics Laboratories' (NAL) new procedure for selecting the gain and frequency response of a hearing aid." *Ear and Hearing* 7:257–65.

BYRNE, D., and D. FIFIELD. 1974. "Evaluation of hearing aid fittings for infants." *British Journal of Audiology* 8:47–54.

BYRNE, D., and N. MURRAY. 1986. "Predictability of the required frequency response characteristic of a hearing aid from the pure tone audiogram." *Ear and Hearing* 7:63–70.

BYRNE, D., and W. TONISSON. 1976. "Selecting the gain of hearing aids for persons with sensorineural hearing impairments." *Scandinavian Audiology* 5:51–59.

CALKINS, E. E. 1969. *And Hearing Not.* New York: Doubleday.

CARHART, R. 1946a. "Selection of hearing aids." *Archives of Otolaryngology* 44:1–18.

———. 1946b. "Tests for selection of hearing aids." *Laryngoscope* 56:780–794.

CARHART, R., and J. JERGER. 1959. "Preferred method for clinical determination of pure tone thresholds." *Journal of Speech and Hearing Disorders* 24:330–45.

CARVER, W. F. 1978. "Loudness balance procedures." In *Handbook of Clinical Audiology*, 2nd ed. Ed. J. Katz. Baltimore: Williams and Wilkins.

CHAIKLIN, J. B., and I. M. VENTRY. 1964. "Spondee threshold measurement: A comparison of 2- and 5-dB methods." *Journal of Speech and Hearing Disorders* 29:47–59.

CHASIN, M. 1985. "Reliability of insertion gain measurements with different earmold configurations." Paper presented at the Annual Convention of the American Speech-Language-Hearing Association, Washington, D.C.

CHRISTIAN, R., and D. BYRNE. 1980. "Variability of MCL measurements: Significance for hearing aid selection." *Australian Journal of Audiology* 2:10–18.

CLARK, W. W., and B. A. BOHNE. 1978. "Animal model for the 4kHz tonal dip." *Annals of Otology, Rhinology and Laryngology* Supp. 51, 87:1—16.

CLARK, W. W., and B. A. BOHNE. 1986. "Cochlear damage: Audiometric correlates?" In *Sensorineural hearing loss: Mechanisms, Diagnosis and Treatment.* Ed. T. Glattke, M. J. Collins, and L. Harker. Iowa City: Iowa University Press.

COHEN, A. B. 1968. *Hi-Fi Loudspeakers and Enclosures*, 2nd ed. New York: Hayden.

COLLINS, M. J. 1985. "Low frequency hearing loss and the frequency response of amplification." Paper presented at a Conference on Hearing Aid Fitting at Washington University School of Medicine, St. Louis, Mo.

CORLISS, E.L.R. 1971. *Facts About Hearing and Hearing Aids.* A consumer guide from the National Bureau of Standards, Washington: U.S. Government Printing Office.

COX, R.M. 1979. "Acoustic aspects of hearing aid/ear canal coupling systems." *Monographs in Contemporary Audiology* 1:1—44.

———. 1981a. "Combined effects of earmold vents and suboscillatory feedback on hearing aid frequency response." *Ear and Hearing* 3:12—17.

———. 1981b. "Using LDLs to establish hearing aid limiting levels." *Hearing Instruments* 32(5): 16, 18, 20.

———. 1983. "Using ULCL measures to find frequency/gain and SSPL 90." *Hearing Instruments* 34(7):17—21, 39.

———. 1985. "Hearing aids and aural rehabilitation: A structured approach to hearing aid selection." *Ear and Hearing* 6:226—39.

COX, R. M., and J. D. BISSET. 1982. "Prediction of aided preferred listening levels for hearing aid gain prescription." *Ear and Hearing* 3:66—71.

COX, R. M., and C. GILMORE. 1986. "Damping the hearing aid frequency response: effects on speech clarity and preferred listening level." *Journal of Speech and Hearing Research* 29:357—65.

COX, R. M., and D. M. MCDANIEL. 1984. "Intelligiblity ratings of continuous discourse: Application to hearing aid selection." *Journal of the Acoustical Society of America* 76:758—66.

COX, R. M., and D. M. RISBERG. 1986. "Comparison of in-the-ear and over-the-ear hearing aid fittings." *Journal of Speech and Hearing Disorders* 51:362—369.

COX, R. M., and G. A. STUDEBAKER. 1980. "Problems in the recording and reproduction of hearing aid-processed signals." In *Acoustical Factors Affecting Hearing Aid Performance.* Ed. G. A. Studebaker and I. Hochberg. Baltimore: University Park Press.

DAVIS, H., and S. R. SILVERMAN. 1978. *Hearing and Deafness.* 4th ed. New York: Holt, Rinehart, and Winston.

DAVIS, H., C. V. HUDGINS, R. J. MARQUIS, R. H. NICHOLS, G. D. PETERSON, D. A. ROSS, and S. S. STEVENS. 1946. "The selection of hearing aids." *Laryngoscope* 56:85—115, 135—63.

DAVIS, J. M., and E. J. HARDICK. 1981. *Rehabilitative Audiology for Children and Adults.* New York: Wiley.

DAWSON, J. K. 1981. "A comparison of physical measurements of pure-tones, third-octave bands of noise and third-octave bands of speech to subjective judgments of audibility threshold, MCL and UCL for three normally hearing listeners." Unpublished independent study. St. Louis, Mo.: Central Institute for the Deaf.

DE VOS, A. W. 1968. "The fitting of hearing aids for babies." *Internat'l Audiology* 7:136—41.

DEMOREST, M. E., and S. A. ERDMAN. 1984. "Applications of self-assessment inventories." *Hearing Instruments* 35(11):32, 36, 38, 40.

———. 1986a. "A database management system for the Communication Profile for the Hearing Impaired." *Journal of the Academy of Rehabilitative Audiology*, in press.

———. 1986b. "Scale composition and item analysis of the communication profile for the hearing impaired." *Journal of Speech and Hearing Research* 29:515—35.

———. 1987. "Development of the communication profile for the hearing impaired." *Journal of Speech and Hearing Disorders* 52: (in press).

DEMOREST, M. E., and B. E. WALDEN. 1984. "Psychometric principles in the selection, interpretation, and evaluation of communication self-assessment inventories." *Journal of Speech and Hearing Disorders* 49:226—40.

DENENBERG, L. J., and M. W. ALTSHULER. 1976. "The clinical relationship between acoustic reflexes and loudness perception." *Journal of the American Auditory Society* 2:79—82.

DILLON, H. 1982. Personal communication.

DILLON, H., and G. WALKER. 1981. "The effect of acoustic environment on the reliability of sound field audiometry." *Australian Journal of Audiology* 3:67—72.

————. 1982a. "Comparison of stimuli used in sound field audiometric testing." *Journal of the Acoustical Society of America* 71:161–72.

————. 1982b. "The selection of modulation waveform for frequency modulated sound field stimuli. *Australian Journal of Audiology* 4(2):56–61.

DIRKS, D., and C. KAMM. 1976. "Psychometric functions for loudness discomfort and most comfortable loudness levels." *Journal of Speech and Hearing Research* 19:613–27.

DIRKS, D. D., D. E. MORGAN, and R. H. WILSON. 1976. "Experimental audiology." In *Handbook of Auditory and Vestibular Research Methods*. Ed. C. A. Smith and J. A. Vernon. Springfield, Ill.: Charles C. Thomas.

DIRKS, D. D., R. W. STREAM, and R. H. WILSON. 1972. "Speech audiometry: Earphones and sound field." *Journal of Speech and Hearing Disorders* 37:162–76.

DUGAL, R. L., L. D. BRAIDA, and N. I. DURLACH. 1980. "Implications of previous research for the selection of frequency-gain characteristics." In *Acoustical Factors Affecting Hearing Aid Performance*. Ed. G. A. Studebaker and I. Hochberg. Baltimore: University Park Press.

ELKINS, E., G. D. CAUSEY, L. D. BECK, D. BREWER, and J. B. DE MOLL. 1975. "Normal and impaired listener performance on the University of Maryland revised CID sentence lists." Unpublished report, University of Maryland.

ENGEBRETSON, A. M., R. E. MORLEY, and G. R. POPELKA. 1987. "Development of an ear-level digital hearing aid and computer assisted fitting procedure." *Journal of Rehabilitative Research and Development* (in press).

ERBER, N. P. 1968. "Variables that influence sound pressure generated in the earcanal by an audiometric earphone." *Journal of the Acoustical Society of America* 44:555–62.

EWERTSEN, H. W., and H. BIRK-NIELSEN. 1973. "Social Hearing Handicap Index: Social handicap in relation to hearing impairment." *Audiology* 12:180–87.

FDA. *See* Food and Drug Administration.

FEATHERSTONE, H. 1978. *A Difference in the Family*. New York: Basic Books.

FERRIS, C. 1980. *A Hug Just Isn't Enough*. Washington: Gallaudet.

FIFIELD, L. B. 1979. "Instructions for three stage ear impression technique using Reprosil materials." Unpublished report. Australia: National Acoustic Laboratories (Address: 5 Hickson Road, Millers Point, N.S.W., 2000).

FLETCHER, H. 1952. "The perception of speech sounds by deafened persons." *Journal of the Acoustical Society of America* 24:490–97.

FLETCHER, H. and R. H. GALT. 1950. "The perception of speech and its relation to telephony." *Journal of the Acoustical Society of America* 22:89–151.

Food and Drug Administration. 1977. "Hearing aid devices: Professional and patient labeling and conditions for sale." *Federal Register* 42 (Feb. 15):9286–96.

FREEMAN, R. D. 1981. *Can't your child hear?* Baltimore: University Park Press.

FRENCH, N.R. and J.C. STEINBERG. 1947. "Factors governing the intelligiblity of speech sounds." *Journal of the Acoustical Society of America* 19:90–119.

GABRIELSSON, A., and H. SJÖGREN. 1979. "Perceived sound quality of sound-reproducing systems." *Journal of the Acoustical Society of America* 65:1019–33.

Gallaudet College Public Service Programs. *Parent Package*. Washington: Gallaudet College.

GIOLAS, T. G., E. OWENS, S. H. LAMB, and E. D. SCHUBERT. 1979. "Hearing performance inventory." *Journal of Speech and Hearing Disorders* 44:169–95.

GLICK, F. P. 1982. *Breaking Silence*. Scottsdale, Pa.: Herald Press.

GREGORY, S. 1976. *The Deaf Child and His Family*. New York: Wiley.

GRIFFIN, B. F. 1980. *Family to Family*. Washington: A. G. Bell.

HAKANSSON, B., A. TJELLSTROM, and U. ROSENHALL. 1984. "Hearing thresholds with direct bone conduction versus conventional bone conduction." *Scandinavian Audiology* 13:3–13.

HAKANSSON, B., A. TJELLSTROM, U. ROSENHALL, and P. CARLSSON. 1985. "The bone-anchored hearing aid: Principal design and a psychoacoustical evaluation." *Acta Otolaryngologica* (Stockholm) 100:229–39.

HALL, J. W., and E. L. DERLACKI. 1986. "The effect of conductive hearing loss and middle ear surgery on binaural hearing." *Annals of Otology, Rhinology and Laryngology* 95:525–30.

HARFORD, E. R. 1980. "The use of a miniature microphone in the ear canal for the verification of hearing aid performance." *Ear and Hearing* 1:329–37.

————. 1981. "A new clinical technique for verification of hearing aid response." *Archives of Otolaryngology* 107:461–68.

HARRIS, G. A. 1983. *Broken Ears, Wounded Hearts*. Washington: Gallaudet.

HAWKINS, D. 1980a. "Loudness discomfort levels: A clinical procedure for hearing aid evaluations." *Journal of Speech and Hearing Disorders* 45:3–15.

————. 1980b. "The effect of signal type on the loudness discomfort level. *Ear and Hearing* 1:38−41.

————. 1983. *Hearing Aid Evaluation and Rehabilitation Strategies.* Unpublished paper.

————. 1985. "Reflections on amplification: Validation of performance." *Journal of the Academy of Rehabilitative Audiology* 18:42−54.

————. 1986. "Selection of hearing aid characteristics." In *Hearing Aid Assessment and Use in Audiologic Habilitation*, 3rd ed. Ed. W. R. Hodgson. Baltimore: Williams and Wilkins, 128−51.

HAWKINS, D. B., and H. G. MUELLER. 1986. 'Some variables affecting the accuracy of probe tube microphone measurements." *Hearing Instruments* 37(1):8−12, 49.

HEINER, M. H. 1949. *Hearing Is Believing.* New York: World.

HELLENBERG, M. M. 1979. *Your Hearing Loss: How to Break the Sound Barrier.* Chicago: Nelson-Hall.

HIGH, W., G. FAIRBANKS, and A. GLORIG. 1964. "Scale for self-assessment of hearing handicap (forms A and B)." *Journal of Speech and Hearing Disorders* 29:215−30.

HODGSON, W. R. 1981a. "Learning hearing aid use." In *Hearing Aid Assessment and Use in Audiologic Habilitation*, 2nd ed. Ed. W. R. Hodgson and P. H. Skinner. Baltimore: Williams and Wilkins.

————. 1986. *Hearing Aid Assessment and Use in Audiologic Habilitation*, 3rd ed. Baltimore: Williams and Wilkins.

————. 1986b. "Special cases of hearing aid assessment." In *Hearing Aid Assessment and Use in Audiologic Habilitation*, 3rd ed. Ed. W. R. Hodgson. Baltimore: Williams and Wilkins.

HODGSON, W. R., and P. H. SKINNER. 1981. *Hearing Aid Assessment and Use in Audiologic Habilitation*, 2nd ed. Baltimore: Williams and Wilkins.

HOUGH, J., J. VERNON, K. DORMER, B. JOHNSON, T. HIMELICK. 1986. "Our experiences with implantable hearing devices and a presentation of a new device." *Annals of Otology, Rhinology and Laryngology.* 95:60−65.

HULL, R. W. 1982. "1975 Unpublished scale (Greeley: University of Northern Colorado)." In *Rehabilitative Audiology.* Ed. R. W. Hull. New York: Grune & Stratton.

HUTTON, C. L. 1980. "Responses to a hearing problem inventory." *Journal of the Academy of Rehabilitative Audiology* 13:133−54.

Illinois Annual School for Mothers of Deaf Children. 1965. *If You Have a Deaf Child.* Champaign, Ill.: University of Illinois.

International Organization for Standardization. 1961. Normal equal-loudness contours for pure tones and normal threshold of hearing under free-field listening conditions (R226-1961). New York: American National Standards Institute.

ISO. *See* International Organization for Standardization.

James B. Lansing Sound, Inc. 1985. Brochure describing JBL loudspeakers. Available from 8500 Balboa Boulevard, Northridge, CA 91329.

JERGER, J., and D. HAYES. "Hearing aid evaluation: Clinical experience with a new philosophy." *Archives of Otolaryngology* 102:214−21.

JERGER, J., and S. JERGER. 1967. "Psychoacoustic comparison of cochlear and VIII N disorders." *Journal of Speech and Hearing Research* 10:659−88.

KALIKOW, D. N., K. N. STEVENS, and L. L. ELLIOTT. 1977. "Speech Perception in Noise Test (SPIN)." *Journal of the Acoustical Society of America* 61:1337−51.

KAMM, C., D. DIRKS, and T. S. BELL. 1985. "Speech recognition and the Articulation Index for normal and hearing-impaired listeners." *Journal of the Acoustical Society of America* 77: 281−88.

KAMM, C., D. DIRKS, and R. MICKEY. 1978. "Effect of sensorineural hearing loss on loudness discomfort level." *Journal of Speech and Hearing Research* 21:668−81.

KAPLAN, H. F. 1982. Facilitating adjustment." In *Rehabilitative Audiology.* Ed. R. W. Hull. New York: Grune & Stratton.

KAPLAN, H., J. FEELEY, and J. BROWN. 1978. "A modified Denver scale: Test-retest reliability." *Journal of the Academy of Rehabilitative Audiology* 11:115−32.

KASTEN, R. N., and J. R. FRANKS. 1986. "Electroacoustic characteristics of hearing aids." In *Hearing Aid Assessment and Use in Audiologic Habilitation*, 3rd ed. Ed. W. R. Hodgson. Baltimore: Williams and Wilkins.

KATZ, J. 1978. *Handbook of Clinical Audiology*, 2nd ed. Baltimore: Williams and Wilkins.

KATZ, J., and T. P. WHITE. 1982. "Auditory impairment versus hearing handicap." In *Rehabilitative Audiology.* Ed. R. H. Hull. New York: Grune & Stratton.

KILLION, M. C. 1978. "Revised estimate of minimum audible pressure: Where is the 'missing 6 dB'?" *Journal of the Acoustical Society of America* 63:1501−8.

———. 1981. "Earmold options for wideband hearing aids. *Journal of Speech and Hearing Disorders* 46:10−20.

———. 1982. "A step-response microphone." I.R.P.I. Report no. 10539−1. Knowles Electronics: Franklin Park, Ill.

———. 1984. "Recent earmolds for wideband OTE and ITE hearing aids." *Hearing Journal* 37(8):15−18, 20−22.

———. 1985. Personal communication.

———. 1986. Personal communication.

KILLION, M. C., C. I. BERLIN, and L. HOOD. 1984. "A low-frequency emphasis open canal hearing aid." *Hearing Instruments* 35(8):30, 32, 34, 66.

KILLION, M. C., and E. L. MONSER. 1980. "Corfig: Coupler response for flat insertion gain." In *Acoustical Factors Affecting Hearing Aid Performance*. Ed. G. A. Studebaker and I. Hochberg. Baltimore: University Park Press.

KILLION, M. C., and G. A. STUDEBAKER. 1978. "A-weighted equivalents of permissible ambient noise during audiometric testing." *Journal of the Acoustical Society of America* 63:1633−35.

KILLION, M. C., L. A. WILBER, and G. I. GUDMUNDSEN. 1985. Insert earphones for more interaural attenuation. *Hearing Instruments* 36(2):34−36.

KIM, D. O. 1984. "Functional roles of the inner- and outer-hair-cell subsystems in the cochlea and brainstem." In *Hearing Science*. Ed. C. Berlin. San Diego: College-Hill Press, 241−62.

KONKLE, D. F., and T. H. TOWNSEND. 1983. "Calibration measurements for speech audiometers." In *Principles of Speech Audiometry*. Ed. D. F. Konkle and W. F. Rintlemann. Baltimore: University Park Press.

KRYTER, K. D. 1962. "Methods for the calculation and use of the articulation index." *Journal of the Acoustical Society of America* 34:1689−97.

KUHN, G. F. 1979. "The pressure transformation from a diffuse sound field to the external ear and to the body and head surface." *Journal of the Acoustical Society of America* 65:991−1000.

KUHN, G. F., and R. M. GUERNSEY. 1983. "Sound pressure distribution about the human head and torso." *Journal of the Acoustical Society of America* 73:95−105.

KWIECINSKI, B. G. 1983. "A study of threshold and loudness summation in normal-hearing listeners." Unpublished independent study. St. Louis: Central Institute for the Deaf.

LAMORE, G. S. 1985. *Now I Understand*. Washington: Gallaudet.

LAMB, S. H., E. OWENS, and E. D. SCHUBERT. 1983. "The revised form of the Hearing Performance Inventory." *Ear and Hearing* 4:169−95.

LEAVITT, R. 1981. "Earmolds: Acoustic and structural considerations." In *Hearing Aid Assessment and Use in Audiologic Habilitation*, 2nd ed. Ed. W. R. Hodgson and P. H. Skinner. Baltimore: Williams and Wilkins.

LEEDS, S. J. 1983. "Predicting auditory dynamic range from threshold measurements." Unpublished independent study. St. Louis: Central Institute for the Deaf.

LEIJON, A. 1983. Personal communication.

LEIJON, A., M. ERIKSSON-MANGOLD, and A. BECH-KARLSEN. 1984. "Preferred hearing aid gain and bass-cut in relation to prescriptive fitting." *Scandinavian Audiology* 13:157−61.

LERMAN, S. R. F. 1980. *Parent Awareness Training: Positive Parenting for the 80's*. New York: A&W Publishers.

LEVITT, H. 1978. "Adaptive testing in audiology." In *Sensorineural Hearing Impairment and Hearing Aids*. Ed. C. Ludvigsen and J. Barfod. *Scandinavian Audiology*, suppl. 6:241−89.

LEVITT, H., M. J. COLLINS, J.R. DUBNO, S. B. RESNICK, R. E. C. WHITE. 1978. *Development of a Protocol for the Prescriptive Fitting of a Wearable Master Hearing Aid*. CSL Research Report No. 11, City University of New York, N.Y.

LIBBY, E. R. 1985a. "State-of-the-art of hearing aid selection procedures." *Hearing Instruments* 36(1):30, 34, 36, 38, 62.

———. 1985b. "The LDL to SSPL90 conversion dilemma." *Hearing Instruments* 36(8):15−16, 68.

———. 1986. "The 1/3-2/3 insertion gain hearing aid selection guide." *Hearing Instruments* 37(3):27−28.

LIBBY, E. R., J. H. JOHNSON, and T. F. LONGWELL. 1981. *Innovative Earmold Coupling Systems: Rationale, Design, Clinical Applications*." Chicago: Zenetron.

LIPPMANN, R. P., L. D. BRAIDA, and N. I. DURLACH. 1981. "Study of multichannel amplitude compression and linear amplification for persons with sensorineural hearing loss." *Journal of the Acoustical Society of America* 69:524–34.

LITCHFIELD, A. 1976. *A Button in Her Ear*. Chicago: Albert Whitman.

LOAVENBRUCK, A. M., and J. R. MADELL. 1981. *Hearing Aid Dispensing for Audiologists*. New York: Grune & Stratton.

LUTERMAN, D. 1976. "The counseling experience." *Journal of the Academy of Rehabilitative Audiology* 9:62–66.

———. 1979. *Counseling Parents of Hearing-Impaired Children*. Boston: Little, Brown.

———. 1984. *Counseling the Communicatively Disordered and Their Families*. Boston: Little, Brown.

LYBARGER, S. F. 1944. U.S. Patent application SN 543,278.

———. 1955. *Basic Manual for Fitting Radioear Hearing Aids*. Pittsburgh: Radioear Corp.

———. 1963. *Simplified Fitting System for Hearing Aids*. Canonsburg, Pa.: Radioear Corporation.

———. 1978a. "Earmolds." In *Handbook of Clinical Audiology*, 2nd ed. Ed. J. Katz. Baltimore: Williams and Wilkins.

———. 1978b. "Selective amplification: A review and evaluation." *Journal of the American Audiological Society* 3:258–66.

———. 1979a. "Controlling hearing aid performance by earmold design." In *Auditory and Hearing Prosthetics Research*. Ed. V. D. Larson, D. P. Egolf, R. L. Kirlin, and S. W. Stile. New York: Grune & Stratton.

———. 1982. "Telephone coupling." In *The Vanderbilt Hearing-Aid Report*. Ed. G. A. Studebaker and F. H. Bess., Upper Darby, Pa.: Monographs in Contemporary Audiology, 91–93.

———. 1983. Unpublished results. In Kuhn, G. F. and R. M. Guernsey. 1983. "Sound pressure distribution about the human head and torso." *Journal of the Acoustical Society of America* 73:95–105.

———. 1985a. "Earmolds." In *Handbook of clinical audiology*, 3rd ed. Ed. J. Katz. Baltimore: Williams and Wilkins, 885–910.

———. 1985b. "The physical and electroacoustic characteristics of hearing aids." In *Handbook of clinical audiology*, 3rd ed. Ed. J. Katz. Baltimore: Williams and Wilkins, 849–884.

MCARTHUR, S. H. 1982. *Raising Your Hearing-Impaired Child: A Guideline for Parents*. Washington: A. G. Bell.

MCCANDLESS, G. A., and P. E. LYREGAARD. 1983. "Prescription of gain/output (POGO) for hearing aids." *Hearing Instruments* 34(1):16–17, 19–21.

MCCANDLESS, G. A., and D. L. MILLER. 1972. "Loudness discomfort and hearing aids." *Hearing Aid Journal* 25:7, 28, 32.

MCCARTHY, P. A., and J. G. ALPINER. 1982. "Remediation process." In *Handbook of Adult Rehabilitative Audiology*, 2nd ed. Ed. J. G. Alpiner. Baltimore: Williams and Wilkins.

———. 1983. "An assessment scale of hearing handicap for use in family counseling." *Journal of the Academy of Rehabilitative Audiology* 16:256–70.

MCLEOD, H. L., and H. J. GREENBERG. 1977. "Relationship between loudness discomfort level and acoustic reflex threshold for normal and sensorineural hearing-impaired individuals." Paper presented at the Annual Convention of the American Speech and Hearing Association, Chicago.

MACRAE, J. 1982. "Acoustical notch filters for hearing aids." *Australian Journal of Audiology* 4:71–76.

———. 1983. "Vents for high-powered hearing aids." *Hearing Journal* 36:13–16.

MADORY, R. D. 1978. "The test-retest reliability of the synthetic sentence identification hearing aid evaluation procedure." Master's thesis. Mount Pleasant: Central Michigan University.

MAHON, W. J. 1985. "1985 U.S. hearing aid sales summary." *The Hearing Journal* 38(12):7–12.

MANTEVANI, M., D. P. PASCOE, and M. W. SKINNER. 1978. "Thresholds of audibility and discomfort, and most-comfortable loudness level of third-octave bands of noise presented in the field." In Central Institute for the Deaf Periodic Progress Report No. 21, St. Louis, Mo.

MANZELLA, D. S., and M. TAIGMAN. 1980. "A hearing screen test for the elderly." *Journal of the Academy of Rehabilitative Audiology* 13:21–28.

MARKLE, D. M., and A. ZANER. 1966. "The determination of gain requirements of hearing aids: A new method." *Journal of Auditory Research* 6:371–78.

MARTIN, M. C., B. C. GROVER, J. J. WORRALL, and V. WILLIAMS. 1976. "The effectiveness of hearing aids in a school population." *British Journal of Audiology* 10:33–40.

MASON, D., and G. R. POPELKA. 1986. "Hearing aid gain with coupler, functional and probe tube measurements." *Journal of Speech and Hearing Research* 29:218–26.

MATSUMOTO, J. 1983. "A study of threshold and loudness summation in listeners with sensorineural hearing impairments." Unpublished independent study. St. Louis: Central Institute for the Deaf.

MEADOW, K. P. 1980. *Deafness and Child Development.* Berkeley: University of California Press.

MELNICK, W. 1979. "Instrument calibration." In *Hearing Assessment.* Ed. W. F. Rintelmann. Baltimore: University Park Press.

MOREST, D. K., and B. A. BOHNE. 1983. "Noise-induced degeneration in the brain and representation of inner and outer hair cells." *Hearing Research* 9:145–51.

MORGAN, D., and D. DIRKS. 1974. "Loudness discomfort level under earphone and in the free field: The effects of calibration methods." *Journal of the Acoustical Society of America* 56:172–78.

MORGAN, D., D. DIRKS, D. BOWER, and C. KAMM. 1979. "Loudness discomfort level and acoustic reflex threshold for speech stimuli." *Journal of Speech and Hearing Research* 22:849–61.

MUELLER, H. G., D. M. SCHWARTZ, and R. K. SURR. 1981. "The use of exponential acoustic horn in an open mold configuration." *Hearing Instruments* 32(10):16–17, 67.

MURPHY, A. T. 1979. *The Families of Hearing-Impaired Children.* Washington: Gallaudet.

NABELEK, A. K. 1982. "Temporal distortions and noise considerations." In *The Vanderbilt Hearing-Aid Report.* Ed. G. A. Studebaker and F. H. Bess. Upper Darby, Pa.: Monographs in Contemporary Audiology, 51–59.

NABELEK, A. K., and P. K. ROBINSON. 1982. "Monaural and binaural speech perception through hearing aids under noise and reverberation with normal and hearing-impaired listeners." *Journal of the Acoustical Society of America* 71:1242–48.

NIEMOELLER, A. F. 1981. "Physical concepts of speech communication in classrooms for the deaf." In *Amplification in Education.* Ed. F. H. Bess, B. A. Freeman, and J. J. Sinclair. Washington: A. G. Bell, 164–179.

NOBLE, W. G., and G. R. C. ATHERLEY. 1970. "The hearing measurement scale: A questionnaire for assessment of auditory disability." *Journal of Auditory Research* 10:229–50.

NORDLUND, B. 1964. "Directional audiometry." *Acta Otolaryngologica* (Stockholm) 57:1–18.

OGDEN, P. W., and S. LIPSETT. 1982. *The Silent Garden.* New York: St. Martin's Press.

OLSEN, W. O., D. NOFFSINGER, and S. KURDZIEL. 1975. "Speech discrimination in quiet and noise by patients with peripheral and central lesions." *Acta Otolaryngologica* (Stockholm) 80: 375–82.

OLSON, A. E., and N. M. HIPSKIND. 1973. "The relation between levels of pure tones and speech which elicit the acoustic reflex and loudness discomfort." *Journal of Auditory Research* 13:71–76.

OWENS, E., and M. RAGGIO. 1987. "Hearing performance inventory for profound and severe loss (PIPSL)." *Journal of Speech and Hearing Disorders* (in press).

OWENS, E. and E. D. SCHUBERT. 1977. "Development of the California Consonant Test." *Journal of Speech and Hearing Research* 20:463–74.

PASCOE, D. P. 1975. "Frequency responses of hearing aids and their effects on the speech perception of hearing-impaired subjects." *Annals of Otology, Rhinology and Laryngology* 84 Supp. 23:1–40.

———. 1978. "An approach to hearing aid selection." *Hearing Instruments* 29(6):12–16, 36.

———. 1980. "Clinical implications of nonverbal method of hearing aid selection and fitting." *Seminars in Speech, Language and Hearing,* 1(3): 217–29.

———. 1985. "Improving the fit of hearing aids." Paper presented at a Conference on Hearing Aid Fitting. St. Louis: Washington University School of Medicine.

———. 1986. "Hearing aid selection procedure used at Central Institute for the Deaf in St. Louis." *Audiological Acoustics* 25(3):90–106.

PASCOE, D. P., J. D. MILLER, M. W. SKINNER, D. ALBEE, D. FREIERT, and Z. HACK. 1980. "Evaluation of the Pascoe Hearing-Aid Selection Procedure." *Central Institute for the Deaf Periodic Progress Report No. 23,* 51.

PAVLOVIC, C. V., G. A. STUDEBAKER, and R. L. SHERBECOE. 1985. "An articulation index based procedure for predicting the speech recognition performance of hearing-impaired individuals." *Journal of the Acoustical Society of America* 80:50–57.

PEARSONS, K. S., R. L. BENNETT, and S. FIDELL. 1976. "Speech levels in various environments." *Bolt Beranek and Newman Report No. 321.* Canoga Park, CA.

PETERSON, J. W. 1977. *I Have a Sister, My Sister Is Deaf.* New York: Harper & Row.
PHONIC EAR, INC. 1984. Descriptive literature on FM communication system. Available from 250 Camino Alto, Mill Valley, CA 94941.
POLLACK, I. 1952. "Comfortable listening levels for pure tones in quiet and noise." *Journal of the Acoustical Society of America* 24:158−62.
POLLACK, M. C. 1980. "Electroacoustic characteristics." In *Amplification for the Hearing-Impaired,* 2nd ed. Ed. M. C. Pollack. New York: Grune & Stratton.
POPELKA, G. R. 1982. *Users Guide for Phase IV; Hearing Aid Evaluation Program (Version 1.1).* St. Louis: Central Institute for the Deaf Press. (Versions for Hewlett Packard, Apple, and IBM microcomputers may be obtained from CID, 818 S. Euclid Ave., St. Louis, MO 63110.)
————. 1983. "Computer assisted hearing aid fitting." Paper presented at the Annual Convention of the American Speech-Language-Hearing Association, Cincinnati.
PUNCH, J. L., and E. L. BECK. 1980. "Low-frequency response of hearing aids and judgments of aided speech quality." *Journal of Speech and Hearing Disorders* 45:325−35.
PUNCH, J. L., and L. B. BECK. 1986. "Relative effects of low-frequency amplification on syllable recognition and speech quality." *Ear and Hearing* 7:57−62.
RAFFIN, M. J. M., and A. R. THORNTON. 1980. "Confidence levels for differences between speech-discrimination scores: A research note." *Journal of Speech and Hearing Research* 23:5−18.
RESNICK, S. B., J. R. DUBNO, S. HOFFNUNG, and H. LEVITT. 1975. "Phoneme errors on a nonsense syllable test." *Journal of the Acoustical Society of America* 58:114.
REZEN, S. V., and C. HAUSMAN. 1985. *Coping with Hearing Loss: A Guide for Adults and Their Families.* New York: Dembner.
ROGERS, C. 1951. *Client Centered Counseling.* Boston: Houghton Mifflin.
————. 1961. *On Becoming a Person.* Boston: Houghton Mifflin.
RUPP, R. R., J. HIGGINS, and J. F. MAURER. 1977. "A feasibility scale for predicting hearing aid use (FSPHAU) with older individuals." *Journal of the Academy of Rehabilitative Audiology* 10:81−104.
SACHS, R. M., and M. D. BURKHARD. 1972. "Earphone pressure response in ears and couplers." Project 20021 for Knowles Electronics, Franklin Park, Ill. Reprinted in *Sensory Aids for the Hearing Impaired.* Ed. H. Levitt, J. M. Pickett, R. A. Houde. New York: IEEE Press, 1980, 130−34.
SANDERS, D. A. 1975. "Hearing aid orientation and counseling." In *Amplification for the Hearing Impaired.* Ed. M. C. Pollack. New York: Grune & Stratton.
SCHARF, B., and M. FLORENTINE. 1982. "Psychoacoustics of elementary sounds." In *The Vanderbilt Hearing-Aid Report.* Ed. G. A. Studebaker and F. H. Bess. Upper Darby, Pa.: Monographs in Contemporary Audiology, 3−15.
SCHARF, B., and R. HELLMAN. 1966. "Model of loudness summation." *Journal of the Acoustical Society of America* 40:71−78.
SCHEIN, J. D. 1985. "Implications of a new generation of hearing aids for consumers." Paper presented at the 10th annual Lexington Hearing Aid Conference, Lexington Hearing and Speech Center, Inc., Jackson Heights, N.Y.
SCHMITZ, H. 1969. "Loudness discomfort level modification." *Journal of Speech and Hearing Research* 12:807−17.
SCHOW, R. L., and M. A. NERBONNE. 1977. "Assessment of hearing handicap by nursing home residents and staff." *Journal of the Academy of Rehabilitative Audiology* 10:2−12.
SCHUKNECHT, H. F. 1974. *Pathology of the Ear.* Cambridge, Ma.: Harvard University Press.
SCHWARTZ, D. M., and B. E. WALDEN. 1980. "Current status of the clinical hearing aid evaluation." In Studies in the use of amplification for the hearing impaired: Proceedings of a symposium. *Excerpta Medica,* 15−28.
————. 1983. "Speech audiometry and hearing aid assessment: A reappraisal of an old philosophy." In *Principles of Speech Audiometry.* Ed. D. F. Konkle and W. F. Rintlemann. Baltimore: University Park Press.
SCHWEITZER, H. C. 1986. "Time: The third dimension of hearing aid performance." *Hearing Instruments* 37(1):17−22.
SCOTT, V. M. 1985. *Belonging.* Washington: Gallaudet.
SEEWALD, R. C., M. ROSS, and M. K. SPIRO. 1985. Selecting amplification charactertistics for young hearing-impaired children." *Ear and Hearing* 6:48−53.

SHAPIRO, I. 1976. "Hearing aid fitting by prescription." *Audiology* 15:163–73.

————. 1979. "Evaluation of relationship between hearing threshold and loudness discomfort level in sensorineural hearing loss." *Journal of Speech and Hearing Disorders* 44:31–36.

SHAW, E. A. G. 1966a. "Earcanal pressure generated by a free sound field." *Journal of the Acoustical Society of America* 39:465–70.

————. 1966b. "Earcanal pressure generated by circumaural and supra-aural earphones." *Journal of the Acoustical Society of America* 39:471–79.

————. 1974a. "Transformation of sound pressure level from the free field to the eardrum in the horizontal plane." *Journal of the Acoustical Society of America* 56:1848–61.

————. 1974b. "The external ear." In *Handbook of Sensory Physiology*, vol. 5(1). Ed. W. D. Keidel and W. E. Neff. Berlin: Springer-Verlag.

————. 1976. "Diffuse field sensitivity of external ear based on reciprocity principles." *Journal of the Acoustical Society of America* 60:S102(A).

SHHH Journal, published by Self-Help for Hard of Hearing People, 4848 Battery Lane, Suite 100, Bethesda, MD. 20814

SILVERMAN, S. R. 1947. "Tolerance for pure tones and speech in normal and defective hearing." *Annals of Otology, Rhinology and Laryngology* 56:658–76.

SKINNER, M. W. 1978. "Hearing of speech during language acquisition." *Otolaryngologic Clinics of North America* 11:631–50.

————. 1979. "Audibility and intelligibility of speech for listeners with sensorineural hearing loss." In *Rehabilitation Strategies for Sensorineural Hearing Loss*. Ed. P. Yanick. New York: Grune & Stratton.

————. 1980. "Speech intelligibility in noise-induced hearing loss: Effects of high-frequency compensation." *Journal of the Acoustical Society of America* 67:306–17.

————. 1984. "Recent advances in hearing aid selection and adjustment." *Annals of Otology, Rhinology and Laryngology*. 93:569–75.

SKINNER, M. W., M. M. KARSTAEDT, and J. D. MILLER. 1982. "Amplification bandwidth and speech intelligibility for two listeners with sensorineural hearing loss." *Audiology* 21: 251–68.

SKINNER, M. W., and J. D. MILLER. 1983. "Amplification bandwidth and intelligibility of speech in quiet and noise for listeners with sensorineural hearing loss. *Audiology* 22:253–79.

SKINNER, M. W., J. D. MILLER, C. L. DEFILIPPO, J. K. DAWSON, and G. R. POPELKA. 1986. "Word identification by listeners with sensorineural hearing loss using four amplification systems." In *Sensorineural Hearing Loss: Mechanisms, Diagnosis, and Treatment*. Ed. T. J. Glattke, M. J. Collins, and L. A. Harker. Iowa City: University of Iowa Press.

SKINNER, M. W., D. P. PASCOE, J. D. MILLER, and G. R. POPELKA. 1982. "Measurements to determine the optimal placement of speech energy within the listener's auditory area: A basis for selecting amplification characteristics." In *The Vanderbilt Hearing-Aid Report*. Ed. G. A. Studebaker and F. H. Bess. Upper Darby, Pa.: Monographs in Contemporary Audiology, 161–169.

SPRADLEY, T. S., and J. P. SPRADLEY. 1985. *Deaf Like Me*. Washington: Gallaudet.

STELMACHOWICZ, P. G., L.L. LARSON, D. E. JOHNSON, and M. P. MOELLER. "Clinical model for the audiological management of hearing-impaired children." *Seminars in Hearing* 6(3): 223–37.

STEPHENS, S. D. G., B. BLEGVAD, and H. J. KROGH. 1977. "The value of some suprathreshold auditory measures." *Scandinavian Audiology* 6:213–21.

STREAM, R. W., and D. D. DIRKS. 1974. "Effects of loudspeaker position on the difference between earphone and free-field thresholds (MAP and MAF)." *Journal of Speech and Hearing Research* 17:549–68.

STUDEBAKER, G. A. 1982. "Hearing aid selection: An overview." In *The Vanderbilt Hearing-Aid Report*. Ed. G. A. Studebaker and F. H. Bess. Upper Darby, Pa.: Monographs in Contemporary Audiology, 147–55.

STUDEBAKER, G. A., R. M. COX, and C. FORMBY. 1980. "The effect of environment on the directional performance of head-worn hearing aids." In *Acoustical Factors Affecting Hearing Aid Performance*. Ed. G. A. Studebaker and I. Hochberg. Baltimore: University Park Press.

SULLIVAN, J. A., A. C. NEUMAN, and H. LEVITT. 1983. "Adaptive estimation of frequency-gain characteristics for binaural hearing aids. "Paper presented at the Annual Convention of the American Speech-Language-Hearing Association, Cincinnati.

SULLIVAN, R. F. 1985. "An acoustic coupling-based classification system for hearing aid fittings." Parts 2 & 3. *Hearing Instruments* 36(12):16, 18−22.

TECCA, J. E., and C. A. BINNIE. 1982. "The application of an adaptive procedure to the California Consonant Test for hearing aid selection. *Ear and Hearing* 3:72−76.

THORNTON, A. R., and M. J. M. RAFFIN. 1978. "Speech-discrimination scores modeled as a binomial variable." *Journal of Speech and Hearing Research* 21:507−18.

TOWNSEND, T. H. 1982. "Revised estimates of hearing aid test system accuracy." *Journal of Speech and Hearing Research* 25:166−70.

TRACOUSTICS. 1982. Brochures on audiometric sound booths and clinical audiometers.

TYLER, R. S., Q. SUMMERFIELD, E. J. WOOD, and M. A. FERNANDES. 1982. "Psychoacoustic and phonetic temporal processing in normal and hearing-impaired listeners." *Journal of the Acoustical Society of America* 72:740−52.

VENTRY, I. M., and J. I. JOHNSON. 1978. "Evaluation of a clinical method for measuring comfortable loudness of speech." *Journal of Speech and Hearing Disorders* 43:149−59.

VENTRY, I. M., and B. E. WEINSTEIN. 1982. "The hearing handicap inventory for the elderly: A new tool." *Ear and Hearing* 3:128−34.

VENTRY, I. M., R. W. WOODS, M. RUBIN, and W. HILL. 1971. "Most comfortable loudness for pure tones, noise and speech." *Journal of the Acoustical Society of America* 49:1805−13.

VICTOREEN, J. A. 1960. *Hearing Enhancement.* Springfield, Ill.: Charles C. Thomas.

WALDEN, B. E., M. E. DEMOREST, and E. L. HEPLER. 1984. "Self-report approach to assessing benefit derived from amplification." *Journal of Speech and Hearing Research* 27:49−56.

WALDEN, B. E., G. I. SCHUHMAN, and R. K. SEDGE. 1977. "The reliability and validity of the comfort level method of setting hearing aid gain." *Journal of Speech and Hearing Disorders* 42:455−61.

WALDEN, B. E., D. M. SCHWARTZ, D. L. WILLIAMS, L. L. HOLUM-HARDEGEN, and J. M. CROWLEY. 1983. "Test of the assumptions underlying comparative hearing aid evaluations." *Journal of Speech and Hearing Disorders* 48:264−73.

WALKER, G., and H. DILLON. 1982. "Compression in hearing aids: An analysis, a review and some recommendations." *National Acoustic Laboratories Report* No. 90, Australian Government Publishing Service, Canberra, Australia.

———. 1983. "The selection of modulation rates for frequency modulated sound field stimuli." *Scandinavian Audiology* 12:151−56.

WALKER, G., H. DILLON, and D. BYRNE. 1984. "Sound-field audiometry: Recommended stimuli and procedures." *Ear and Hearing* 5(1):13−21.

WALLENFELS, H. G. 1967. *Hearing Aids on Prescription.* Springfield, Ill.: Charles C. Thomas.

WARD, W. D. 1976. "A comparison of the effects of continuous, intermittent and impulse noise." In *Effects of Noise on Hearing.* Ed. D. Henderson, R. P. Hamernik, D. S. Dosanjh, J. H. Mills. New York: Raven Press, 407−19.

WARFIELD, F. 1957a. *Cotton in My Ears.* New York: Viking.

———. 1957b. *Keep Listening.* New York: Viking.

WATSON, N. A., and V. O. KNUDSEN. 1940. "Selective amplification in hearing aids." *Journal of the Acoustical Society of America* 11:406−19.

WIGHTMAN, F. L., T. MCGEE, and M. C. KRAMER. 1977. "Factors influencing frequency selectivity in normal and hearing-impaired listeners." In *Psychophysics and Physiology of Hearing.* Ed. E. F. Evans and J. P. Wilson. London: Academic Press 295−306.

WILSON, R. H., and R. H. MARGOLIS. 1983. "Measurements of auditory thresholds for speech stimuli." In *Principles of Speech Audiometry.* Ed. D. F. Konkle and W. F. Rintlemann. Baltimore: University Park Press.

WILSON, R. H., D. E. MORGAN, and D. D. DIRKS. 1973. "A proposed SRT procedure and its statistical precedent." *Journal of Speech and Hearing Disorders* 38:184−91.

WITTING, E. G., and W. HUGHSON. 1940. "Inherent accuracy of a series of repeated clinical audiograms." *Laryngoscope* 50:259−69.

WYLDE, M. A. 1982. "The remediation process: Psychologic and counselling aspects." In *Handbook of Adult Rehabilitative Audiology,* 2nd ed. Ed. J. G. Alpiner. Baltimore: Williams and Wilkins.

ZARNOCH, J. M., and J. G. ALPINER. 1982. "The Denver scale of communication function for senior citizens living in retirement centers." In *Handbook of Adult Rehabilitative Audiology,* 2nd ed. Ed. J. P. Alpiner. Baltimore: Williams and Wilkins.

ZWISLOCKI, J. J. 1970. "An acoustic coupler for earphone calibration." Special Report LSC S-7. Laboratory of Sensory Communication, Syracuse, N.Y.

INDEX

AUTHOR INDEX

373

SUBJECT INDEX

Acoustic damper, 109–11, 228
Acoustic feedback, 98, 107, 111, 334
  at earmold vent, 271
  in hearing aid, 236, 284–85
Acoustic parameters of speech, 14–16
Acoustic reverberation. *See* Reverberation
Actual rear-eal gain. *See also* Functional gain; Insertion gain
Adaptive procedure, for audiometric testing, 122
Adjustment of hearing aid, 11–12
AGC circuits. *See* Compression circuits
Air-conduction hearing aid, 209–12
Ambient noise
  obtaining threshold in, 38–40
  in sound-pressure level measurements, 85
American National Standards Institute (ANSI), 38
Amplification system, effective bandwidth of, 32–33
Amplifier, 58
Amplitude-modulated (AM) tones, 46
Anechoic chamber, 40
ANSI. *See* American National Standards Institute
Articulation Index, 33–35
Ascending approach, 122–25
Attack time, 221
Audibility of speech, 28–29
Audiological evaluation, reasons for, 3
Audiometer
  Békésy, 129
  calibrating earphone output of, 75–77
  calibrating, for insert earphone, 81–82
  required capabilities of, 55
Audiometric testing
  adaptive procedure for, 122–29
  ascending approach to, 122–25
  bracketing approach to, 127
  clinician-controlled presentation in, 122–29
  clinician proficiency in, 131
  descending approach to, 125–27
  diversity of clinical situations for, 38
  dizziness during, 203
  equipment for, 9, 55–70, 83–85
  instructions in, 130–31
  listener-controlled presentation in, 129–30
  method of adjustment in, 127
  in noise, 38–40
  nystagmus during, 203
  and rating loudness of sounds, 127
  reliability of measures in, 131–36
  room for, 9, 38–45
  simple up-down procedure for, 127
  stimuli for, 45–55
  validity of measures in, 136–39
Auditoriums, hearing in. *See* Speech in reverberant rooms
Auditory area
  defined, 119, 194
  determining, 120–22, 139–48
  reliability of measures of, 132–36
  thresholds and comfort levels in determining, 121–22

validity of measures of, 136–39
Auditory brainstem response (ABR), 245
Auditory processing capability, 20–25
  with cochlear hearing impairment, 21, 24
  with conductive hearing impairment, 21
  for frequency selectivity, 23
  for frequency and timing resolution, 22
  for intensity resolution, 22–23
  with neural hearing impairment, 24–25
  normal filtering of sounds, 23–24
  with normal hearing, 20–21
Aural atresia, 242
Aural rehabilitation
  group, 7
  importance of hearing aid to, 4
  recommending, 321–22
  using results of audiological assessment for planning, 3
Automatic gain control (AGC), 221–22
Azimuth
  angles for SPL measurement, 90–92
  defined, 90
  effect of, on sound-field thresholds, 93–97

Balance, of speech energy frequencies, 29–30
Bandwidth
  critical, 23
  effective, 32
  of loudspeakers, 58–60
  recommended, for hearing aid evaluation, 49
Bass-reflex loudspeaker enclosure, 61–62
Batteries, for hearing aid, 324, 332
Behind-the-ear hearing aid, 99, 105, 106, 111, 209–11, 235
Békésy audiometer, 129
Bell Telephone Laboratories, 33
Berger, Hagberg, and Rane procedure, 159–61, 186, 198–99, 202
BICROS fitting. *See* CROS fittings
Binaural hearing aids,
  advantages of, 239
  criteria for gain and SSPL90 for, 241
  vs. monaural, 239–40
  sequence of fitting, 241
Binaural hearing condition
  creating, 240–41
  normal, 238
Binaural summation, 239, 241
Body hearing aid, 99, 106, 209
Body-baffle effect, 106, 209
Bone-conduction hearing aid, 209, 212–19
Bracketing approach, 122, 127
Brainstem-electric-response audiometry (BERA), 143
Byrne and Dillon procedure, 165–70, 186
Byrne procedure, 200, 202
Byrne and Tonisson procedure, 162–65, 186

California Consonant Test, 53, 300
Canal hearing aid, 211–12
Cassette player, 63–64
Central Institute for the Deaf (CID), 50
Cerumen, effects of, 114
Chair, in testing room, 65

reaction to, 5–7, 310–11
Hearing impairment, compensating for,
  by attitudes, 345–46
  with cognitive skills, 344–45
  environmental factors in, 341
  help of associates in, 346–47
  by lipreading, 343–44
  techniques for talkers for, 341–42
Helmholz resonance, 228
Helping relationship, 307–11
High-frequency gain, preserving, with earmold,
  228–31
Horn enclosure, for loudspeaker, 61
Hughson-Westlake procedure, 122–25
Human dimension in hearing aid evaluation, 2–8
Human-potential approach to counseling, 307–8

Implanted post, for bone-conduction vibrator, 219
Industrial Acoustics Company, 38
Infants. *See* Children
Input compression, 221
Insert earphone, measuring SPL output of, 81–82
Insertion gain
  defined, 9, 113, 115, 150, 276
  measuring, 276–77
  procedure for measuring, 278–79
Instruction procedure, in testing, 130–31
Intensity resolution, 22–23
International Organization for Standardization, 93
International Standards Organization (ISO), 38
Interview, evaluation, 312
In-the-ear hearing aid, 105–6, 211–12
IROS fittings, 233, 235, 236, 237
ISO. *See* International Standards Organization

KEMAR. *See* Knowles Electronics Manikin for Au-
  ditory Research
Knee point, 221
Knowles Electronics Manikin for Auditory
  Research (KEMAR), 111–12

Leijon procedure, 199, 202
Lesions, neural, 24
Libby horn, 226, 227
Libby procedure, 186
Libby third-gain rule, 179, 186
Limiter compression, 221
Lipreading, 343–44
Listener
  effect of, on sound field, 90–92
  position of, in testing room, 44
Listener-controlled attenuator, for audiometer,
  129
Listener-controlled presentation, 129–30
Listening comfort levels, instructions for obtain-
  ing, 36
Listening condition, for speech, 16–20
Live voice testing, 53, 120
Long-term listening range, 177
Loudness discomfort level (LDL). *See* Uncomfort-
  able listening level
Loudness recruitment, 22–23
Loudness summation, 23–24, 286
  and hearing aid adjustment, 196
Loudspeaker
  arrangement of, in testing room, 58–60

azimuth, in SPL measurement, 90
bandwidth, 58–60
choosing type of, 62–63
desirable qualities of, 58
distortion control in, 62
efficiency of, 62
enclosures, 61–62
frequency response of, 60–61
harmonic distortion in, 45
location of, in testing room, 83–84
position of listener to, 10
Low-frequency gain, controlling, with earmold
  vents, 233–35
Lybarger half-gain rule, 157
Lybarger one-quarter gain formula, 157, 165

MAF. *See* Minimum audible field
MAP. *See* Minimum audible pressure
Masking noise
  contralateral, for pure-tone testing, 50
  and frequency selectivity, 23
  and threshold testing, 40
Maximum acoustic output. *See* Saturation sound-
  pressure level
Maximum power output (MPO). *See* Saturation
  sound-pressure level
MCL. *See* Most comfortable loudness level
Medical examination
  FDA requirement for, 2
  reasons for, 2–3
Ménière's disease, 135, 286
Method of adjustment, 127, 129–30
Microphone
  control, 113
  direct audio input, 222
  field, 84–85
  of hearing aid, 105–7, 222
  probe and probe-tube, 69, 70, 78, 113–16
  reference, 113
  systems, for hearing aid evaluation, 68–70
  systems, for measuring insertion gain, 277–78
MIL. *See* Most intelligible listening level
Minimum audible field (MAF), 93
Minimum audible pressure (MAP), 77
Modified Carhart approach, to hearing aid
  evaluation, 150
Modulation rate, 46
Monaural hearing aid fitting, 239–40
Most comfortable listening level (MCL). *See* Most
  comfortable loudness level
Most comfortable loudness level, 36, 121
Most intelligible listening level (MIL). *See also*
  Hearing aid comparison instructions for
  obtaining, 36
MPO. *See* Maximum power output
Multiple sclerosis, 24

Narrow bands of noise
  bandwidth of, 50
  digitally-filtered, 51
  for sound-field uniformity, 43
  stimulus skirts of, 50
  as testing stimuli, 50–52
National Acoustics Laboratories, 49, 151
National Association of Broadcasters, 63, 64
National Hearing Survey, 4

measuring, 10
resonances and antiresonances, in testing
rooms, 40
reverberation, 18–20, 40–44
Sound booth, 40. *See also* Room for audiometric
testing
Sound energy of speech. *See* Speech, acoustic
parameters of
Sound field
calibrating, 95
differences in, at hearing aid input and output,
105–11
direct, 41
effect of listener on, 90–92
at hearing aid microphone, 105
locating loudspeaker and listener in, 83–85
near, 41
normal thresholds in, 93–97
reverberant, 41
sound-pressure level measurements in, 85–90
testing, lack of standards for, 94
uniformity, 42–43, 45–46, 47, 52
Sound reflection, 18–20
Sound-level meter, 65–66, 85
Sound-pressure level (SPL)
reducing variations in, 43
for testing in noise, 39–40
Sound-pressure level measurements
comparing values of, 82
at eardrum vs. in coupler, 82
estimating level of broad-band sounds for, 89
with KEMAR, 111–12
measuring calibration signal for, 89–90
microphone position for, 85
with probe and probe-tube microphones, 112–
16
sound field vs. eardrum, 90–97
sound field vs. eardrum, estimating, 97
Sound-pressure level measurements, in sound
field, 83–97
calibrating frequency-specific sounds for,
85–88
measuring ambient noise in, 85
position of loudspeaker and listener for, 83–85
position of microphone for, 85
speech and competing sounds in, 88–90
Sound-pressure level measurements, using insert
earphone
correction factors for ER-3A earphone for,
81–82
procedure for, 81–82
and residual earcanal volume, 82
Sound-pressure level measurements, using supra-
aural earphones
earcanal SPL variability in, 79–80
eardrum vs. 6-cc coupler SPL in, 77–80
eardrum vs. Zwislocki coupler SPL in, 80–81
standard procedure for, 75
Sound-treated room, 40. *See also* Room for audiometric testing
Speech
acoustic parameters of, 14–16
amplitude levels, 193–94
audibility of, 28–29
balance of frequencies in, 29–30

context of, 20
listening conditions for, 16–20
in noise, 16–18
normal energy range of, 15–16
recorded, in hearing aid evaluations, 53
in reverberant rooms, 18–20
Speech energy
balance, between low- and high-frequency, 177
relation of dynamic range to, 25–35
Speech intelligibility, 20, 299
Speech Perception Test in Noise (SPIN), 54
Speech recognition
effect of hearing impairment on, 9
tests of, 299–301
Speech sounds, identification of, 28
Speech spectrum, in prescribing real-ear gain,
151–52
Speech stimuli, in hearing aid evaluations, 52–54
Speech-reception threshold (SRT), 53, 125–26
Speech-shaped noise, 54, 55
as competing signal, 90
SPL. *See* Sound-pressure level
Spondaic words. *See* Spondee
Spondee, 53, 120
Square-wave modulation of tones, 46
Squeal. *See also* Acoustic feedback
cause of, 107
preventing, 236
Squelch effect, 239
SRT. *See* Speech-reception threshold
SSPL90. *See* Saturation sound-pressure level
Stepped-bore tubing, 226–27
Stimuli
for determining auditory area, 122–39
in hearing aid evaluation, 45–55
modes for presenting, 139
for obtaining thresholds and comfort levels,
120–21
for sound-field uniformity, 45–46
Stimulus skirts, 46, 50, 51
Strial atrophy (strial presbycusis), 24
Summation of loudness, 239, 241
Supra-aural earphone, measuring sound from,
75, 77–81
Sweep-frequency trace, 129
Synthetic Sentence Identification test, 54

Table, in testing room, 65
Technical dimensions of hearing aid evaluation,
8–12
Telecoil, 222–25, 340
Teleloop, 223
Telephone, using, with hearing aid, 222–25
Television, enhanced with hearing aid, 223–25
Temporal distortion of sound, 221
Test box, 98
Third-gain rule, 179
Third-octave FM tones, for sound-field unifor-
mity, 52
Three-speaker array (of loudspeakers), 59–60
Thresholds. *See also* Auditory area
criteria for judging, 121
defined, 121
detection, 121

380

as factor in prescribing real-ear gain, 155
obtaining children's, 127–29
obtaining, for preselection of hearing aid and
    earmold, 243–46
procedures for obtaining, 120–22
recognition, 121
sound-field, prescribing, 248
Threshold of discomfort (TD). *See* Uncomfortable
    listening level
Time smearing, 19
Timing and frequency resolution, 22
Tone control, of hearing aid, 219
Tracoustics, Inc., 38
Triangular modulation of tones, 46
Tubing, 225, 226–27
2-cc coupler gain, predicting, 250–54

UCL. *See* Uncomfortable listening level
ULCL. *See* Upper limit of comfortable loudness
Unaided speech-reception threshold, prescription
    procedures based on, 170
Uncomfortable listening level (UCL), 30–31
defined, 121–22
individual choice of, 197
measuring, 197–98
Uncomfortable listening level, procedure for
    prescribing
Berger, Hagberg, and Rane, 198–202
Byrne, 200, 202
for children, 203–5
Cox, 201, 202–3

Hawkins, 201, 203
Leijon, 199, 202
Pascoe, 200, 202
POGO, 199, 202
Skinner, 203
Uncomfortable loudness level. *See* Uncomfortable
    listening level
Undisturbed field, 90
U.S. Food and Drug Administration (FDA) hear-
    ing aid regulations, 2–3
Upper limit of comfortable loudness (ULCL),
    126–27
Use-gain
defined, 10
setting, of hearing aid, 278

Vents, 231–35
adjustable diameter, 233
as cause of feedback, 98
parallel, 231
side-branch, 231
Vibrator, of hearing aid, 209, 335

Warble tones. *See* Frequency-modulated tones
White noise, 54, 55
as competing signal, 90
Wilson, Morgan, and Dirks procedure, 125–26
WIPI lists, 53
Women, adjusting SPL values for, 79–80
Word and sentence lists, 53–54

Zwislocki coupler, 80–81, 99